AF790521

Paper-Based Diagnostic Devices for Infectious Diseases

Online at: https://doi.org/10.1088/978-0-7503-5820-0

IOP Series in Global Health and Radiation Oncology

Series editor

Wilfred Ngwa
Dana-Farber/Harvard Cancer Center, University of Massachusetts Lowell, Johns Hopkins University, USA

Editor biography

Wilfred Ngwa is the Director of the Global Health Catalyst, a cross-institutional collaboration initiative launched at Harvard to catalyze high impact collaborations in global health. He currently serves as Adjunct Professor at the University of Massachusetts, as Associate Professor of Radiation Oncology at Johns Hopkins University and as ICTU Distinguished Professor of Public Health. He is a chair of the Lancet Oncology Commission for Sub-Saharan Africa, has published three books on global health and serves on the editorial board of a number journals, including ASCO's *Journal of Global Oncology, Ecancermedicalsciences*, and *Frontiers in Oncology*. He has won many awards from Harvard, the USA National Institutes of Health, and international professional organizations for his innovations and his leading work in global health to address disparities both in the USA and globally.

Aims and scope

This series includes books in the emerging area of global radiation oncology and its applications in global health. Building on the published book by the series editor entitled *Emerging Models for Global Health in Radiation Oncology*, it will further detail the work being done globally to promote cancer research and awareness, particularly in lower-income countries.

Paper-Based Diagnostic Devices for Infectious Diseases

Edited by
Nidhi Puranik
Department of Biochemistry & Genetics, Barkatullah University, Bhopal, India

Arpana Parihar
CSIR-Advanced Materials and Processes Research Institute (AMPRI), India

Raju Khan
CSIR-Advanced Materials and Processes Research Institute (AMPRI), India
and
Academy of Scientific and Innovative Research (AcSIR), India

IOP Publishing, Bristol, UK

© IOP Publishing Ltd 2023

All rights reserved. No part of this publication may be reproduced, stored in a retrieval system or transmitted in any form or by any means, electronic, mechanical, photocopying, recording or otherwise, without the prior permission of the publisher, or as expressly permitted by law or under terms agreed with the appropriate rights organization. Multiple copying is permitted in accordance with the terms of licences issued by the Copyright Licensing Agency, the Copyright Clearance Centre and other reproduction rights organizations.

Permission to make use of IOP Publishing content other than as set out above may be sought at permissions@ioppublishing.org.

Nidhi Puranik, Arpana Parihar and Raju Khan have asserted their right to be identified as the editors of this work in accordance with sections 77 and 78 of the Copyright, Designs and Patents Act 1988.

ISBN 978-0-7503-5820-0 (ebook)
ISBN 978-0-7503-5817-0 (print)
ISBN 978-0-7503-5818-7 (myPrint)
ISBN 978-0-7503-5819-4 (mobi)

DOI 10.1088/978-0-7503-5820-0

Version: 20230501

IOP ebooks

British Library Cataloguing-in-Publication Data: A catalogue record for this book is available from the British Library.

Published by IOP Publishing, wholly owned by The Institute of Physics, London

IOP Publishing, No.2 The Distillery, Glassfields, Avon Street, Bristol, BS2 0GR, UK

US Office: IOP Publishing, Inc., 190 North Independence Mall West, Suite 601, Philadelphia, PA 19106, USA

Dedicated to Almighty, who gave us the strength to complete this work.

Contents

Preface

Point-of-care testing devices for early detection, screening, and diagnosis have been proven to significantly improve patient survival rates and quality of life, as well as significantly reduce the cost and complexity of disease treatment. This has proven to be particularly applicable to appropriate environments within low-income and developing nations. In this context, paper-based diagnostic tools have gained significant popularity due to their cost effectiveness, ability to integrate with various platforms, capacity for multiplexing, and their utility in various domains under pointof-care testing setups. From a biomedical standpoint, paper-based biosensor assays are used for the qualitative and quantitative detection of a wide variety of antigens, antibodies, DNA, RNA, miRNA.

Providing a timely update on the current understanding of paper-based biosensors, this book aims to deal with the current state-of-the-art of paper-based biosensors technology and addresses its future prospects for the detection of infectious diseases, with particular relevance and applications for low-income and developing countries. Owing to the advantages offered by paper-based biosensors, such as lowcost platforms for fast and easy detection of a biomarker in the field of clinical diagnostics, this book focuses on the design and fabrication strategies of paper-based devices for the detection of various biomolecules in biomedicine. This is further illustrated with the inclusion of specific case studies as applications within each appropriate chapter.

This comprehensive research and reference text would be suitable for researchers, scholars, and manufacturers in medical device design, biomaterials, bioengineering, materials science, nanobiotechnology, and biochemistry.

With Warm Regards
Nidhi Puranik
Arpana Parihar
Raju Khan

Acknowledgement

All contributors of the respective chapters in this book are thankfully acknowledged by the editors. Their honest efforts, hard work, and analytical approach have been well appreciated and recognized. The editors are thankful to Director, CSIR-AMPRI, Bhopal, MP, India, for his invaluable advice and direction. Dr. Arpana Parihar is thankful to the Department of Science and Technology, Government of India, for providing her fellowship (DST/WOSB/HN-4/2021) under DST-WoS-B Scheme. Dr. Raju Khan acknowledges funding from SERB (IPA/2020/000130).

Editor biographies

Dr Nidhi Puranik is a faculty in the Department of Biochemistry and Genetics at Barkatullah University in Bhopal, India. She has published over 30 articles and peerreviewed journal articles pertaining to paper-based diagnostics. Her current research is focused on this technology with an emphasis on early cancer diagnostics, with extensive in-field applications and instruction. She has been awarded the prestigious GATE, CSIR-NET, ICAR-NET, DRDO Junior research fellowship, MPCST Young Scientist award, MPCST Young Scientist training fellowship and Young investigator award. She has published over 40 research articles with high citation scores.

Dr Arpana Parihar is working as a DST Women Scientist B at CSIR-Advanced Materials and Research Institute, in Bhopal, India. She did her Ph.D. at Raja Rammana Centre for Advanced Technology, Indore, and postdoctoral research work at the Centre for Biomedical Engineering (CBME), Indian Institute of Technology (IIT) Delhi. Dr. Parihar is awarded prestigious GATE, CSIR-NET, DST-WoS A, and WoS B fellowships. She has more than 8 years of research and teaching experience in the field of disease therapeutics and diagnostics. Her research work in the field of cancer therapeutics and Fabrication technologies (Micro/Nano-fabrication) for Bio-devices/bio-medical POCT Devices for early diagnosis of cancer and infectious disease gained considerable attention. She has been awarded with prestigious GATE, CSIR-NET, and DST-WoS B fellowships. She has published over 45 articles and three edited books with Elsevier and written 21 book chapters in a number of published referenced works with the reputed publisher.

Dr Raju Khan, FRSC is currently working as a Principal Scientist and Associate Professor at CSIR-AMPRI Bhopal, Madhya Pradesh, India. He has more than 15 years of experience in electrochemistry, and development of biosensors-based diagnostics. He is a member of the International Advisory Committee, World Academy of Science, Engineering and Technology, and a Fellow of the Royal Society of Chemistry. He has published more than 90 research articles with high citation scores. He has edited 20 books with various reputed publishers. He has several ongoing/completed projects including National/International scientific collaborations with the USA, Czech Republic, and Russia.

List of contributors

Ruchira Chaudhary
Barkatullah University, Bhopal, India

Pallavi Singh Chauhan
Amity Institute of Biotechnology, Amity University Madhya Pradesh, India

Sonu Gandhi
DBT-National Institute of Animal Biotechnology (NIAB), Hyderabad, India

Jyoti Jain
Gajra Raja Medical College Gwalior, Madhya Pradesh, India

Meenu Jain
Gajra Raja Medical College Gwalior, Madhya Pradesh, India

Savita Bharat Jain
Gajra Raja Medical College Gwalior, Madhya Pradesh, India

Urmila Jarouliya
Jiwaji University, Gwalior (M.P.), India

Brijendra Kashyap
Department of Biotechnology Engineering, Institute of Engineering & Technology, Bundelkhand University, Jhansi, India

Raju Khan
Advanced Materials and Processes Research Institute (AMPRI), Academy of Scientific and Innovative Research (AcSIR), India

Vedika Khare
School of Nanotechnology, UTD, RGPV Campus, India

Rishika Khetan
Gajra Raja Medical College Gwalior, Madhya Pradesh, India

Pramod Kumar
ICMR-National Institute of Cancer Prevention and Research (NICPR), I-7, Sector-39, Noida 201301, National Capital Region, India

Meerambika Mishra
Department of Infectious Diseases and Pathology, University of Florida, USA

Vaibhav Misra Misra
Gajra Raja Medical College Gwalior, Madhya Pradesh, India

Sagar Narlawar
DBT-National Institute of Animal Biotechnology (NIAB), Hyderabad, India

Bijayananda Panigrahi
Biopioneer Private Limited, India

Rachna Parashar
All India Institute of Medical Sciences, Bhopal, India

Arpana Parihar
Advanced Materials and Processes Research Institute (AMPRI), India

Tanusha Pathak
All India Institute of Medical Sciences, Bhopal, India

Nidhi Puranik
Department of Biochemistry & Genetics, Barkatullah University, Bhopal, India

Preeti Puranik
Department of Computer Sciences, Shri Jain Diwakar College, India

Aushtosh Singh Raghuvanshi
AcSIR, India

Pragati Raghuwanshi
All India Institute of Medical Sciences, Bhopal, India

Aditya Raj
Hari Singh Gaur University, Sagar, India

Bandi Lokesh Reddy
Department of Biotechnology Sri Venkateshwara University, India

Riya Sharma
DBT-National Institute of Animal Biotechnology (NIAB), Hyderabad, India

Sushil Kumar
Sharma Defence Research & Development Establishment, Gwalior (M.P.), India

Ankit Sharma
LabyRx Immunologic Therapeutics Pvt Ltd, USA

Arun Sharma
Department of Chemistry, MITS Group of Institutions, India

Neha Sharma
Amity Institute of Biotechnology, Amity University Madhya Pradesh, India

Rohit Kumar Singh
Ben Gurion University of the Negev, Israel

Agrata Singh
Amity Institute of Biotechnology, India

Rajesh Singh Tomar
Amity Institute of Biotechnology, Amity University Madhya Pradesh, India

Ayushi Singhal
Advanced Materials and Processes Research Institute (AMPRI) Academy of Scientific and Innovative Research (AcSIR), India

Uday Suryakant
School of Biotechnology, India

Shiv Kumar Yadav
Department of Zoology, Government Lal Bahadur Shastri College, India

Chapter 1

Paper-based biosensors: overview from past to future

Narlawar Sagar Shrikrishna, Riya Sharma and Sonu Gandhi

Paper-based biosensors offer a prudent platform for medical diagnostics. In the past, filter paper has been used as a substrate for fabrication of litmus paper strips, which is an example of a primitive chemical sensor. But recently paper-based biosensors have evolved to the extent that they can detect many diseases and their associated biomarkers. Many applications in the field of point-of-care (POC) diagnostics use paper-based materials as a substrate for fabricating various biosensors. Since paper is versatile, porous and flexible it can serve as a substrate for the construction of various biosensors. This tunable porosity facilitates the capillary action-governed movement of the fluids. Hence, paper is also a great material to fabricate microfluidic devices. Recently, paper-based biosensors have started emerging and are still evolving. Various formats of these biosensors such as lateral flow assay devices (LFAs), microfluidic paper-based analytical devices (μPADs) and dipsticks were developed in the past and are still improving. This chapter will briefly focus on the journey of paper-based biosensors since their inception to recent advancements in the field.

1.1 Introduction

Paper can be thought of as a flattened cellulose matrix. Paper manufacturing has a long history that dates back to the second century AD in China (Hu *et al* 2014). Paper has been used by humans for a variety of purposes. However, the majority of its use is for writing purposes. The pH strip, invented in 1958 (Frazer 1958), was the first report of employing paper as a sensor. Many years after its discovery, paper has been employed to develop suitable biosensors; otherwise, many crude biosensors have been fabricated.

Biosensors are the sensors which specifically contain any of the biomolecules (nucleic acid, carbohydrate, protein or lipid) as a biorecognition element and with the help of their integrated transducing elements detect the analyte (figure 1.1).

doi:10.1088/978-0-7503-5820-0ch1

© IOP Publishing Ltd 2023

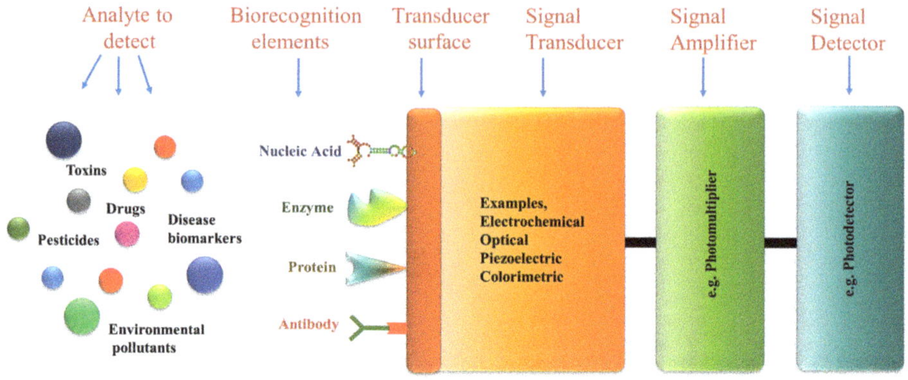

Figure 1.1. Construction, design and various components of a biosensor.

Aanalytes could be anything ranging from environmental pollutants (Shrikrishna *et al* 2021), drugs (Gandhi *et al* 2009), disease biomarkers (Narlawar *et al* 2022, Banga *et al* 2019), pesticides (Islam *et al* 2019, Talan *et al* 2018, Raman Suri *et al* 2009, 2008) or toxins (Kasoju *et al* 2020a, 2020b). Figure 1.1 represents a schematic and overall design of a biosensor. Biosensors can be fabricated on a variety of substrates. Paper, being one of the cheapest among other substrates, is utilized extensively to fabricate biosensors. But, the key question besides its cost is, why there is a dire need for the fabrication of paper-based biosensors? The following section will deal with this question.

Deadly and infectious diseases, such as acquired immunodeficiency syndrome (AIDS), malaria, and tuberculosis (TB) kill over 15 million people each year, accounting for almost 25% of all fatalities globally (Morens *et al* 2004, Bissonnette and Bergeron 2010). Because of the scarcity of cost-effective medical interventions, over 95% of the fatalities happen in underdeveloped and economically weaker countries (Lee *et al* 2010, Yager *et al* 2006). To alleviate this problem clinical diagnostics has become a major tool to identify the root cause of the symptoms in patients, assess therapy effectiveness, and screen for probable ailments in asymptomatic but individuals at high risk of disease (Hay Burgess *et al* 2006). As a result, clinical diagnosis has become critical in the healthcare industry. Thus, clinical diagnosis has a significant role in clinical and epidemiological decision-making. Malaria, for example, takes the life of a child every 40 s equating to almost a million infants each year in Africa (Sachs and Malaney 2002). But, in fact malaria can be prevented and at the same time could also be cured if timely diagnosis is available. Because quick medical treatment is essential, once symptoms appear, then fast and accurate diagnosis of malaria is essential for its prevention and treatment. In resource-constrained situations, however, the clinical diagnosis is frequently reliant on the medical examiner's experience rather than laboratory proof. If a quick test kit for malaria diagnosis is available which is affordable, easy to use, and accurate, it can be a life saver. This is the area where paper-based biosensors played an essential role in diagnosis. Therefore, efforts have been made in the past and will continue to take place in the future.

Advanced technology like polymerase chain reaction (PCR) has been adopted by developed countries but its use is still limited in developing and underdeveloped countries because of the lack of laboratory infrastructure, financial resources and availability of skilled personnel. It is the same with techniques like enzyme linked immuno sorbent assay (ELISA) (Yager *et al* 2008, Mabey *et al* 2004). To trouble-shoot the above mentioned problems, POC diagnostics became an easier, faster, more cost-effective and ideal way for resource-constrained environments (Tabak 2007). As a result, POCs are critical for launching and scaling up on-site medical care facilities for prevention and control of the infectious diseases (Hauck *et al* 2010, Wang *et al* 2010, Lee *et al* 2010).

Because of its obvious benefits, microfluidic technologies have been extensively used in the fabrication of POC to solve global health challenges (Hawkins and Weigl 2010). Microfluidic devices can operate with small amounts of liquids when connected with various operating units such as reactors, valves and pumps and when incorporated into a miniature analytical system (Hawkins and Weigl 2010, Chin *et al* 2007). As a result, microfluidic devices considerably minimize sample and reagent usage, the complexity of operating processes, and the duration of assay without sacrificing sensitivity and specificity (Laksanasopin *et al* 2009, Chin *et al* 2007, Whitesides 2006). Most microfluidic devices apart from paper-based micro-fluidics have been constructed using glass slides, silicon materials, and polymers such as poly(methyl methacrylate) (PMMA) and poly(dimethyl siloxane) (PDMS) and so require both complex production methods and external equipment, rendering them unfit for POC testing/on-site testing (Nilghaz *et al* 2012). In contrast, paper-based microfluidics have great potential to deliver POC diagnostics to developing countries in terms of being **a**ffordable, **s**ensitive, **s**pecific, **u**ser-friendly, **r**apid and robust, **e**quipment-free, and **d**eliverable to end-users (ASSURED) (Huang *et al* 2010, Hawkins and Weigl 2010)'. The following section deals with the classification of these paper-based biosensors and their usage in various fields.

1.2 Classification of paper-based biosensors

Paper-based biosensors can be classified into three types based on their operating formats. These are microfluidics biosensors or microfluidic paper-based analytical devices (μPADs), dipstick tests strips or simply dipsticks and lateral flow assays (LFA) paper-based biosensors. μPADs are the devices containing single/multi-hydrophilic channels surrounded by hydrophobic area. Dipsticks, as the name suggests, are the strips of filter paper loaded with the reagents/chemicals to detect specific analytes. LFAs are self-contained devices made up of various capillary flow directing components. These biosensors can also be classified in another way based on its detection principles viz., colorimetric biosensors, fluorescence-based biosensors, electrochemical biosensors, etc. Details of these biosensors are given in the later sections of this chapter.

Initially, commercial dipstick tests were used to assess some of the clinical samples containing different biomarkers of diseases, blood, protein and urine samples (Vuljanić *et al* 2019). The dipstick tests were straightforward and easy to evaluate;

nonetheless, the primary drawbacks were inaccuracy and lengthy analysis. As a result, numerous LFAs were explored in order to improve analytical performance utilizing vertical flow immunoassays, which are commonly employed for quick identification of disease biomarkers (Posthuma-Trumpie *et al* 2009). LFAs are even employed in pregnancy testing (Yetisen *et al* 2013). LFAs are now used as a routine test in various clinical diagnostics, for example, in studies involving screening of blood coagulation. The sample in the LFA flows horizontally towards a detection zone, whereas the sample in the vertical flow immunoassays flows vertically to a detection line (Kuswandi *et al* 2017). Direction of flow of the sample is the evident difference among these tests, but the vertical flow of the sample provides for faster detection and better sensitivity in ng/mL concentrations. Furthermore, the higher concentration of antibodies in lateral flow tests might hinder the agglutination, which could result in incorrect interpretation of the test and this problem could be avoided in vertical flow assays systems (Fu and Downs 2017). As a result, modern advancements utilize largely the 'vertical flow' test format for the identification of biomarkers. For example, a lateral flow test with vertical flow setting has been employed for the analysis of DNA microarrays for *Neisseria meningitidis* (Rivas *et al* 2018).

There are various constraints on the analytical performance of paper-based biosensors in spite of their potential applications. These constraints are with the sensitivity of the test, accuracy and simultaneous detection of several biomarkers. Electrochemical methods are among the other methods of detection which have been employed in the biomarker detection in addition to optical detections. Despite the fact that these detection approaches had been applied in development of μPAD, they had their own drawbacks in terms of sensitivity and simplicity (Liana *et al* 2012). Such disadvantages need a strategic rethinking of the existing state of paper-based biosensors, as well as the possibilities of improving their performance and commercialization in future endeavours. This viewpoint aims to answer such a critical need.

The major interest in paper-based biosensor devices is the intricacy of response processes in the detection zone. Various prototypes for fluid-handling have been produced, including 'self-wicking' basic types and more advanced types such as fluid-guided handling employing microfluidics. These methods of handling fluids gave rise to the classification of paper-based biosensors to three distinct categories, namely the dipsticks test, LFA, and μPADs. All these categories are summarized below. The merits and demerits of each type of biosensor are outlined in table 1.1.

1.2.1 Microfluidic biosensors

As defined earlier, paper is a matrix of cellulose which is porous and hydrophilic, making it an ideal material for creating microfluidic channels. Generally, microfluidic biosensors are called μPADs. 'μ' stands for microfluidic and 'PAD' stands for paper-based analytical devices. Whitesides *et al* initiated the development of μPADs in 2007 (Mao and Huang 2012). They fabricated the 2D (figure 1.2(d)) and 3D (figure 1.2(e)) microfluidics paper devices by patterning a paper with channel forming reagents with different assay designs (Nilghaz *et al* 2012). The fabricated μPADs rely mostly on the force developed by capillary action through the pores of filter paper (Martinez *et al* 2009). 2D μPADs are

Table 1.1. Classification, merits and demerits of paper-based biosensors.

Type	Principle of detection	Merits	Demerits
Microfluidic biosensors (μPADs)	Optical detection Colorimetric Detection Electrochemical detection	All types of detection possible	Tedious optimization and need of expert are required
Dipstick tests	Optical detection	Simple to fabricate and quick standardization possible	Only qualitative analysis and optical mode of analysis is possible
Lateral flow assays	Optical detection Colorimetric Detection Electrochemical detection	Quantitative analysis is possible	Take a very long time for optimization and is difficult to fabricate

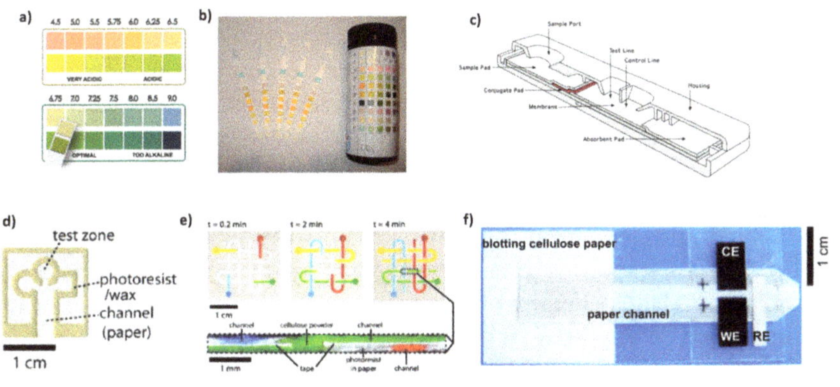

Figure 1.2. Various forms of paper-based biosensors: ((a) and (b)) dipstick assay strips, (c) lateral flow assay strips, ((d) and (e)) microfluidic paper-based analytical devices (μPAD), and (f) microfluidic paper-based electrochemical devices (μPED). Reprinted from reference Hu *et al* (2014) with permission of Elsevier.

generally fabricated by two lithographic techniques, in one a physical barrier and in another a chemical barrier is generated to create the microfluidic channels (Cassano and Fan 2013). To build channels and barriers in paper, several technologies such as wax printing, inkjet printing, photolithography and plasma etching have been recently developed (Martinez *et al* 2010a). The wicking rate of fluid can be influenced by the size of the resulting fabricated channels, as well as the quality of the paper and the external conditions such as temperature and humidity (Martinez *et al* 2010b). Hand dispensing chemicals or inkjet printing can be used to immobilize reagents for biological processes on the filter paper with various designs such as a dumbbell pattern or a clover leaf pattern (Pelton 2009, Sicard and Brennan 2013). After patterning, once the chemicals have dried, these μPADs can be utilized for biochemical research. For the fabrication of 3D μPADs, stacking of the layers of patterned paper is required so that the channels in neighbouring layers of paper can connect (Martinez *et al* 2008). Both the μPADs can be used for the chromatographic separation of samples, e.g., used for filtering of samples. But 3D μPAD is beneficial due to its capacity to incorporate a complex network of microchannels (Martinez *et al* 2010a).

One variation of microfluidic paper-based analytical devices (μPADs) with the incorporation of electrodes is called the microfluidic paper-based electrochemical device (μPED). μPED provides the electrochemical signals as opposed to colorimetric in conventional μPAD. The electrodes in the μPED can be created using screen printing technology (Nie *et al* 2010), with the help of an inkjet printer (Kit-Anan *et al* 2012), or simply hand drawing with a pencil (Dossi *et al* 2013) on filter paper using conducting inks. A typical μPED is comprised of three electrodes, these are the counter electrode (CE), reference electrode (RE) and working electrode (WE) (figure 1.2(f)) (Nie *et al* 2010). To provide a sensitive and specialized sensing function, the working electrode has been modified biologically or chemically. Specificity of μPED is obtained in the same way by procedures employed in μPADs, these are enzymatic reactions, an antibody–antigen reaction, or a nucleic acid hybridization reaction. These reactions employed in μPEDs, unlike colorimetric tests, are primarily the oxidation–reduction reactions. Materials used to build a working electrode surface of μPED are gold nanoparticles, graphene materials and carbon nanotubes. These nanomaterials are used to change the working electrode surface to provide better sensitivity of the electrochemical processes (Wang *et al* 2012b, Yan *et al* 2012, Lu *et al* 2012).

μPADs have unlocked a plethora of paper-based biosensors to address the multiple disadvantages of lateral flow assays. They have not only provided the benefit of assay multiplexing but also provided a window for quantitative analysis (Dincer *et al* 2017). Numerous μPADs variations have been created, with detection methods including electrochemical (Dungchai *et al* 2009), optical (Liu *et al* 2016), chemiluminescence (Wang *et al* 2016), and 'piezo-resistive micro-electromechanical system (MEMS)' (Liu and Crooks 2011). Furthermore, many μPADs have been fabricated for the measurement of biomarkers such as glucose in the blood and uric acid in the body fluids (Fischer *et al* 2016, Nery and Kubota 2016). μPAD-based enzyme biosensors have served as an effective clinical diagnostic tool (Santhiago *et al* 2014). But, they do, however, suffer from thermal instability, necessitating particular storage conditions. Furthermore, μPADs are not only compatible with optical or colorimetric detection (Dungchai *et al* 2009) but also with the electrochemical detections (Wang *et al* 2018, Ge *et al* 2014). The merits and demerits of μPADs are listed in table 1.1.

1.2.2 Dipstick tests

Dipsticks are the simplest form of paper-based microfluidics. A typical example of dipsticks are pH strips. In general, pH strips are prepared by drenching filter paper strips in a solution of pH indicators in appropriate concentrations. Then filter paper is loaded with the specific identification reagent. The identification reagent then reacts with the provided analyte (H^+) ions and develops the colour. Then a standard indicator card can be used for the measurement of pH of the resulting solution and then the amount of H^+ can be semi-quantified. Furthermore, pH strips have been used to assess the pH of saliva and urine (figure 1.2(a)) in order to get general health information about the body. These pH strips (esparticularly pH indicators) can also be used to identify potassium acetate, lead acetate and other contaminants (Hu *et al* 2014). Correspondingly, test strips have been developed for the detection of urine (figure 1.2(b)) and for the identification of the metabolic products in urine, and they have evolved into fundamental diagnostic tools for indicating pathological alterations. A conventional urine test strip, for example, can identify metabolic products in urine from patients with diabetic and related disorders.

The dipstick test strip-based biosensor is a basic analytical instrument made up of immobilized chemicals that is used for qualitative analysis. There are certain dipstick test examples accessible today, such as test strips for the detection of uric acid and detection of glucose (Kuswandi *et al* 2005), pathogen detection strips (Nurul Najian *et al* 2016), and so forth. For quick detection of the novel coronavirus, **r**everse **t**ranscription **r**ecombinase **a**ided **a**mplification (RT-RAA) technique was used along with lateral flow dipstick (LFD) wherein the nucleocapsid (N) gene was targeted along with its related primers and probe sequences. With this assay LOD obtained was 1 copy/µl (Zheng *et al* 2021). More information on such techniques where PCR is involved could be found in chapter 9. Because the dipstick assay strips are simple to fabricate, they have enormous potential for commercial enterprises. The fundamental disadvantage of the dipstick assay strip is with the quantitative analysis which as of now cannot be done. High popularity of dipsticks is due to the easy and simple colour change observed after the addition of the analyte. Since it is useful only for qualitative analysis, it cannot be used for the quantitative analysis of biomarkers. As a consequence, this kind of test is ideal for obtaining quick and reliable results. The merits and demerits of dipsticks-based biosensors are described in table 1.1.

1.2.3 Lateral flow assay

As the name suggests, lateral flow is the flow of sample along the paper-based device. In simple terms, LFAs are modified and advanced dipstick strips, they are usually comprised of a sample pad, absorbent pad (also called a wicking pad), backing pad and a nitrocellulose membrane (Mansfield 2007) (figure 1.2(c)). The role of the absorbent pad is to generate the capillary action which is needed for the generation of fluid flow. The backing pad provides strength to the overall device. The role of the nitrocellulose membrane is to provide a platform for the reaction and detection of the assay (Mansfield 2007). On the surface of the nitrocellulose membrane, the captured molecules such as antibodies can be coated to generate test and control lines (Mansfield 2007). In order to synchronize the capillary flow of the fluid, the two neighbouring components overlap by a small amount. At the time of assay running, a small amount of the sample is placed on the designated sample pad. The sample pad is prepared in the appropriate buffer in an order which is compatible with the test reagents/analyte being added, which could improve their compatibility (Wong and Tse 2009). When the mixture flows along the pad, it carries the conjugated particle which had been previously loaded on the conjugated pad. There are numerous plasmonic nanoparticles such as upconversion nanoparticles and gold nanoparticles which have been used for the development of LFA (Lin *et al* 2012).

There are two modes of LFA, one is called the sandwich LFA and the other is the competitive (or inhibitory) LFA (Wong and Tse 2009). In the sandwich mode of LFA, if an analyte is present then the conjugated nanoparticles react with the analyte to form the analyte–nanoparticle complex. The formed complexes are then caught in the test line because of the interaction of the analyte with the appropriate capturing molecules. The test line can be exceeded by obsessive conjugated particles that are analyte-free. These particles are subsequently trapped by a different sort of capturing molecule, forming a control line. On the other hand, in the competitive format of LFA, the conjugated nanoparticles may react with capturing molecules placed at both the test and control lines. The result of this is the analyte competes for binding sites at the test line with the capturing molecules, resulting in non-aggregation of conjugated particles at the test line. This scenario changes in the absence of the analyte of interest, in that case, conjugated nanoparticles can be collected at both the test and control lines (Wong and Tse 2009).

The LFA paper-based biosensor is a more advanced variant of a dipstick which allows regulated migration of the sample along the pad. Because of these advances, it is now viable to construct multistep assays which otherwise are difficult to perform. LFA consists of four major components: a sample pad (where sample application takes place), a conjugation pad (used to store reagents), a detection pad (where detection of analyte takes place), and an absorbent pad (which makes the sample flow). Despite the fact that LFA strips have a greater level of sample handling complexity, correct quantification requirements exist in this kind (Moghadam *et al* 2015). LFA strips have particularly been developed for the detection of COVID-19 where these detect IgG and IgM in various clinical samples such as serum, plasma and whole blood of patients (Sheridan 2020, Li *et al* 2020). Recently LFA based biosensors for COVID-19 detection can also be found in the literature cited here (Roberts *et al* 2021). Moreover, chapter 7 will deal with paper-based diagnostics for the SARS-CoV-2 detection. The merits and demerits of LFA given in the table 1.1.

1.3 Overview of the microfluidic devices from the past

In the previous sections we have shown what the paper-based microfluidics are and their types. In this section we are going to describe efforts from the past to build paper-based microfluidic system. As described earlier, any biosensors can have different transducing elements, e.g., colorimetric, electrochemical, fluorescence etc. This section gives an overview of advances in each detection system.

1.3.1 Overview of colorimetric biosensors

Colorimetric detection of analytes present in the sample is one of the most extensively used detection methods for paper-based biosensors. The reason behind this is the clear visual signal, distant areas of application, efficient detection of analyte, simple operation, and high stability (Fu and Wang 2018, Aparna *et al* 2018, Mohammadi and Yaghoubi 2017, Dai *et al* 2017). Colorimetric detection of any analyte involves the passive flow of the test compound of interest to the test line of device via capillary action, where the colorimetric reaction takes place due to reaction with loaded assay reagents. The result of this is the detection of change in colour at the site of the detection area of μPAD (Arrastia *et al* 2015, Cardoso *et al* 2017a). These colour changes at the detection zones of μPAD had been captured using smartphone cameras (Nuchtavorn and Macka 2016, Ortiz-Gomez *et al* 2016), or CMOS (complementary metal–oxide–semiconductor) cameras (Boonsri *et al* 2017, Meelapsom *et al* 2016), and then uploaded to a personal computer (PC)/smartphone for further investigation. Liu and Gomez fabricated a μPAD, working on the principle of colorimetric detection and used scanning device for measuring acetylcholinesterase (AChE) activity and for the screening of inhibitors (figure 1.3(a)). They fabricated the μPAD with the help of a wax printer, in which hydrophobic wax was layered on the surface of chromatographic paper in order to build microchannels. They had put the solutions of 5,5-dithiobis-(2-nitrobenzoic acid) (DTNB) and samples containing AChE and acetylthiocholine iodide (ATC) directly onto the surface of μPAD throughout the detection procedure. Their device displayed the high sensitivity for detection AChE activity, indicating that it has substantial potential for quantifying neurotransmitter activity (Liu and Gomez 2017). The same group (Arrastia *et al* 2015, Gonzalez *et al* 2016, Avoundjian *et al* 2017) worked on the alternative μPAD for the examination of IgG antibodies as well as glucose detection. IgG detection used the colorimetric principle while the glucose sensor used a scanning device. Cardoso *et al* employed the novel idea of metal stamping technology to detect nitrites from food and environmental samples via μPAD (Cardoso *et al* 2015). Later, the other group published a

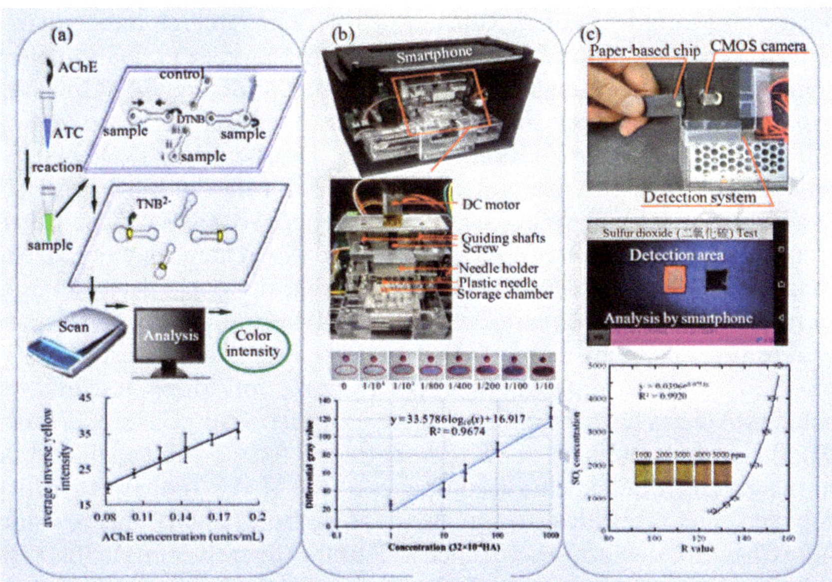

Figure 1.3. Paper-based colorimetric biosensors from the past: (a) AchE detection by wax printed μPAD, (b) colorimetric detection of Influenza-A using smartphone, (c) colorimetric detection of SO_2 by fabricated microfluidic chip. Reprinted from reference Fu and Wang (2018) with permission of Elsevier.

number of μPAD based on the principle of colorimetry for the detection of numerous analytes such as bilirubin, urea, glucose, etc, in the samples (Gabriel *et al* 2017, Cardoso *et al* 2017b, 2015). Mujawar *et al* used chromogenic reagents to colorimetrically detect various ions present in wastewater as well as drinking water. Ions such as Fe^{3+}, Ni^{2+}, Co^{2+}, Zn^{2+}, and Hg^{2+} were detected using μPAD which was made up of thick filter sheets of paper using a chemical vapour deposition (CVD) technique. Their fabricated μPAD had a very good detection limit for Hg^{+} ions. It could detect 0.5 parts per billion (ppb) of Hg^{+} ions (Mujawar *et al* 2016). Many ideas for using mobile smartphones to conduct colorimetric detection on μPAD platforms may be found in some of the papers cited here (Yang *et al* 2016, Choi *et al* 2015, Nuchtavorn and Macka 2016). Wu *et al*, for example, developed a Dot-ELISA for the sensitive detection of influenza-A. They fabricated this system using the common components of LFA, i.e., nitrocellulose membrane functionalized with specific antibodies. Photos of nitrocellulose membranes were taken with the help of smartphone specified technique (figure 1.3(b)) and the concentration of influenza-A was calculated by inspecting the image's differential grey value. Their experimental findings demonstrated an outstanding linearity ($R^2 = 0.9937$) using known influenza-A and proper controls (Wu *et al* 2017). Lopez-Ruiz *et al* had demonstrated a colorimetric biosensor made of paper (μPAD) for the determination of nitrite content. It could simultaneously determine the nitrite content and the pH of the water samples. Their μPAD had four areas for measuring pH and two areas for the detection of nitrite along with a single area for the reference. For detection of pH, they could achieve 0.04 units of resolution with the accuracy of 0.009 units. The achieved resolution was superior to that of conventional pH testing using the pH strips. They could also achieve a good limit of detection (LOD) for nitrite, i.e., 0.52 mg l^{-1} (Lopez-Ruiz *et al* 2014). The research on the detection of nitrite content further continued and as a result, Ortiz-Gomez *et al* also detected the nitrite content in the water samples but with a different approach, i.e., Griess reaction. For this purpose, they used the smartphone camera to detect nitrite content of water with the LOD of 1.30 μM (Ortiz-Gomez *et al* 2016). Dong *et al* used gold nanoparticles linked with anti-CRP (C-reactive protein) antibodies for the colorimetric detection of CRP. They fabricated the microfluidic immunoassay chip based on the paper substrate for the purpose of the detection of CRP. They paired this system with a smartphone for further analysis. The fabricated system was affordable and could detect 54 ng ml^{-1} of CRP (Dong *et al* 2017). Colorimetric detection of different analytes using asmartphone or a digital cameras coupling with μPADs have been extensively researched across the breadth of diagnostic applications. As a result of that, research on the colorimetric μPAD has further expanded, as an example of this, Liu *et al* demonstrated the system for the measurement of SO_2 concentration from commercial food samples. They fabricated microfluidic chip using paper and PMMA (poly(methyl methacrylate)) polymer. The fabricated system used the complementary metal–oxide–semiconductor (CMOS) camera as a colorimetric detector (figure 1.3(c)). In this system the sample was loaded on a short strip of filter paper which was previously coated with acid–base indicator in the suggested device, and the paper was then put into a PMMA microchip. The CMOS camera was used to examine the following reaction-induced colour shift, and the reaction picture data were sent to a mobile phone. Finally, using self-written RGB analysis software, the SO_2 concentration was calculated from the picture intensity data (Liu *et al* 2017). Chaiyo *et al* developed the µPADs using a wax printing approach for the electrochemical as well as colorimetric detection of three distinct ions: Cu^{2+}, Pb^{2+}, and Cd^{2+}. In this, silver (Ag) nanoparticles modified with cetyltrimethylammonium bromide (CTAB) were used at the detection zone which is further etched by thiosulfate to create-modified Ag nanoparticles which were then introduced to the detecting zone and etched by thiosulfate to create smaller silver nanoparticles under the effects of oxidation for the Cu^{2+} device. The findings of the tests indicated that the device has a detection limit of about 4.12×10^{-3} ppm (Chaiyo *et al* 2016). Gandhi *et al* fabricated the strip-based LFA based on the immunochromatographic principle for the detection of morphine drug in urine samples with a LOD of 2.5 ng ml^{-1} (Gandhi *et al* 2009). More information on paper-based immunochromatographic assays can be found in chapter 3. Colorimetric paper-based biosensors are not only limited to detecting chemical agents, drugs and ions but also for the detection of different types of diseases and their associated pathogens. For instance, Yen *et al* developed colorimetric LFA for the detection of yellow fever, dengue and the ebola virus with a LOD for all viral protein 150 ng ml^{-1} (Yen *et al* 2015). Another LFA for the detection of *Campylobacter jejuni* had been developed by He *et al C. jejuni* is a causative agent for common food poisoning. The proposed LFA based biosensor was fabricated using platinum coated gold nanorods working on a principle of surface enhanced Raman scattering (SERS) with a LOD of 50 cfu ml^{-1} (He *et al* 2019). The more information on SERS based biosensors could be found in chapter 4. Recently, the COVID-19 pandemic has created havoc worldwide. To detect the deadly coronavirus responsible for the pandemic, Liu *et al* came up with a novel idea of integrating colorimetric dipsticks into a PMMA based microfluidic device. With this device 30 copies of viral RNA per sample can be detected (Liu *et al* 2021). Such integration of a microfluidic technology with a paper-based platform can be found with more details in chapter 11. With further advancements in the colorimetric dipsticks, Zheng *et al* developed dipsticks with a LOD of 1 copy/µl which was explained in the dipstick assay section earlier (Zheng *et al* 2021). See table 1.2 for the expanded list on colorimetric biosensors.

1.3.2 Overview of fluorescence-based biosensors

µPADs that use fluorescence detection make use of the fluorophores (fluorescent dyes) and interaction chemistry amid the target (analyte of interest) and fluorescent dyes (Boonsri *et al* 2017, İncel *et al* 2017). There are three phases of the fluorescent detection phase. These are excitation, excited-state lifetime and fluorescence emission. To generate luminescence of the fluorophores, a light source of a suitable wavelength is used in the sensing process. Then the resultant light is separated by filtering out emission photons from excited photons. Then it is quantified and utilized for the calculation of the concentration of the target analyte. There are many fluorescence and paper-based biosensors that have been developed in the past and these are described below.

Noor *et al* fabricated the µPAD-based system for ratiometric detection of nucleic acid hybridization. In this system they take advantage of fluorescence resonance energy

Table 1.2. Paper-based biosensors from the past showing the format and mode of detection.

Format of paper-based biosensor	Mode of detection	Analyte/target molecule	Limit of detection	Reference
Dipstick	Colorimetric	Bovine serum albumin (BSA) and glucose	2.5 mM (glucose) 0.38 μM (BSA)	Martinez *et al* (2007)
Dipstick	Colorimetric	N-acylhomoserine lactones	1×10^{-8} M	Struss *et al* (2010)
Dipstick	Colorimetric	RNA particles	1 copy/μl	Liu *et al* (2021)
Dipstick	Colorimetric	Influenza-A virus	Qualitative	Jeong *et al* (2017)
μPAD	Colorimetric	Pentachlorophenol	0.01–100 ng ml^{-1}	Sun *et al* (2014)
μPAD	Chemiluminescence	Glucose, uric acid	0.14 mmol l^{-1} (Glucose) 0.52 mmol l^{-1} (Uric acid)	Yu *et al* (2011)
μPAD	Electrochemical (redox signal)	Glucose, uric acid	3.81×10^{-5} M (glucose)	Chen *et al* (2012)
μPAD (Hybrid)	Fluorescence quenching	*Lactobacillus acidophilus*	11.0 cfu ml^{-1}	Zuo *et al* (2013)
μPAD	Colorimetric	Influenza-A (H1N1 virus)	2.7×10^3 PFU ml^{-1}	Lei *et al* (2015)
μPAD (3D)	Colorimetric	*Mycobacterium tuberculosis*	1.27 nM	Teengam *et al* (2017b)
μPED	Electrochemical	Glucose	4.9 mM (glucose)	Dungchai *et al* (2009)
μPED	Electrochemical	Cancer markers (CA125 and CEA)	0.2 mU ml^{-1} (CEA125), 0.01 ng ml^{-1}	Wang *et al* (2012a)
μPED (ePAD)	Electrochemical	Antibodies	0.96 ng ml^{-1} (IgG), 0.14 ng ml^{-1} (IgM)	Yakoh *et al* (2021)
LFA	Colorimetric	*Escherichia coli*	10 cfu ml^{-1} (PBS)	Choi *et al* (2010)
LFA	Colorimetric	Ebola virus, dengue virus and yellow fever virus	150 ng ml^{-1} (for all viruses)	Yen *et al* (2015)
LFA	Colorimetric	HIV	0.8 pg ml^{-1}	Loynachan *et al* (2018)
LFA	Colorimetric	*Staphylococcus aureus*	10^4 CFU ml^{-1}	Lu *et al* (2019)

transfer (FRET) properties of immobilized quantum dots (QD). Quantum dots serve as doners in this system. The paper substrate in the μPAD served here as the FRET signal amplifier and the LOD in this process could reach up to 450 pmol (Noor and Krull 2014). In subsequent research, the same group could bring down the LOD to 37 zmol under ultraviolet light illumination (figure 1.4(a)). To achieve this low LOD, they used the same assay format as described above, but they used the thermophilic helicase dependant amplification phase (Noor *et al* 2015). The same group also developed the device for the detection of cancer biomarkers. They developed the μPAD based on the FRET principle to detect the biomarkers (Das and Krull 2017). Later, Liang *et al* introduced a μPAD system in which multiplexed monitoring of cancerous cells was possible. They used the aptamer modified QDs immobilized on silica nanoparticles. Aptamers are the small fragment/stretches of DNA (deoxyribose nucleic acid) or RNA (ribose nucleic acid) of nucleic acids which fold into tertiary 3D structures and bind to the target with high affinity (Narlawar and Gandhi 2021). More information on aptamer and paper-based biosensors can be found in chapter 6. In this system the fluorescence of the QDs was suppressed by FRET after absorption by graphene oxide (GO), but it was restored after exposure to the target cells. Interestingly, by simply altering the aptamer and/or colour of the QDs, the device may identify additional target cancer cells. The feasibility of the suggested device was proved by determining three distinct cancer cells at the same time, namely MCF-7, HL-60 and K562. The resulting limits of detection for these cells were found to be 62, 70 and 65 cells/ml, respectively (Liang *et al* 2016b). The same group also developed a 3D paper-based device for the sensitive detection of hydrogen peroxide (H_2O_2) produced from liver cancer cells. They also utilized the QD and GO as a FRET pair. The fluorescence of the QDs was suppressed by FRET after absorption by GO, but restored upon exposure to

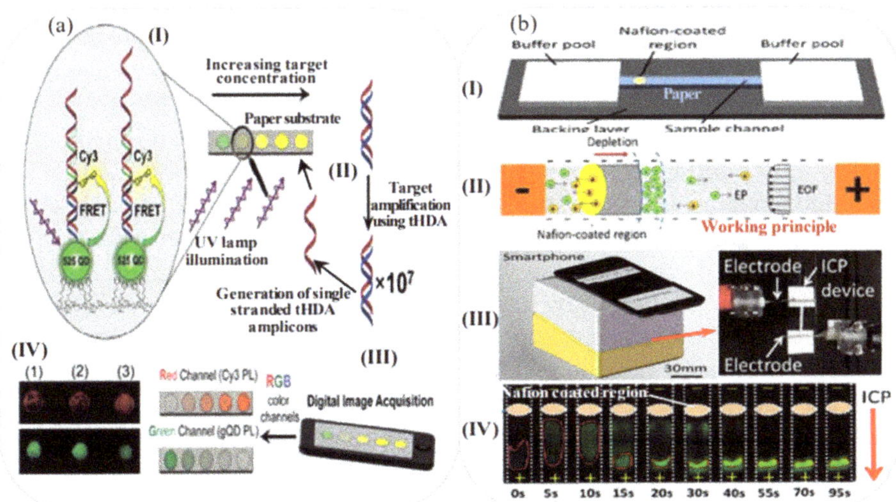

Figure 1.4. Paper-based fluorescent biosensors from the past: (a) fluorescent, paper-based detection of nucleic acid hybridization, (b) ion concentration polarization (ICP) generation mechanism. Reprinted from reference Fu and Wang (2018) with permission of Elsevier.

the target cells (Liang *et al* 2017, 2016a). Several fluorescent-based μPAD approaches for detecting trace quantities of heavy metal ions have been suggested. Zhang *et al*, for example, developed a μPAD for the multiplexed and simultaneous detection of several heavy metal contaminants in food. They utilized graphene oxide modified by fluorescent Cy5-labelled single-stranded DNA. With this system they could detect Hg (II), Ag(I), and NEO ion with the limit of detection of 121 nM, 47 nM and 153 nM, respectively. Further the Bian *et al* used fluorescent gold (Au) nanocluster-based test sheets to detect Hg^{2+} and Pb^{2+} ions in recyclable form. When the testing paper sheet was exposed to Hg^{2+} an evident fluorescence quenching was seen. But then a considerable fluorescent increase was found in the presence of Pb^{2+}. Furthermore, the limit of detection for Hg^{2+} ions and Pb^{2+} ions were determined to be 5 μM and 50 μM, respectively (Bian *et al* 2017). Later, Qi *et al* developed the multiplex detection system for the Cu^{2+} and Hg^{2+} ions. They used cadmium telluride (CdTe) quantum dots as a fluorescent system and fabricated the 3D μPAD for the multiplexing assay. With this system they could get a LOD of 0.035 g l^{-1} and 0.056 g l^{-1} for Cu^{2+} and Hg^{2+} ions respectively (Qi *et al* 2017). As a result of such systems, numerous paper-based methods have been developed for concentrating the material prior to detection utilizing an ion concentration polarization (ICP) mechanism (Li *et al* 2016, Gong *et al* 2015). Li *et al* developed an ICP using nitrocellulose membrane which were coated with nafion perfluorinated resin and put at one end of a detector channel to generate an ICP (figure 1.4(b)). This technology obtained a 28-fold maximal concentration augmentation of fluorescent dye samples in 70 seconds, according to the experimental data (Li *et al* 2016). Gong *et al* also demonstrated a paper-based ICP device for direct DNA analysis. The device was constructed with a sample channel, two reservoirs, and an area covered with nanoporous Nafion. In this device, with the introduction of external voltage supply the electroendosmotic flow (EOF) and electrophoretic migration (EPH) were generated. Result of which is the movement of anions in the sample solutions. The suggested device was utilized to detect human hepatitis-B (HBV) DNA in the blood. This device was also utilized to assess the integrity of sperm DNA in raw human sperm. Without preceding viral load amplification, a detection limit of 150 copies/ml was attained, validating the device's potential for early HBV diagnosis (Gong *et al* 2015). Additional information on the paper-based early diagnostic system in medical science can be found in chapter 2. Yang's group also introduced the nafion-based ICP devices developed by printing wax on both sides of μPAD. The result of which is the improvement in ICP concentration effect (Yang *et al* 2015). Phan *et al* suggested the μPAD based on the ICP using nanoporous polymer matrix. Within 200 seconds, the device increased the concentration of fluorescent dye samples by 60 times (Phan *et al* 2016). Those were the fluorescence and paper-based biosensors from the past. Considering the 21st century as the era of Internet of Things (IoT), various fluorescence-based biosensors utilizing this technology have been developed recently. For instance, Guo *et al* developed the paper-based fluorescent biosensors to quantitatively detect spike and nucleocapsid protein of SARS-CoV-2 with the LOD of 1.6 and 2.2 ng ml^{-1} respectively (Guo *et al* 2021). More information on IoT based biosensors can be found in chapter 12.

1.3.3 Overview of electrochemical biosensors

Electrochemical paper-based biosensors are more sensitive biosensors than colorimetric biosensors. Electrochemical biosensors based on paper in general are called 'paper-based electrochemical devices' (μPEDs). μPEDs are cost effective to fabricate, portable, they confer good selectivity and sensitivity towards the analyte. As a result they are the μPAD of the electrochemical biosensors (Scordo *et al* 2018, Bhardwaj *et al* 2017). The various electrochemical systems used in conjugation with μPEDs are flow injection, microelectrodes, ion-exchange membrane, convective mass transfer, etc. Furthermore, the electrochemical methods for the analysis are potentiometry, cyclic voltammetry, amperometry and coulometry. Voltammetry is one of the most widely used methods coupled with μPEDs (Cuartero *et al* 2015, Cinti *et al* 2017). Cuartero *et al* for example, demonstrated a μPED for the detection of halides (Cl^-, Br^-, I^-) from a variety of water samples as well as from dietary supplements. The fabricated μPED comprised of a cation exchange Donnan exclusion membrane and a Ag-foil working electrode (figure 1.5(a)). Cyclic voltammetry was employed in the detection method to execute successive oxidation/plating of the halide ions at the Ag electrode, followed by regeneration with an inverted potential. The suggested device's viability was tested using a combination of Cl^-, Br^- and I^- ions generated in concentrations ranging from 104.8 to 0.1 μM for Br and I and from 104.5 to 0.6 μM for Cl. The detection limit was discovered to be of the order of 105 μM (Cuartero *et al* 2015). Further, Teengam *et al* developed the electrochemical detection system for the detection of human

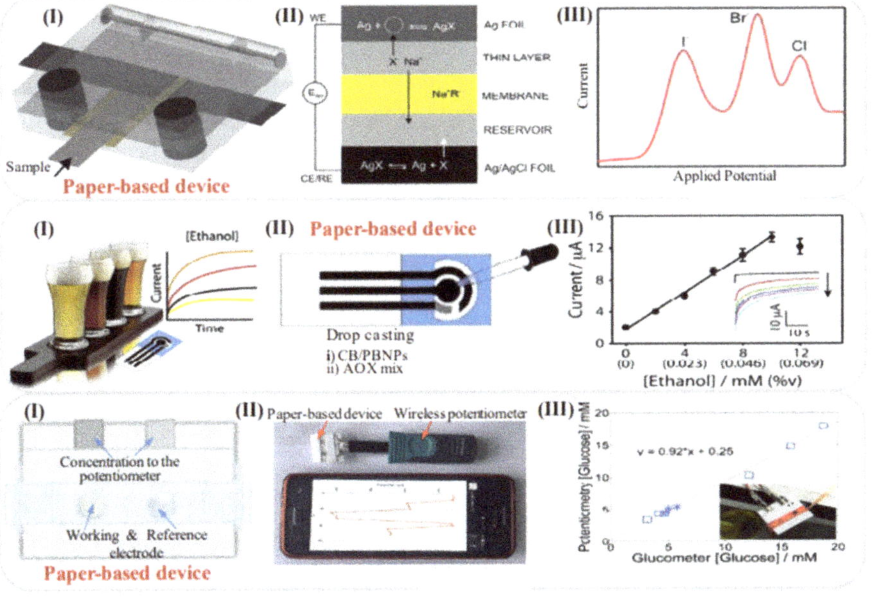

Figure 1.5. Paper-based electrochemical biosensors from the past: (a) electrochemical detection of halide ions by paper-based device coupled with cyclic voltammetry, (b) detection of alcohol in beer samples using screen-printed electrode, and (c) blood glucose monitoring by potentiometric method. Reprinted from reference Fu and Wang (2018) with permission of Elsevier.

papillomavirus (HPV). In this, they have fabricated the graphene-polyaniline (G-PANI) electrode which was modified by anthraquinone-labelled pyrrolidinyl peptide nucleic acid (acpcPNA) probe (AQ-PNA). This probe was patterned using inkjet printing (Teengam *et al* 2017a). In a further step, Tian *et al* developed an electrochemical system for the detection of a lung cancer biomarker. The proposed electrochemical biosensor had the limit of detection of 0.167 nM (Tian *et al* 2017). These were the few paper-based electrochemical biosensors (μPEDs) which used cyclic voltammetry for electrochemical analysis. But there are several μPEDs which used the amperometry as a electrochemical analytical method, these could be found in the literature cited here (Burrs *et al* 2016, Dias *et al* 2016). A good example for the amperometry is the Cinti *et al* group's electrochemical biosensor consisting of a paper-based screen-printed electrode. This electrode was fabricated by drop casting for the detection ethanol in beer samples (figure 1.5(b)(I)). The working electrode area of the electrode had carbon black (CB) and Prussian blue nanoparticles (PBNPs) which were used as an electrocatalyst in the proposed device to detect the hydrogen peroxide produced by the enzymatic interaction between alcohol oxidase (AOx) and ethanol (figure 1.5(b)(II)). The developed system had the sensitivity of 9.13 $\mu A\ mM^{-1}\ cm^{-2}$ and the limit of detection of 0.52 mM. The suggested biosensor enabled a simple measurement of ethanol in beer up to the concentration of 10 mM (figure 1.5(c)(III)) (Cinti *et al* 2017). Later on, Dias *et al* used a 3D printed batch injection analysis (BIA) cell for the detection of glucose in human blood serum. In this system they paired the BIA cell with screen-printed electrodes to fabricate a paper-based enzymatic device. This device used amperometry as the electrochemical analytical method of detection for determining glucose concentrations in human blood serum. The limit of detection of blood glucose in the serum with this system was 110 μM (Dias *et al* 2016). Furthermore, Burrs *et al* demonstrated cyclic voltammetry and DC potential amperometry based electrochemical system for the detection of glucose. They fabricated the paper with graphene and fractal platinum nanocauliflowers. The limit of detection for the glucose by this system was 0.08 μM (Burrs *et al* 2016). Apart from the voltammetry and amperometry, potentiometric detection of analyte using electrochemical paper-based biosensors could be found in the literature cited here (Cánovas *et al* 2017, Sjöberg *et al* 2016, Parrilla *et al* 2017). For example, Cánovas *et al* developed a small and sensitive wireless paper-based potentiometric technology for precise glucose monitoring in the blood. The platform, as illustrated in figure 1.5(c), was primarily comprised of a paper-based potentiometric chip, a wireless potentiometer, and a commercial glucometer. The potentiometric chip's working electrode was a strip of platinized filter paper covered with a nafion membrane to entrap the enzyme glucose oxidase. The reference electrode, on the other hand, was made of a polyvinylbutyral-based membrane cast onto conductive paper. In the range of 0.33 mM, the device attained a sensitivity of 95.9% (Cánovas *et al* 2017). In another potentiometric approach, Hu *et al*'s group developed the system for the detection of several ions. In this, they have fabricated the paper-based potentiometric ion-sensing devices with Ag/AgCl electrodes using an inkjet printing process. It was demonstrated that unaltered Ag/AgCl electrodes could detect chloride, but electrodes modified with ionophore-doped PVC membranes could detect Cl^-, K^+, Na^+ and Ca^{2+} ions. The detection technique in all circumstances required the employment of a reference electrolyte (aqueous KCl solution) in the actual sample solution (Hu *et al* 2016). Similarly, some researchers (Lisak *et al* 2015, Ruecha *et al* 2017) employed the interesting technique of inkjet printing for the fabrication of electrochemical paper-based potentiometric devices for ion detection. One distinct area of electrochemistry, i.e., photoelectrochemistry has also been used for the detection of various analytes. Photoelectrochemical (PEC) detection (Hasanzadeh and Shadjou 2016) is distinguished by its ease of use, low cost, high sensitivity, and selectivity, making it excellent for high-throughput tests. Ge *et al* created a paper-based PEC detection system for sensitive and specific POC diagnostics, using a porous Ag-paper working electrode as a sensor platform and multilabeled nanoporous gold-carbon nanospheres as tracers. The immunological device's great sensitivity, obtained by improved electrochemiluminescence (ECL) emission and the high catalytic efficiency of the porous Ag-paper working electrode, enables it to identify cancer markers virtually immediately in serum samples with short incubation durations and low detection limits. The detection limits for the three tumour markers (CEA, CA125, and AFP) in animal serum were 1.0 pg ml^{-1}, 1.6 mU ml^{-1} and 1.8 pg ml^{-1}, respectively (Ge *et al* 2015). Recently, a label free paper-based electrochemical biosensor was developed by Yakoh *et al* for the detection of SARS-CoV-2 antibodies. In this sensor, an electrochemical paper-based analytical device (ePAD) was fabricated using wax printing technology and the LOD measured using the same was 0.96 and 0.14 ng ml^{-1} for IgG and IgM respectively (Yakoh *et al* 2021). Similarly, screen-printed electrode-based detection of Nucleocapsid protein of SARS-CoV-2 was developed by Eissa and Zourob. The developed biosensor showed good LOD for the Nucleocapsid protein i.e. 0.8 pg ml^{-1} (Eissa and Zourob 2021). More information on label free paper-based devices can be found in chapter 5. So, these were the paper-based electrochemical biosensors from the past and they will be further improving in the future and may open doors for very sensitive analyte detection systems. See the table 1.2 for the expanded list on electrochemical biosensors.

1.4 Paper-based microfluidics/biosensors-future perspective

The future of frugal microfluidics technology will be in paper-based technologies. This is evident from the extensive use of μPADs in the development of POCs. Since μPADs are easy to develop, have scale-up ability and a multi-functional role in the medical diagnostics system, they will be more common in the near future. Moreover, the accuracy and sensitivity of μPADs is already improving, so in the near future it will be even more accurate and sensitive. Therefore, more appropriate diagnosis of the disease/disorders will be possible.

Since paper is a flexible material, it can also be used in wearable biosensors. Wearable biosensors/devices are already on trend due to the health-conscious behaviour of the current generation. Since paper is cheap, it can be used for developing cost-effective wearable biosensors. Therefore, paper has enormous scope in the near future.

One of the areas in medical industry, i.e., telemedicine plays a vital role in enhancing the healthcare service especially in the underdeveloped and developing countries where resources are limited. Paper-based biosensors coupled with smartphones can provide great help to those countries in the future. Nevertheless, the promises of paper-based POCs will not be realized until the additional parts of POCs, such as sample pre-treatment, plasma separation (from blood) and nucleic acid isolation and amplification, are accomplished on paper. These considerations are critical for paper-based biosensors, which outperform traditional immunoassays especially in terms of its sensitivity and specificity. With the further optimization and improvement in those technologies, we believe that paper-based biosensors/microfluidics may play a significant role in the development of paper-based POCs.

1.5 Conclusion

In this chapter we have summarized the major findings on paper-based biosensors largely classified into three modes, i.e., μPAD, LFA and dipsticks. Among all the modes, the μPADs were widely used for POC due to its benefits over the others. All these modes of paper-based microfluidics/biosensors could be coupled with different ways of detection such as colorimetric, fluorescence and electrochemical detection. We have thoroughly summarized those ways of detection in this chapter. We also described the need of paper-based biosensors for the cost-effective clinical diagnostics and POC applications.

Conflict of interest

The authors declare no conflict of interest.

Acknowledgement

Authors would like to thank Grant Number CRG/2020/003014 from Science and Engineering Research Board (SERB), New Delhi for kind support and Indian Council of Medical Research (ICMR), New Delhi.

References

Aparna R S, Anjali Devi J S, Sachidanandan P and George S 2018 Polyethylene imine capped copper nanoclusters—fluorescent and colorimetric onsite sensor for the trace level detection of TNT *Sensors Actuators* B **254** 811–9

Arrastia M, Avoundjian A, Ehrlich P S, Eropkin M, Levine L and Gomez F A 2015 Development of a microfluidic-based assay on a novel nitrocellulose platform *Electrophoresis* **36** 884–8

Avoundjian A, Jalali-Heravi M and Gomez F A 2017 Use of chemometrics to optimize a glucose assay on a paper microfluidic platform *Anal. Bioanal. Chem.* **409** 2697–703

Banga I, Tyagi R, Shahdeo D and Gandhi S 2019 *Biosensors and their application for the detection of avian influenza virus* (Nanotechnology in Modern Animal Biotechnology: Concepts and Applications) (Amsterdam: Elsevier), 1–16

Bhardwaj J, Devarakonda S, Kumar S and Jang J 2017 Development of a paper-based electrochemical immunosensor using an antibody-single walled carbon nanotubes bio-conjugate modified electrode for label-free detection of foodborne pathogens *Sensors Actuators* B **253** 115–23

Bian R X, Wu X T, Chai F, Li L, Zhang L Y, Wang T T, Wang C G and Su Z M 2017 Facile preparation of fluorescent Au nanoclusters-based test papers for recyclable detection of Hg^{2+} and Pb^{2+} *Sensors Actuators* B **241** 592–600

Bissonnette L and Bergeron M G 2010 Diagnosing infections—current and anticipated technologies for point-of-care diagnostics and home-based testing *Clin. Microbiol. Infect.* **16** 1044–53

Boonsri M, Vongnam K, Namuangruk S, Sukwattanasinitt M and Rashatasakhon P 2017 Pyrenyl benzimidazole-isoquinolinones: aggregation-induced emission enhancement property and application as TNT fluorescent sensor *Sensors Actuators* B **248** 665–72

Burrs S L, Bhargava M, Sidhu R, Kiernan-Lewis J, Gomes C, Claussen J C and McLamore E S 2016 A paper based graphene-nanocauliflower hybrid composite for point of care biosensing *Biosens. Bioelectron.* **85** 479–87

Cánovas R, Parrilla M, Blondeau P and Andrade F J 2017 A novel wireless paper-based potentiometric platform for monitoring glucose in blood *Lab Chip* **17** 2500–7

Cardoso T M G, Garcia P T and Coltro W K T 2015 Colorimetric determination of nitrite in clinical, food and environmental samples using microfluidic devices stamped in paper platforms *Anal. Methods* **7** 7311–7

Cardoso T M G, Channon R B, Adkins J A, Talhavini M, Coltro W K T and Henry C S 2017a A paper-based colorimetric spot test for the identification of adulterated whiskeys *Chem. Commun.* **53** 7957–60

Cardoso T M G, de Souza F R, Garcia P T, Rabelo D, Henry C S and Coltro W K T 2017b Versatile fabrication of paper-based microfluidic devices with high chemical resistance using scholar glue and magnetic masks *Anal. Chim. Acta* **974** 63–8

Cassano C L and Fan Z H 2013 Laminated paper-based analytical devices (LPAD): fabrication, characterization, and assays *Microfluid. Nanofluidics* **15** 173–81

Chaiyo S, Apiluk A, Siangproh W and Chailapakul O 2016 High sensitivity and specificity simultaneous determination of lead, cadmium and copper using μPAD with dual electrochemical and colorimetric detection *Sensors Actuators* B **233** 540–9

Chen X, Chen J, Wang F, Xiang X, Luo M, Ji X and He Z 2012 Determination of glucose and uric acid with bienzyme colorimetry on microfluidic paper-based analysis devices *Biosens. Bioelectron.* **35** 363–8

Chin C D, Linder V and Sia S K 2007 Lab-on-a-chip devices for global health: past studies and future opportunities *Lab Chip* **7** 41–57

Choi D H, Lee S K, Oh Y K, Bae B W, Lee S D, Kim S, Shin Y B and Kim M G 2010 A dual gold nanoparticle conjugate-based lateral flow assay (LFA) method for the analysis of troponin I *Biosens. Bioelectron.* **25** 1999–2002

Choi S, Kim S K, Lee G J and Park H K 2015 Paper-based 3D microfluidic device for multiple bioassays *Sensors Actuators* B **219** 245–50

Cinti S, Basso M, Moscone D and Arduini F 2017 A paper-based nanomodified electrochemical biosensor for ethanol detection in beers *Anal. Chim. Acta* **960** 123–30

Cuartero M, Crespo G A and Bakker E 2015 Paper-based thin-layer coulometric sensor for halide determination *Anal. Chem.* **87** 1981–90

Dai G, Hu J, Zhao X and Wang P 2017 A colorimetric paper sensor for lactate assay using a cellulose-Binding recombinant enzyme *Sensors Actuators* B **238** 138–44

Das P and Krull U J 2017 Detection of cancer biomarker protein on modified cellulose paper by fluorescence using aptamer-linked quantum dots *Analyst* **142** 3132–5

Dias A A, Cardoso T M G, Cardoso R M, Duarte L C, Muñoz R A A, Richter E M and Coltro W K T 2016 Paper-based enzymatic reactors for batch injection analysis of glucose on 3D printed cell coupled with amperometric detection *Sensors Actuators* B **226** 196–203

Dincer C, Bruch R, Kling A, Dittrich P S and Urban G A 2017 Multiplexed point-of-care testing—xPOCT *Trends Biotechnol.* **35** 728–42

Dong M, Wu J, Ma Z, Peretz-Soroka H, Zhang M, Komenda P, Tangri N, Liu Y, Rigatto C and Lin F 2017 Rapid and low-cost CRP measurement by integrating a paper-based microfluidic immunoassay with smartphone (CRP-Chip) *Sensors* **17** 684

Dossi N, Toniolo R, Pizzariello A, Impellizzieri F, Piccin E and Bontempelli G 2013 Pencil-drawn paper supported electrodes as simple electrochemical detectors for paper-based fluidic devices *Electrophoresis* **34** 2085–91

Dungchai W, Chailapakul O and Henry C S 2009 Electrochemical detection for paper-based microfluidics *Anal. Chem.* **81** 5821–6

Eissa S and Zourob M 2021 Development of a low-cost cotton-tipped electrochemical immunosensor for the detection of SARS-CoV-2 *Anal. Chem.* **93** 1826–33

Fischer C, Fraiwan A and Choi S 2016 A 3D paper-based enzymatic fuel cell for self-powered, low-cost glucose monitoring *Biosens. Bioelectron.* **79** 193–7

Frazer S C 1958 Laboratory trial of a paper strip test for proteinuria *Br. Med. J.* **1** 981

Fu E and Downs C 2017 Progress in the development and integration of fluid flow control tools in paper microfluidics *Lab Chip* **17** 614–28

Fu M and Wang Y-N 2018 Detection methods and applications of microfluidic paper-based analytical devices *TrAC Trends Anal. Chem.* **107** 196–211

Gabriel E F M, Garcia P T, Lopes F M and Coltro W K T 2017 Paper-based colorimetric biosensor for tear glucose measurements *Micromachines* **8** 104

Gandhi S, Caplash N, Sharma P and Raman Suri C 2009 Strip-based immunochromatographic assay using specific egg yolk antibodies for rapid detection of morphine in urine samples *Biosens. Bioelectron.* **25** 502–5

Ge L, Yu J, Ge S and Yan M 2014 Lab-on-paper-based devices using chemiluminescence and electrogenerated chemiluminescence detection *Anal. Bioanal. Chem.* **406** 5613–30

Ge S, Li W, Yan M, Song X and Yu J 2015 Photoelectrochemical detection of tumor markers based on a CdS quantum dot/ZnO nanorod/Au@Pt-paper electrode 3D origami immunodevice *J. Mater. Chem.* B **3** 2426–32

Gong M M, Nosrati R, San Gabriel M C, Zini A and Sinton D 2015 Direct DNA analysis with paper-based ion concentration polarization *J. Am. Chem. Soc.* **137** 13913–9

Gonzalez A, Estala L, Gaines M and Gomez F A 2016 Mixed thread/paper-based microfluidic chips as a platform for glucose assays *Electrophoresis* **37** 1685–90

Guo J, Chen S, Tian S, Liu K, Ni J, Zhao M, Kang Y, Ma X and Guo J 2021 5G-enabled ultra-sensitive fluorescence sensor for proactive prognosis of COVID-19 *Biosens. Bioelectron.* **181** 113160

Hasanzadeh M and Shadjou N 2016 Electrochemical and photoelectrochemical nano-immune-sensing using origami paper based method *Mater. Sci. Eng.* C **61** 979–1001

Hauck T S, Giri S, Gao Y and Chan W C W 2010 Nanotechnology diagnostics for infectious diseases prevalent in developing countries *Adv. Drug Deliv. Rev.* **62** 438–48

Hawkins K R and Weigl B H 2010 Microfluidic diagnostics for low-resource settings *Proc. SPIE: BioMEMs, and Medical Microsystems* **7593** 163–77

Hay Burgess D C, Wasserman J and Dahl C A 2006 Global health diagnostics *Nature* **444** 1–2

He D, Wu Z, Cui B, Xu E and Jin Z 2019 Establishment of a dual mode immunochromatographic assay for *Campylobacter jejuni* detection *Food Chem.* **289** 708–13

Hu J, Stein A and Bühlmann P 2016 A disposable planar paper-based potentiometric ion-sensing platform *Angew. Chem.-Int. Ed.* **55** 7544–7

Hu J, Wang S Q, Wang L, Li F, Pingguan-Murphy B, Lu T J and Xu F 2014 Advances in paper-based point-of-care diagnostics *Biosens. Bioelectron.* **54** 585–97

Huang C J, Lin H I, Shiesh S C and Bin L G 2010 Integrated microfluidic system for rapid screening of CRP aptamers utilizing systematic evolution of ligands by exponential enrichment (SELEX) *Biosens. Bioelectron.* **25** 1761–6

İncel A, Akın O, Çağır A, Yıldız Ü H and Demir M M 2017 Smart phone assisted detection and quantification of cyanide in drinking water by paper based sensing platform *Sensors Actuators* B **252** 886–93

Islam S, Shukla S, Bajpai V K, Han Y-K, Huh Y S, Ghosh A and Gandhi S 2019 Microfluidic-based graphene field effect transistor for femtomolar detection of chlorpyrifos *Sci. Rep.* **9** 1–7

Jeong J, Cho E, Yun D, Kim T, Lee I S and Jung S 2017 Label-free colorimetric detection of influenza antigen based on an antibody-polydiacetylene conjugate and its coated polyvinylidene difluoride membrane *Polymers* **9** 127

Kasoju A, Shahdeo D, Khan A A, Shrikrishna N S, Mahari S, Alanazi A M, Bhat M A, Giri J and Gandhi S 2020a Fabrication of microfluidic device for Aflatoxin M1 detection in milk samples with specific aptamers *Sci. Rep.* **10** 1–7

Kasoju A, Shrikrishna N S, Shahdeo D, Khan A A, Alanazi A M and Gandhi S 2020b Microfluidic paper device for rapid detection of aflatoxin B1 using an aptamer based colorimetric assay *RSC Adv.* **10** 11843–50

Kit-Anan W, Olarnwanich A, Sriprachuabwong C, Karuwan C, Tuantranont A, Wisitsoraat A, Srituravanich W and Pimpin A 2012 Disposable paper-based electrochemical sensor utilizing inkjet-printed polyaniline modified screen-printed carbon electrode for ascorbic acid detection *J. Electroanal. Chem.* **685** 72–8

Kuswandi B, Gani A A and Ahmad M 2017 Immuno strip test for detection of pork adulteration in cooked meatballs *Food Biosci.* **19** 1–6

Kuswandi B, Ratnasari I and Gani A A 2005 Optical detection of uric acid based on immobilised ferriin onto modified PVA membrane *2005 Asian Conf. Sensors Int. Conf. New Tech. Pharm. Biomed. Res.—Proc.* pp 107–10

Laksanasopin T, Chin C D, Moore H, Wang J, Cheung Y K and Sia S K 2009 Microfluidic point-of-care diagnostics for resource-poor environments *Proc. 31st Annual Int. Conf. IEEE Eng. Med. Biol. Soc. Eng. Futur. Biomed. EMBC* pp 1057–9

Lee W G, Kim Y G, Chung B G, Demirci U and Khademhosseini A 2010 Nano/microfluidics for diagnosis of infectious diseases in developing countries *Adv. Drug Deliv. Rev.* **62** 449–57

Lei K F, Huang C H, Kuo R L, Chang C K, Chen K F, Tsao K C and Tsang N M 2015 Paper-based enzyme-free immunoassay for rapid detection and subtyping of influenza A H1N1 and H3N2 viruses *Anal. Chim. Acta* **883** 37–44

Li X, Niu Y, Chen Y, Wu D, Yi L and Qiu X 2016 Microfluidic paper-based sample concentration using ion concentration polarization with smartphone detection *Micromachines* **7** 199

Li Z *et al* 2020 Development and clinical application of a rapid IgM-IgG combined antibody test for SARS-CoV-2 infection diagnosis *J. Med. Virol.* **92** 1518–24

Liana D D, Raguse B, Justin Gooding J and Chow E 2012 Recent advances in paper-based sensors *Sensors (Switzerland)* **12** 11505–26

Liang L, Lan F, Li L, Su M, Ge S, Yu J, Liu H and Yan M 2016a Fluorescence 'turn-on' determination of H_2O_2 using multilayer porous SiO2/NGQDs and PdAu mimetics enzymatic/oxidative cleavage of single-stranded DNA *Biosens. Bioelectron.* **82** 204–11

Liang L, Lan F, Yin X, Ge S, Yu J and Yan M 2017 Metal-enhanced fluorescence/visual bimodal platform for multiplexed ultrasensitive detection of microRNA with reusable paper analytical devices *Biosens. Bioelectron.* **95** 181–8

Liang L, Su M, Li L, Lan F, Yang G, Ge S, Yu J and Song X 2016b Aptamer-based fluorescent and visual biosensor for multiplexed monitoring of cancer cells in microfluidic paper-based analytical devices *Senors Actuators* B **229** 347–54

Lin M, Zhao Y, Wang S Q, Liu M, Duan Z F, Chen Y M, Li F, Xu F and Lu T J 2012 Recent advances in synthesis and surface modification of lanthanide-doped upconversion nanoparticles for biomedical applications *Biotechnol. Adv.* **30** 1551–61

Lisak G, Cui J and Bobacka J 2015 Paper-based microfluidic sampling for potentiometric determination of ions *Sensors Actuators* B **207** 933–9

Liu C C, Wang Y N, Fu L M and Yang D Y 2017 Rapid integrated microfluidic paper-based system for sulfur dioxide detection *Chem. Eng. J.* **316** 790–6

Liu C and Gomez F A 2017 A microfluidic paper-based device to assess acetylcholinesterase activity *Electrophoresis* **38** 1002–6

Liu D, Shen H, Zhang Y, Shen D, Zhu M, Song Y, Zhu Z and Yang C 2021 A microfluidic-integrated lateral flow recombinase polymerase amplification (MI-IF-RPA) assay for rapid COVID-19 detection *Lab Chip* **21** 2019–26

Liu H and Crooks R M 2011 Three-dimensional paper microfluidic devices assembled using the principles of origami *J. Am. Chem. Soc.* **133** 17564–6

Liu S, Su W and Ding X 2016 A review on microfluidic paper-based analytical devices for glucose detection *Sensors (Basel)* **16** 2086

Lopez-Ruiz N, Curto V F, Erenas M M, Benito-Lopez F, Diamond D, Palma A J and Capitan-Vallvey L F 2014 Smartphone-based simultaneous ph and nitrite colorimetric determination for paper microfluidic devices *Anal. Chem.* **86** 9554–62

Loynachan C N *et al* 2018 Platinum nanocatalyst amplification: redefining the gold standard for lateral flow immunoassays with ultrabroad dynamic range *ACS Nano* **12** 279–88

Lu C, Gao X, Chen Y, Ren J and Liu C 2019 Aptamer-based lateral flow test strip for the simultaneous detection of *Salmonella typhimurium*, *Escherichia coli* O157:H7 and Staphylococcus aureus**53** 646–59

Lu J, Ge S, Ge L, Yan M and Yu J 2012 Electrochemical DNA sensor based on three-dimensional folding paper device for specific and sensitive point-of-care testing *Electrochim. Acta* **80** 334–41

Mabey D, Peeling R W, Ustianowski A and Perkins M D 2004 Diagnostics for the developing world *Nat. Rev. Microbiol.* **2** 231–40

Mansfield M A 2007 The use of nitrocellulose membranes in lateral-flow assays *Drugs of Abuse* 71–85

Mao X and Huang T J 2012 Microfluidic diagnostics for the developing world *Lab Chip* **12** 1412–6

Martinez A W, Phillips S T, Butte M J and Whitesides G M 2007 Patterned paper as a platform for inexpensive, low-volume, portable bioassays *Angew. Chem.* **119** 1340–2

Martinez A W, Phillips S T and Whitesides G M 2008 Three-dimensional microfluidic devices fabricated in layered paper and tape *Proc. Natl Acad. Sci. USA* **105** 19606–11

Martinez A W, Phillips S T, Whitesides G M and Carrilho E 2009 Diagnostics for the developing world: microfluidic paper-based analytical devices *Anal. Chem.* **82** 3–10

Meelapsom R, Jarujamrus P, Amatatongchai M, Chairam S, Kulsing C and Shen W 2016 Chromatic analysis by monitoring unmodified silver nanoparticles reduction on double layer microfluidic paper-based analytical devices for selective and sensitive determination of mercury(II) *Talanta* **155** 193–201

Moghadam B Y, Connelly K T and Posner J D 2015 Two orders of magnitude improvement in detection limit of lateral flow assays using isotachophoresis *Anal. Chem.* **87** 1009–17

Mohammadi A and Yaghoubi S 2017 A new dual colorimetric chemosensor based on quinazolinone for CN^-, AcO^- and Cu^{2+} ions *Sensors Actuators* B **241** 1069–75

Morens D M, Folkers G K and Fauci A S 2004 The challenge of emerging and re-emerging infectious diseases *Nature* **430** 242–9

Mujawar L H, Felemban A A and El-Shahawi M S 2016 Hexamethyldisilazane modified paper as an ultra-sensitive platform for visual detection of Hg^{2+}, Co^{2+}, Zn^{2+} and the application to semi-quantitative determination of Hg^{2+} in wastewater *Anal. Sci.* **32** 491–7

Narlawar S, Coudhury S and Gandhi S 2022 Magnetic properties-based biosensors for early detection of cancer *Biosensor Based Advanced Cancer Diagnostics* 165–78

Narlawar S S and Gandhi S 2021 Fabrication of graphene nanoplatelets embedded 'partition cartridge' for efficient separation of target-bound ssDNA during SELEX *Mater. Today Adv.* **12** 100174

Nery E W and Kubota L T 2016 Evaluation of enzyme immobilization methods for paper-based devices-a glucose oxidase study *J. Pharm. Biomed. Anal.* **117** 551–9

Nie Z, Nijhuis C A, Gong J, Chen X, Kumachev A, Martinez A W, Narovlyansky M and Whitesides G M 2010 Electrochemical sensing in paper-based microfluidic devices *Lab Chip* **10** 477–83

Nilghaz A, Wicaksono D H B, Gustiono D, Abdul Majid F A, Supriyanto E and Abdul Kadir M R 2012 Flexible microfluidic cloth-based analytical devices using a low-cost wax patterning technique *Lab Chip* **12** 209–18

Noor M O, Hrovat D, Moazami-Goudarzi M, Espie G S and Krull U J 2015 Ratiometric fluorescence transduction by hybridization after isothermal amplification for determination of zeptomole quantities of oligonucleotide biomarkers with a paper-based platform and camera-based detection *Anal. Chim. Acta* **885** 156–65

Noor M O and Krull U J 2014 Camera-based ratiometric fluorescence transduction of nucleic acid hybridization with reagentless signal amplification on a paper-based platform using immobilized quantum dots as donors *Anal. Chem.* **86** 10331–9

Nuchtavorn N and Macka M 2016 A novel highly flexible, simple, rapid and low-cost fabrication tool for paper-based microfluidic devices (μPADs) using technical drawing pens and in-house formulated aqueous inks *Anal. Chim. Acta* **919** 70–7

Nurul Najian A B, Engku Nur Syafirah E A R, Ismail N, Mohamed M and Yean C Y 2016 Development of multiplex loop mediated isothermal amplification (m-LAMP) label-based gold nanoparticles lateral flow dipstick biosensor for detection of pathogenic Leptospira *Anal. Chim. Acta* **903** 142–8

Ortiz-Gomez I, Ortega-Muñoz M, Salinas-Castillo A, Álvarez-Bermejo J A, Ariza-Avidad M, de Orbe-Payá I, Santoyo-Gonzalez F and Capitan-Vallvey L F 2016 Tetrazine-based chemistry for nitrite determination in a paper microfluidic device *Talanta* **160** 721–8

Parrilla M, Cánovas R and Andrade F J 2017 Paper-based enzymatic electrode with enhanced potentiometric response for monitoring glucose in biological fluids *Biosens. Bioelectron.* **90** 110–6

Pelton R 2009 Bioactive paper provides a low-cost platform for diagnostics *TrAC Trends Anal. Chem.* **28** 925–42

Phan D T, Shaegh S A M, Yang C and Nguyen N T 2016 Sample concentration in a microfluidic paper-based analytical device using ion concentration polarization *Sensors Actuators* B **222** 735–40

Posthuma-Trumpie G A, Korf J and Van Amerongen A 2009 Lateral flow (immuno)assay: its strengths, weaknesses, opportunities and threats. A literature survey *Anal. Bioanal. Chem.* **393** 569–82

Qi J, Li B, Wang X, Zhang Z, Wang Z, Han J and Chen L 2017 Three-dimensional paper-based microfluidic chip device for multiplexed fluorescence detection of Cu^{2+} and Hg^{2+} ions based on ion imprinting technology *Sensors Actuators* B **251** 224–33

Raman Suri C, Boro R, Nangia Y, Gandhi S, Sharma P, Wangoo N, Rajesh K and Shekhawat G S 2009 Immunoanalytical techniques for analyzing pesticides in the environment *TrAC Trends Anal. Chem.* **28** 29–39

Raman Suri C, Kaur J, Gandhi S and Shekhawat G S 2008 Label-free ultra-sensitive detection of atrazine based on nanomechanics *Nanotechnology* **19** 235502

Rivas L, Reuterswärd P, Rasti R, Herrmann B, Mårtensson A, Alfvén T, Gantelius J and Andersson-Svahn H 2018 A vertical flow paper-microarray assay with isothermal DNA amplification for detection of *Neisseria meningitidis Talanta* **183** 192–200

Roberts A, Chouhan R S, Shahdeo D, Shrikrishna N S, Kesarwani V, Horvat M and Gandhi S 2021 A recent update on advanced molecular diagnostic techniques for COVID-19 pandemic: an overview *Front. Immunol.* **12** 5316

Ruecha N, Chailapakul O, Suzuki K and Citterio D 2017 Fully inkjet-printed paper-based potentiometric ion-sensing devices *Anal. Chem.* **89** 10608–16

Sachs J and Malaney P 2002 The economic and social burden of malaria *Nature* **415** 680–5

Santhiago M, Nery E W, Santos G P and Kubota L T 2014 Microfluidic paper-based devices for bioanalytical applications *Bioanalysis* **6** 89–106

Scordo G, Moscone D, Palleschi G and Arduini F 2018 A reagent-free paper-based sensor embedded in a 3D printing device for cholinesterase activity measurement in serum *Sensors Actuators* B **258** 1015–21

Sheridan C 2020 Fast, portable tests come online to curb coronavirus pandemic *Nat. Biotechnol.* **38** 515–8

Shrikrishna N S, Mahari S, Abbineni N, Eremin S A and Gandhi S 2021 New trends in biosensor development for pesticide detection *Biosensors in Agriculture: Recent Trends and Future Perspectives. Concepts and Strategies in Plant Sciences* (Cham: Springer) 137–68

Sicard C and Brennan J D 2013 Bioactive paper: biomolecule immobilization methods and applications in environmental monitoring *MRS Bull.* **38** 331–4

Sjöberg P, Määttänen A, Vanamo U, Novell M, Ihalainen P, Andrade F J, Bobacka J and Peltonen J 2016 Paper-based potentiometric ion sensors constructed on ink-jet printed gold electrodes *Sensors Actuators* B **224** 325–32

Struss A, Pasini P, Ensor C M, Raut N and Daunert S 2010 Paper strip whole cell biosensors: a portable test for the semiquantitative detection of bacterial quorum signaling molecules *Anal. Chem.* **82** 4457–63

Sun G, Wang P, Ge S, Ge L, Yu J and Yan M 2014 Photoelectrochemical sensor for pentachlorophenol on microfluidic paper-based analytical device based on the molecular imprinting technique *Biosens. Bioelectron.* **56** 97–103

Tabak L A 2007 Point-of-care diagnostics enter the mouth *Ann. N. Y. Acad. Sci.* **1098** 7–14

Talan A, Mishra A, Eremin S A, Narang J, Kumar A and Gandhi S 2018 Ultrasensitive electrochemical immuno-sensing platform based on gold nanoparticles triggering chlorpyrifos detection in fruits and vegetables *Biosens. Bioelectron.* **105** 14–21

Teengam P, Siangproh W, Tuantranont A, Henry C S, Vilaivan T and Chailapakul O 2017a Electrochemical paper-based peptide nucleic acid biosensor for detecting human papillomavirus *Anal. Chim. Acta* **952** 32–40

Teengam P, Siangproh W, Tuantranont A, Vilaivan T, Chailapakul O and Henry C S 2017b Multiplex paper-based colorimetric DNA sensor using pyrrolidinyl peptide nucleic acid-induced AgNPs aggregation for detecting MERS-CoV, MTB, and HPV oligonucleotides *Anal. Chem.* **89** 5428–35

Tian T, Liu H, Li L, Yu J, Ge S, Song X and Yan M 2017 Paper-based biosensor for noninvasive detection of epidermal growth factor receptor mutations in non-small cell lung cancer patients *Sensors Actuators* B **251** 440–5

Vuljanić D *et al* 2019 Analytical verification of 12 most commonly used urine dipsticks in croatia: comparability, repeatability and accuracy *Biochem. Med.* **29** 123–32

Wang C C, Hennek J W, Ainla A, Kumar A A, Lan W J, Im J, Smith B S, Zhao M and Whitesides G M 2016 A paper-based pop-up electrochemical device for analysis of beta-hydroxybutyrate *Anal. Chem.* **88** 6326–33

Wang D, Liu C, Liang Y, Su Y, Shang Q and Zhang C 2018 A simple and sensitive paper-based bipolar electrochemiluminescence biosensor for detection of oxidase-substrate biomarkers in serum *J. Electrochem. Soc.* **165** B361

Wang P, Ge L, Yan M, Song X, Ge S and Yu J 2012a Paper-based three-dimensional electrochemical immunodevice based on multi-walled carbon nanotubes functionalized paper for sensitive point-of-care testing *Biosens. Bioelectron.* **32** 238–43

Wang S, Ge L, Song X, Yu J, Ge S, Huang J and Zeng F 2012b Paper-based chemiluminescence ELISA: lab-on-paper based on chitosan modified paper device and wax-screen-printing *Biosens. Bioelectron.* **31** 212–8

Wang S Q, Xu F and Demirci U 2010 Advances in developing HIV-1 viral load assays for resource-limited settings *Biotechnol. Adv.* **28** 770–81

Whitesides G M 2006 The origins and the future of microfluidics *Nature* **442** 368–73

Wong R and Tse H 2009 Quantitative, false positive, and false negative issues for lateral flow immunoassay as exemplified by onsite drug screens *Lateral Flow Immunoassay* 1–19

Wu D *et al* 2017 A paper-based microfluidic Dot-ELISA system with smartphone for the detection of influenza A *Microfluid. Nanofluid.* **21** 1–9

Yager P, Domingo G J and Gerdes J 2008 Point-of-care diagnostics for global health *Annu. Rev. Biomed. Eng.* **10** 107–44

Yager P, Edwards T, Fu E, Helton K, Nelson K, Tam M R and Weigl B H 2006 Microfluidic diagnostic technologies for global public health *Nature* **442** 412–8

Yakoh A, Pimpitak U, Rengpipat S, Hirankarn N, Chailapakul O and Chaiyo S 2021 Paper-based electrochemical biosensor for diagnosing COVID-19: detection of SARS-CoV-2 antibodies and antigen *Biosens. Bioelectron.* **176** 112912

Yan M, Zang D, Ge S, Ge L and Yu J 2012 A disposable electrochemical immunosensor based on carbon screen-printed electrodes for the detection of prostate specific antigen *Biosens. Bioelectron.* **38** 355–61

Yang K, Peretz-Soroka H, Liu Y and Lin F 2016 Novel developments in mobile sensing based on the integration of microfluidic devices and smartphones *Lab Chip* **16** 943–58

Yang R J, Pu H H and Wang H L 2015 Ion concentration polarization on paper-based microfluidic devices and its application to preconcentrate dilute sample solutions *Biomicrofluidics* **9** 014122

Yen C W, De Puig H, Tam J O, Gómez-Márquez J, Bosch I, Hamad-Schifferli K and Gehrke L 2015 Multicolored silver nanoparticles for multiplexed disease diagnostics: distinguishing dengue, yellow fever, and Ebola viruses *Lab Chip* **15** 1638–41

Yetisen A K, Akram M S and Lowe C R 2013 Paper-based microfluidic point-of-care diagnostic devices *Lab Chip* **13** 2210–51

Yu J, Ge L, Huang J, Wang S and Ge S 2011 Microfluidic paper-based chemiluminescence biosensor for simultaneous determination of glucose and uric acid *Lab Chip* **11** 1286–91

Zheng Y Z *et al* 2021 Reverse transcription recombinase-aided amplification assay with lateral flow dipstick assay for rapid detection of 2019 Novel Coronavirus *Front. Cell. Infect. Microbiol.* **11** 24

Zuo P, Li X, Dominguez D C and Ye B C 2013 A PDMS/paper/glass hybrid microfluidic biochip integrated with aptamer-functionalized graphene oxide nano-biosensors for one-step multiplexed pathogen detection *Lab Chip* **13** 3921–8

Chapter 2

Paper-based biosensor as an early diagnostic system in medical sciences

Tanusha Pathak, Rachna Parashar, Pragati Raghuwanshi and Aushtosh Singh Raghubanshi

The last decade has marked various advancements in the medical and healthcare sectors. Various devices have been developed to improve point of care and standard treatment. In order to cure any disease timely diagnosis of the disease is the key. Diagnostic technologies existing earlier were complex and expensive; with the aim to make diagnosis easier, efficient and inexpensive, extensive research has been carried out across the globe. Paper can be considered as an ideal diagnostic tool due to its simple texture, abundance in nature, biocompatibility and cost-effective production. Researchers across the globe have devised various diagnostic assays using paper such as dipsticks, lateral flow assays and microfluidic paper-based analytical devices (μpads). Quantitative analysis can be done using techniques such as colorimetry, electrochemical analysis, chemiluminescence, electrochemiluminescence and electrical conductivity. Despite these advancements and advantages, paper-based diagnostic devices are not yet completely ideal for diagnosis purposes. This chapter will discuss various types of paper-based devices, their principle of working and applications and will also list the limitations and further advancements in paper-based diagnostic devices.

2.1 Introduction

Health-related difficulties are a silent and gloomy reality that humanity faces all around the world. According to the World Health Organization (WHO), deprived/inadequate healthcare services have resulted in morbidity among millions of people. It has been heavily counted as a result of the presence of many contagious and non-contagious diseases such as diabetes, cancer, malaria, chronic lung diseases, and other ailments, with an estimated death rate of 56 million people each year. Because of the severity and prevalence of these diseases, researchers from all over the world have worked to improve healthcare and medical facilities [1].

doi:10.1088/978-0-7503-5820-0ch2

© IOP Publishing Ltd 2023

The availability of diagnoses is critical to the clinical treatment and management of all kinds of health issues. Traditional diagnostics for such tasks are quite effective; yet, most of them are restricted by time-consuming methods and greater test sample volumes, among other things. Statistical assessments conducted by numerous public and private entities have demonstrated that incorrect diagnoses not only place an economic strain on the patient, they moreover increase the possibility of health complications occurring [2]. In traditional settings, diseased patients diagnosed utilizing high-tech instruments often found in specialized laboratories, where molecular and microbiology-based methods are commonly used [3]. In such scenarios the patient develops a serious illness by the time clinical diagnostics are established. These tactics are extremely potent and precise, but they are typically time-consuming, making them unsuitable in a lot of circumstances, particularly in emergencies, ambulatory, and distant contexts. To address these difficulties, extensive efforts have been made to develop alternative and innovative diagnostic strategies.

Biomedical diagnostic researches are becoming increasingly important in the modern medical profession. Infectious illness screening, early detection, chronic disease therapy, health management, and well-being tracking are all applications for biosensors. Improved biosensor technology allows for the detection of disease and the monitoring of the body's reaction to treatment. Sensor technology is essential for a wide range of low cost and improved-form-factor medical devices. Biosensors offer a lot of potential because they are simple, scalable, and efficient to manufacture [4].

2.1.1 Biosensors: as advancement in medical sciences

A biosensor is an analytical device that detects changes in biological processes and turns them into an electric signal. The output of the transducer will be either current or voltage depending on the type of enzyme and materials used in the biological element (electric form) [4]. It uses a physicochemical detector as well as a bio-recognition element to detect analytes. Bio-recognition element, transducer, amplifier, and detector are the major components of a biosensor (figure 2.1) [1].

As illustrated in figure 2.1, analyte, bioreceptor, transducer, electronics, and reader display are some of the parts or components of a biosensor. For the results display, the display reading device utilized in the biosensor is normally coupled with the accompanying electronics or signal processors. Biosensor readers are often custom-designed and built to accommodate the different operating mechanisms of biosensors. As the sensor analyses the consumer under numerous stimuli, the transducer logs the data and converts the stimulus into an electrical signal that can be quantified as output data [5].

2.1.2 Biosensors in healthcare

Biosensors have found their most effective applications in a wide range of industries, the most prominent of which being medical, healthcare, and clinical services. The capabilities of biosensors that fulfils the requirement of healthcare and linked services are explored in figure 2.2. Disease diagnosis, retinal prostheses, contrast

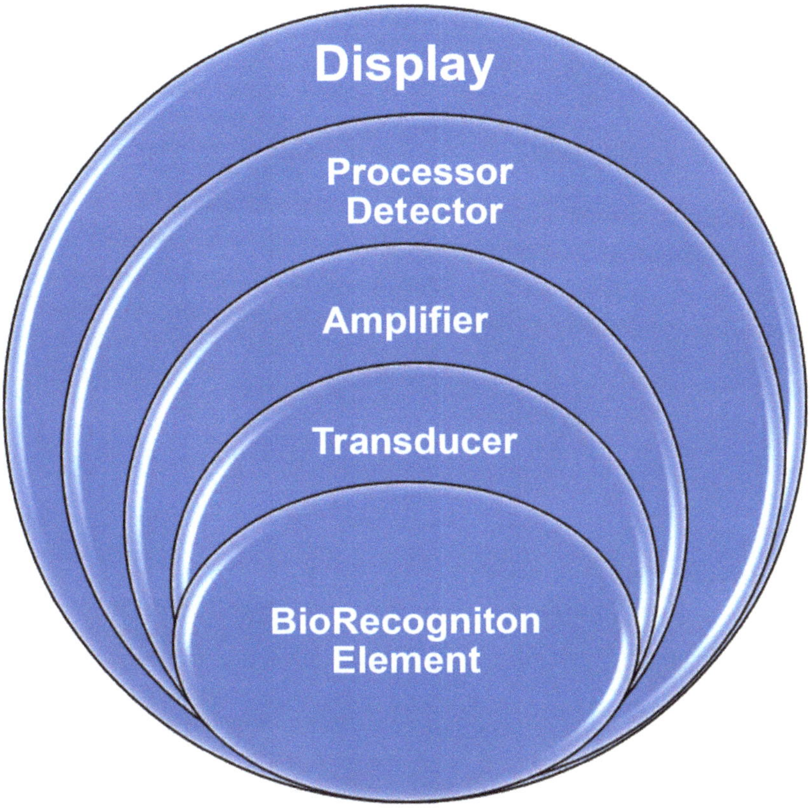

Figure 2.1. Components of a biosensor.

imaging during radiodiagnosis, cardiac diagnostics, medical mycology, health monitoring, and other broad groups of biosensor applications are adequately addressed [6]. In the recent scenario, COVID-19 is a highly infectious pandemic caused by a newly discovered coronavirus that has spread over the world. In recent years, numerous infectious diseases such as avian influenza, SARS, Hendra, Nipah, and others have sparked major attention. As a result, biosensors offer enormous potential and capability for detecting viral and/or disease outbreaks. Another important feature of the biosensor is its capacity to diagnose heart problems. Cardiovascular illnesses are the leading cause of death worldwide, claiming the lives of nearly 17 million people each year. The use of biomarkers in biosensors is critical in the cardiovascular disease diagnostic revolution. For the precise diagnosis of cardiac disorders, the design and development of highly sensitive and specific biosensors using practical surface chemistries and non-material is critical [4].

2.2 Paper-based biosensors

Because of the low cost and flexibility of paper as a substrate, paper-based sensors are an innovative alternative technology for fabricating simple, low cost, portable,

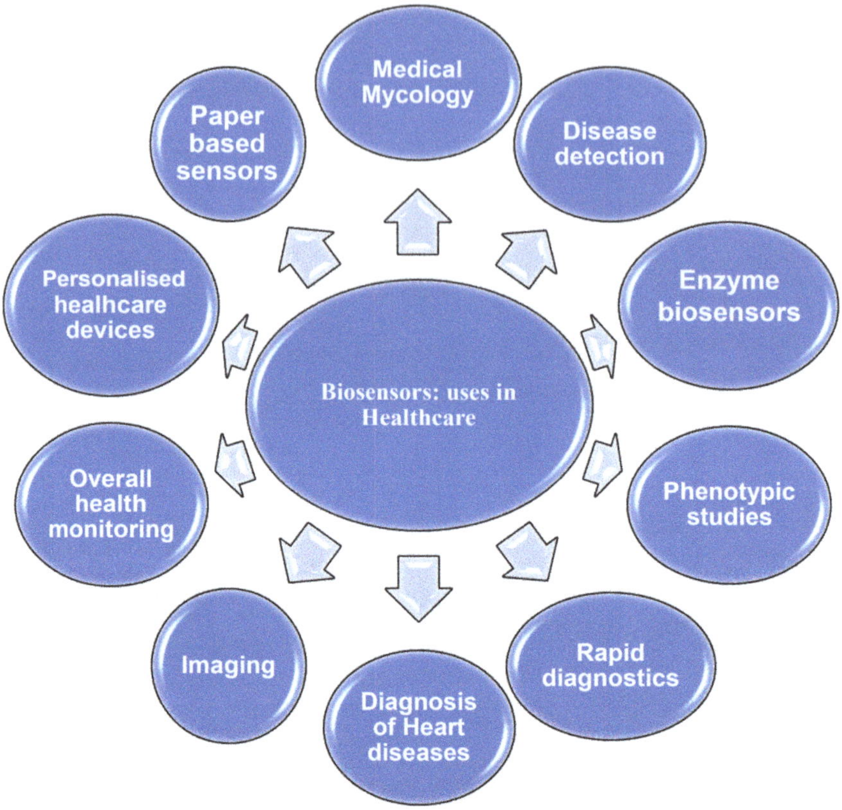

Figure 2.2. Applications of biosensors in healthcare.

and disposable analytical instruments for a number of applications such as clinical diagnosis, food quality control, and environmental monitoring. Certain unique properties of paper as a sensing platform, are its abilities to allow passive liquid movement and compliance with chemicals/biochemicals, are the main benefits of employing paper in sensory applications. Varying as per the end-user, goal to be achieved in paper-based sensors, the building methods and analysis methodologies can be adjusted or manipulated to fit the needs. Current paper-based sensors are focused on microfluidic solutions to the detecting site, on the other hand more advanced designs combine complex 3D geometries based on the similar microfluidic principles. Although paper-based sensors offer a lot of potential, they have several limitations, such as precision and specificity. More fresh and novel discoveries in paper-based sensing are expected to provide further proression, thanks to advancements in manufacturing and analytical methodologies. These sensors could help assuage the present aims of a pocket-friendly, portable device with excellent specificity and sensitivity, as well as multiple analyte discrimination [7].

Paper is a low cost, easily accessible soft matrix with many capillaries that allow fluid to self-pump when it comes into direct contact. Paper has become a viable alternative to self-powered microfluidics for next-generation tailored biosensing due to these features. Martin and Synge were the first to employ paper as a diagnostic platform to access chromatographic procedures, they were awarded the Nobel Prize in 1952. Paper has since been utilized as a simple and reliable platform for a variety of analytical and bioanalytical procedures [2].

2.2.1 Properties of paper as a sensory device

Jute, wood, flax, cotton, sisal, hemp, ramie, bamboo, bassage, and other plant materials are used in commercial paper sheet production, depending on the necessary qualities and categories [2, 8]. The chromophoric intrinsic component lignin is present in wood-made paper that makes it unfit for spectroscopic characterizations of paper-based diagnostic equipment. Despite the fact that lignin content is more likely to be destroyed in downstream processing, even a minimal amount can have a major influence on the efficiency of optical paper-based diagnostics. As a result, lignin-free cotton-made chromatographic filter sheets of higher quality are chosen for this application [2, 9].

2.2.2 Advantages and properties of paper-based diagnostic devices

Some of the advantages of paper-based diagnostic devices are:

- *Flexibility*

  Due to paper's ability to be moulded and reconfigured into a variety of shapes, sizes, it can be utilized in many diagnostic devices. Chemically, paper is also a stable compound which eliminates the risk of reacting or damaging the diagnostic samples.
- *Cost-effective*

  Paper is readily available and extremely easy to manufacture which makes paper-based diagnostic tools a pocket-friendly healthcare option.
- *Eco friendly*

  With increasing advancements in healthcare facilities, medical or bio-waste has emerged as major concern for environmentalists all across the globe. Paper's biodegradable nature and easily disposable qualities make it an environment friendly option.
- *Biocompatible*

  As discussed above, paper is biodegradable and easy to dispose of which makes it a biocompatible diagnostic option.

Paper has been employed in analytical and bioanalytical equipment for over a century due to the advantage of low cost and natural properties. Paper is one of the most versatile substrates for the construction of low cost disposable devices and sensing platforms, due to its biodegradability, biocompatibility, global abundance, chemical stability, and three-dimensional fibrous structure.

Features and properties of paper-based diagnostic devices are illustrated in figure 2.3.

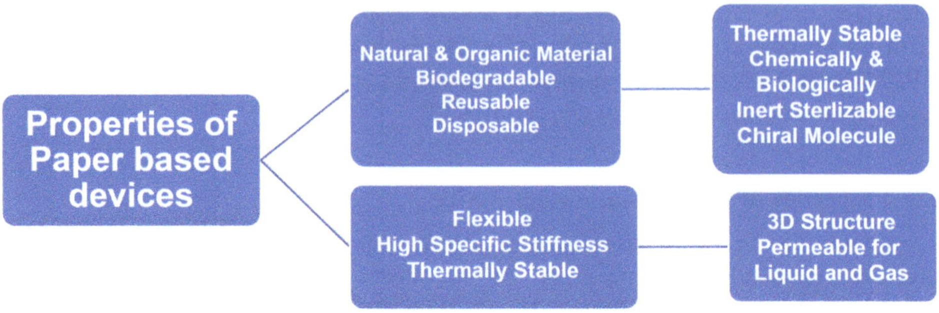

Figure 2.3. Properties of paper-based devices.

2.3 Types of paper-based devices

As described in the earlier sections, the intricacy of the reaction processes of detection is a fundamental challenge in paper-based microfluidic devices, as described in earlier sections. Several ideas have been presented to provide handling capacity, ranging from simple self-wicking to barrier directed fluid handling in complicated microfluidic chips. Because of these difficulties, paper-based biosensors have been divided into several categories, including dipsticks, lateral flow assays (LFA), and μ-PADs, which are discussed in this section [2].

2.3.1 Dipstick type paper-based biosensor

Dipstick biosensors are a simple diagnostic instrument that uses pre-deposited chemicals to detect qualitatively. pH strips, uric acid strips, pathogen detection strips, glutathione strips, and other dipstick sensors have been used for diagnostic purposes [2, 10, 11].

These are simple to make and are suitable for commercial projects. However, one of the biggest drawbacks is the inability to give quantitative data. Otherwise, when it comes to qualitative detection, when it is not critical to know the precise concentration of analyte, the dipstick format is the ideal option for quick and reliable findings [2].

The first paper device for the semi-quantitative detection of glucose in urine was presented in 1956 [12], which evolved into immunochromatographic paper test strips (also known as lateral flow or dipstick tests). The pregnancy test kits are very good examples of dipstick tests [13]. These immunoassays are composed of a strip of paper with a sample pad (for introducing the sample), a reagent pad (containing antibodies coupled to a signalling indicator that are specific to the target molecule), and a test line (for evaluating the outcomes) (capture antibodies immobilized on the surface). When a sample is placed on the specimen pad, it is drawn along the paper strip through capillary forces, where the antigen presents in the sample binds to the signal antibody. The formed antigen/signal antibody continues to flow down the paper strip, where it would be captured by the capture antibody at the surface, leading to a positive result. Coloured latex microspheres or gold nanoparticles are commonly used as signal indicators [7, 14]. These simple and low cost devices are often limited in their ability to provide a qualitative 'yes/no' sort of detection, despite their reliability [7].

2.3.2 Paper devices based on LFA

LFAs made of paper are a more enhanced form of dipstick that permit for controlled fluid flow. The test strips have improved to the point where they may now be used to introduce complicated designs for multistep assays.

The four integral parts of LFA strips are: the (i) sample pad, (which is made of cellulose and separates impurities and stores dried buffer); (ii) conjugation pad (which is made of glass fibre and is used for dry reagent storage); (iii) detection pad (made of nitrocellulose and captures reagent to generate signals), and (iv)absorbent pad (again made of cellulose that absorbs reagent and provides a driving force for flow). Although LFA strips have acquired a higher level of complexity, quantification restrictions remain in these systems [15]. The flow of reagents and samples blend in the conjugation pad, activating reactions that finally forms a detectable band in the existence of analyte [16, 17]. Apart from that, LFA provides superior sample handling, as well as sample pre-treatment to screen out interfering molecules [2].

Many successful LFAs are designed for use at the point of care. Some places where LFAs are used can be a doctor's examination room, an emergency room in a general hospital, toxic compound testing labs on food or feed. These can also be used to the presence or absence of infectious diseases, or adulteration with harmful chemicals in the food/feed sectors. This format is frequently used for testing pertaining to biological warfare, law enforcement agencies, and forensics. Other regulatory organizations can frequently demand that samples that test positive undergo an independent test. LFA tests can be employed for preliminary screening at the point of care/need in this situation [15].

2.3.3 Microfluidic paper-based analytical device

The use of microfluidics-based technologies has revealed a variety of hidden potentials of paper-based devices for overcoming LFA's varied constraints. Microfluidic paper-based analytical device (μ-PAD) not only improved flow, but also allowed for multiplexing and quantitative analysis [18].

So far, chemiluminescence [19, 20], electrochemical [21], spectroscopy [22], and peizo-resistive micro-electro mechanical system (MEMS) [23] based sensing have been reported for paper-based microfluidic devices. Additionally, several paper-based biosensors have been used to enable colorimetric biosensing processes. These biosensors primarily provide two techniques, which are classified as enzyme mimic systems or enzyme aided systems. These enzyme-assisted systems are associated with superior specificity and sensitivity, whereas enzyme mimic systems are recognized for their large range of high temperature sensitivity [2].

Various biosensors have been developed for detection of various analytes using body fluids such as uric acid, saliva, glucose etc [2, 24–27]. A paper-based enzyme linked immunoassay assay with comparable sensitivity for the detection of rabbit IgG with a DL of 54 fM was developed by Cheng *et al* (2010). This same group later enhanced efficacy of the μ-PAD by reducing level of paper borne interfering agents [28].

2.3.4 Smart accessories-based paper bio-analyser

For quantitative or semi-quantitative estimation, paper-based biosensors are supported by various smart devices such as smartphones, strip readers, dedicated electronic signal processing modules, and so on [29]. Because of their ease of use, tunability, and simplicity for end users, smartphones are outperforming all other paper-based smart devices. Furthermore, because the end-user is already habituated to one or more smartphones in the present worldwide scenario, the initial investment in those diagnostic kits is minimal. As a consequence, the research potential of smartphone-assisted paper-based point of care treatment (POCT) has been boosted [2]. Smartphone assisted LFA analyser is developed by You *et al* [30] and electrochemical sensors are developed by Wang and team in [31]. The main benefits of employing these systems are that they provide rigid, authenticated, ordered data at a lower cost for future reference. Because of the commercial potential of smartphone-assisted paper-based biosensing modules, various collaborations have begun to develop such models with the support of top smartphone manufacturers and healthcare behemoths. As a result, a flood of smartphone-based diagnostic gadgets for general healthcare has emerged. Table 2.1 summarizes features of various paper based biosensors.

Table 2.1. Summary of all four kinds of paper-based biosensors with advantages and disadvantages.

Type of device	Advantage	Disadvantage
Dipstick	• Simple design • Fast standardization • Easy to handle • Qualitative analysis • Low cost • Readily available	• Supports one step • process • Optical mode of detection, novariation in read-outis possible • Does not give quantitative data
LFA	• Adaptable sample movement • Electrochemical recognition modepossible • Quantitative analysis possible	• Extendedoptimization process • Time consumingfabrication procedure • Reasonably low volume handling • Trained personnel needed
μPAD	• Provides flexible flow of sample • Various methods for Quantitative detections	• Very low sample volume (less than 10 ml), does not support mass production in large volumes • Long optimization time • Expert personnel needed

2.4 Quantitative analysis via paper-based biosensors

Paper-based sensors are simple, mass-scalable devices at low cost. However, to produce an efficient and accurate analytical device, appropriate transduction procedures are required, which may need the use of additional reagents, materials, and instrumentation, all of which add to the cost and complexity. With the aim of maintaining affordability and simplicity of the device, low-power approaches, such as optical and wireless, are used as transducers. The five most frequently mentioned methods are colorimetric, electrochemiluminescence, electrochemical, electrical conductivity and chemiluminescence which are briefly discussed below.

2.4.1 Colorimetric analysis

Colorimetric detection is often utilized when a semi-quantitative result is sufficient for analysis. Martinez *et al* [32] were the first to show paper-based microfluidic systems for colorimetric glucose and protein detection. The investigation was based on a colour change that occurred after the sample was introduced and filled the reaction zone. In the case of the glucose assay, a positive result was drawn when the colour changed from clear to brown which can be explained by the enzymatic oxidation of iodide to iodine, on the other hand for the protein assay, a positive result was observed by a colour change of tetrabromophenol blue from yellow to blue. The inferences drawn in these investigations were based on change of colour [32]. However, these techniques cannot be compared accurately to advanced techniques such as UV–visible spectroscopy and atomic absorption because the human eye interprets colour and intensity differently depending on the individual, ambient light conditions, and the quality of the paper substrate whether dry or wet [7].

2.4.2 Electrochemical detection

A three-electrode system, consisting of a counter electrode, a reference electrode, and a working electrode, is frequently used in electrochemical techniques. A three-electrode setup is duplicated on paper to create a paper-based electrochemical sensor. This means that a sensor like this might be used instead of the usual electroanalytical approach, which requires expensive solid-state electrodes [7]. On many substrates, including paper, a variety of inks can be employed to make electrodes. For the working and counter electrodes, carbon inks are commonly employed, whereas the reference electrode is made with silver/silver chloride ink [33, 34]. Dungchai *et al* [33] used a paper-based electrode for the electrochemical analysis for the detection of glucose, lactate and uric acid on paper-based electrodes for the first time.

2.4.3 Electrical conductivity

This technique involves measuring changes in conductance of any material under the influence of any chemical species. However, this technique hasn't been used commonly and has limited applications in gas phase only [35, 36].

2.4.4 Chemiluminescent and electrochemiluminescent detection

Chemiluminescence and electrochemiluminescence are simple, low cost and highly sensitive. A device made by Yu *et al* [37] employed a microfluidic paper-based device for the detection of glucose and uric acid via a chemiluminescence reaction between a rhodamine derivative and hydrogen peroxide.

The combination of electrochemical methods with chemiluminescence developed a novel technique called electrochemiluminescence. The combination of the two techniques provides more selectivity along with an increase in the dynamic range of concentration. Delaney *et al* constructed paper microfluidic devices based on this analysis method [38].

2.5 Applications of paper-based biosensors

Paper-based detection systems are a viable tool that can be used in a variety of fields, including health diagnostics, environmental monitoring and food quality control. Paper offers a number of advantages over plastic and glass substrates, including being inexpensive, disposable, abundant, and easy to transport. Until recently, researchers have concentrated on designing paper-based sensors with simpler fabrication techniques and functioning that may be employed in developing-world applications that require simple and easy-to-use devices [7].

Some of the most common applications of paper-based biosensors are discussed below.

2.5.1 Health diagnostics

As prospective lab-on-a-chip (LOC) devices, paper sensing devices are appealing. The major goals of LOC are to reduce the number of laboratory tests required and to allow for portable POC diagnostics and on-site detection [39].

Several research efforts employing paper-based sensors for the detection of various types of analytes for clinical diagnosis have been undertaken using human samples such as urine, saliva, and blood. Various analytes have been explored, including glucose, lactate, nitrate, ketone, nucleic acid, cholesterol, uric acid protein.

- Reaction of paper with various biological samples:

  a. *Blood/blood serum or plasma*

  The most common sample used for clinical, pathological, and research and development laboratory diagnostic is blood. Blood is a type of connective tissue that aids in the body's important functions. Physiologically, it transports oxygen and nutrients to every cell in the body, as well as collecting carbon dioxide produced during the cellular process. Blood has a complex composition, with corpuscles and plasma including amino acids, proteins, fatty acids, lipids, vitamins, metabolites, and glucose, as well as trace amounts of important ions. All corpuscles (red and white) and platelets are found in the colloid (or suspended) fraction of the blood and play a role in the formation of clots to reduce blood loss in injuries. This is why samples are drawn directly from patients. Clogging of blood usually hampers blood flow and may result in incorrect results. Contributing to the above-mentioned factors, the physical nature of blood contributes to some of the fluid flow obstruction via the paper-based substrate in diagnostic tests. Viscosity and granularity of blood also hinder the specificity of these devices [40].

b. *Urine*

Urine, an excretory filtrate watery volume comprised of numerous small molecules and sometimes proteins under clinical circumstances, is another commonly utilized clinical sample. Due to its non-invasive methods of sample collection, that enables safe handling, urine is commonly used in clinical contexts.

However, disparities in constitution that varies from one individual to another, analyte concentrations, and colour (all of which are dependent on the individual) are some of the major reasons for inconsistencies in analytical signalling [40].

2.5.2 Food quality control

Food quality control is critical in the food sector, from the production process to the packaging stage, before a product may be sold. It is also crucial to keep track of how long a product lasts after it is on the shelf. A paper sensing device integrated with a commercial glucometer was utilized as a potential device for electrochemical analysis. The employment of glucometer as an electrochemical reader allows on-site detection of ethanol instead of a laboratory-based analysis. The sensor detected enzymatic action alcohol dehydrogenase on ethanol in the presence of β-NAD+ and ferricyanide played an important role in electron transfer [7, 41].

Another application was to detect the presence of pesticides in the food and beverage industry. A sensor composed of acetylcholinesterase enzyme and indophenyl acetate reagent imparted a blue colour. A decline in intensity of the blue colour indicated the presence of pesticides followed by interpretation via a digital camera [42].

2.5.3 Environment monitoring

Because of increased pollutants in immediate environments in urban areas especially in metro cities. detection of various hazardous pollutants like carbon monoxide (CO), sulphur-di-oxide (SO_2), nitrogen dioxide (NO_2) etc it is must to control allergic and respiratory ailments bronchial asthma, COPD, and lung cancer. Real-time detection of heavy metals and other pollutants is critical in environmental monitoring since sample conditions can change during the day as a result of industrial effluents, as well as during the collection and transit back to the lab. As a result, sensors that can detect and accurately monitor environmental variables on-site are in high demand [7].

2.6 Challenges in paper-based diagnostic devices

While paper has a lot of potential as a platform for LOC devices, current developments in fabrication and analysis techniques are still needed to match the performance of traditional analytical approaches. One of the most common limitations is the device's overall sensitivity. This is usually owing to how the sample is applied to the paper, which can be done at a significant distance from the detecting zone. The local analyte concentration may drop when the analyte is conveyed across the paper as a result of solution spreading, and it may also evaporate if the distance and time of transit are far from the point of introduction. The problem of evaporation can be solved by encasing the paper or the paper's peripheral border with sticky tape or by sandwiching the porous paper substrate between vinyl and polyester plastic films [43].

Another major issue with paper-based devices is that it requires a large volume of samples which makes it unsuitable for many diagnostic procedures [40]. The inconsistencies in thickness of paper-based sensors which eventually is one of major limitations of these devices. It alters the bed volume leading to false results especially in cases with low analyte concentration [44].

Paper-based devices cannot be pre-conditioned hence they are not suitable for samples that require preconditioning sensitive screening of analytes and removal of non-significant moieties present in the clinical samples which might have negative effect on signal generation, and also prevents the fouling of sensing surface [45].

2.7 Recent advancements and developments

Some of the very recent developments for biosensors are listed below.

Great advancements are being made in paper-based biosensors. These range from dipsticks to origami-based sensors. The evolution of the very simplistic dipstick type strips to the origami-based complex features. With the addition of higher complexity paper-based biosensors can now be used for multistep detection [40].

Paper-based biosensors have also been advanced to fulfil the aim of semi--quantitative and sometimes quantitative detections via the incorporation of the peripherals/accessories which has also added to their accuracy, easy fabrication, and low cost nature. Now, these paper-based biosensors have been employed in various detection/diagnostic assays that monitor clinically molecules and biomarkers via metabolites and salt concentration [46].

The latest development in paper-based biosensing devices is the manipulation of these devices using origami-based modules that enable them to detect disease biomarkers and clinically significant metabolites. For example, detection of carcinoembryonic antigen (CEA) via photo-electrochemical paper and doping of N-carbon dots/TiO_2–Pt-nanocomposite [47].

Another research has reported a three-dimensional microfluidic origami device has been developed using the Ag-nanosphere impregnated paper which detects the CEA in clinical samples. The Ag paper is utilized as working electrode and Au nanocages have been utilized as tris-(bipyridine)—ruthenium (ii) (Ru(bpy)32+) is employed as ECL amplifier molecules [48].

2.8 Conclusions

In the current world scenario we are surrounded by all kinds of health hazards and new diseases. Due to pollution, global warming, exploitation of natural resources, lack of waste disposal techniques, increased risks of wars etc humanity has become more prone to health issues both mentally and physically. More and more people are experiencing physical sickness in some form or other. However, in order to prevent sickness from becoming further complicated proper healthcare is needed and it is safe to say that correct diagnosis is the first step towards beating disease. For better and earlier diagnosis of any disease, accurate and sensitive diagnostic systems are needed. This chapter has discussed various properties and features of paper as a diagnostic device. It also lists the types of these devices and various types of methods employed for detection. It is of no doubt that paper can be referred to as one of the best diagnostic tools due to its abundance, simplicity, cost-effectiveness and inertness towards various biological samples. However, there are certain short-comings in using paper-based devices for diagnosis that will be resolved with time.

References

[1] Mahato K, Maurya P K and Chandra P 2018 Fundamentals and commercial aspects of nanobiosensors in point-of-care clinical diagnostics *3 Biotech.* **8** 1–14

[2] Mahato K, Srivastava A and Chandra P 2017 Paper based diagnostics for personalized health care: emerging technologies and commercial aspects *Biosens. Bioelectron.* **96** 246–59

[3] Chandra P, Tan Y N and Singh S P (ed) 2017 *Next Generation Point-of-Care Biomedical Sensors Technologies for Cancer Diagnosis* vol 10 (Singapore: Springer Singapore)

[4] Haleem A, Javaid M, Singh R P, Suman R and Rab S 2021 Biosensors applications in medical field: a brief review *Sens. Int.* **2** 100100

[5] Bansal S, Jyoti A, Mahato K, Chandra P and Prakash R 2017 Highly sensitive *in vitro* biosensor for enterotoxigenic *Escherichia coli* detection based on ssDNA anchored on PtNPs-chitosan nanocomposite *Electroanalysis* **29** 2665–71

[6] Tan T-H, Gochoo M, Chen Y-F, Hu J-J, Chiang J Y, Chang C-S, Lee M-H, Yung-Nian Hsu and Hsu J-C 2017 Ubiquitous emergency medical service system based on wireless biosensors, traffic information, and wireless communication technologies: development and evaluation *Sensors* **17** 202

[7] Liana D D, Raguse B, Gooding J J and Chow E 2012 Recent advances in paper-based sensors *Sensors* **12** 11505–26

[8] Dang H S and Roberts B P 1996 Radical-chain reactions of sulfonyl azides and of ethyl azidoformate with allylstannanes: homolytic allylation at nitrogen *J. Chem. Soc., Perkin Trans.* **1** 1493–8

[9] Academy P 2016 *Fibrous Materials for Paper* (Minia: Paper Academy)

[10] Najian A N, Syafirah E E N, Ismail N, Mohamed M and Yean C Y 2016 Development of multiplex loop mediated isothermal amplification (m-LAMP) label-based gold nanoparticles lateral flow dipstick biosensor for detection of pathogenic leptospira *Anal. Chim. Acta* **903** 142–8

[11] Singh P, Nath P, Arun R K, Mandal S and Chanda N 2016 Novel synthesis of a mixed Cu/CuO-reduced graphene oxide nanocomposite with enhanced peroxidase-like catalytic activity for easy detection of glutathione in solution and using a paper strip *RSC Adv.* **6** 92729–38

[12] Comer J P 1956 Semiquantitative specific test paper for glucose in urine *Anal. Chem.* **28** 1748–50

[13] Von Lode P 2005 Point-of-care immunotesting: approaching the analytical performance of central laboratory methods *Clin. Biochem.* **38** 591–606

[14] Zhao W, Ali M M, Aguirre S D, Brook M A and Li Y 2008 based bioassays using gold nanoparticle colorimetric probes *Anal. Chem.* **80** 8431–7

[15] Posthuma-Trumpie G A, Korf J and van Amerongen A 2009 Lateral flow (immuno) assay: its strengths, weaknesses, opportunities and threats. A literature survey *Anal. Bioanal.Chem.* **393** 569–82

[16] Bahadır E B and Sezgintürk M K 2016 Lateral flow assays: principles, designs and labels *TrAC, Trends Anal. Chem.* **82** 286–306

[17] Koczula K. M. and Gallotta A 2016 Lateral flow assays. *Essays Biochem.* **60** 111–20

[18] Rezk A R, Qi A, Friend J R, Li W H and Yeo L Y 2012 Uniform mixing in paper-based microfluidic systems using surface acoustic waves *Lab Chip* **12** 773–9

[19] Shi C G, Shan X, Pan Z Q, Xu J J, Lu C, Bao N and Gu H Y 2012 Quantum dot (QD)-modified carbon tape electrodes for reproducible electrochemiluminescence (ECL) emission on a paper-based platform *Anal. Chem.* **84** 3033–8

[20] Wang S, Ge L, Song X, Yu J, Ge S, Huang J and Zeng F 2012 Paper-based chemiluminescence ELISA: lab-on-paper based on chitosan modified paper device and wax-screen-printing *Biosens. Bioelectron.* **31** 212–8

[21] Nie Z, Nijhuis C A, Gong J, Chen X, Kumachev A, Martinez A W, Narovlyansky M and Whitesides G M 2010 Electrochemical sensing in paper-based microfluidic devices *Lab Chip* **10** 477–83

[22] Ellerbee A K, Phillips S T, Siegel A C, Mirica K A, Martinez A W, Striehl P, Jain N, Prentiss M and Whitesides G M 2009 Quantifying colorimetric assays in paper-based microfluidic devices by measuring the transmission of light through paper *Anal. Chem.* **81** 8447–52

[23] Liu H and Crooks R M 2011 Three-dimensional paper microfluidic devices assembled using the principles of origami *J. Am. Chem. Soc.* **133** 17564–6

[24] Fischer C, Fraiwan A and Choi S 2016 A 3D paper-based enzymatic fuel cell for self-powered, low-cost glucose monitoring *Biosens. Bioelectron.* **79** 193–7

[25] Nery E W and Kubota L T 2016 Evaluation of enzyme immobilization methods for paper-based devices—a glucose oxidase study *J. Pharm. Biomed. Anal.* **117** 551–9

[26] Soni A and Jha S K 2015 A paper strip based non-invasive glucose biosensor for salivary analysis *Biosens. Bioelectron.* **67** 763–8

[27] Yin H, Wang M, Li B, Yang Z, Zhou Y and Ai S 2015 A sensitive electrochemical biosensor for detection of protein kinase A activity and inhibitors based on phos-tag and enzymatic signal amplification *Biosens. Bioelectron.* **63** 26–32

[28] Cheng C M, Martinez A W, Gong J, Mace C R, Phillips S T, Carrilho E, Mirica K A and Whitesides G M 2010 Paper-based ELISA *Angew. Chem.* **122** 4881–4

[29] Carvalhal R F, Simão Kfouri M, de Oliveira Piazetta M H, Gobbi A L and Kubota L T 2010 Electrochemical detection in a paper-based separation device *Anal. Chem.* **82** 1162–5

[30] You D J, San Park T and Yoon J Y 2013 Cell-phone-based measurement of TSH using Mie scatter optimized lateral flow assays *Biosens. Bioelectron.* **40** 180–5

[31] Wang X, Gartia M R, Jiang J, Chang T W, Qian J, Liu Y, Liu X and Liu G L 2015 Audio jack based miniaturized mobile phone electrochemical sensing platform *Sens. Actuators* B **209** 677–85

[32] Martinez A W, Phillips S T, Butte M J and Whitesides G M 2007 Patterned paper as a platform for inexpensive, low-volume, portable bioassays *Angew. Chem.* **119** 1340–2
[33] Dungchai W, Chailapakul O and Henry C S 2009 Electrochemical detection for paper-based microfluidics *Anal. Chem.* **81** 5821–6
[34] Arena A, Donato N, Saitta G, Bonavita A, Rizzo G and Neri G 2010 Flexible ethanol sensors on glossy paper substrates operating at room temperature *Sens. Actuators* B **145** 488–94
[35] Steffens C, Manzoli A, Francheschi E, Corazza M L, Corazza F C, Oliveira J V and Herrmann P S P 2009 Low-cost sensors developed on paper by line patterning with graphite and polyaniline coating with supercritical CO_2 *Synth. Met.* **159** 2329–32
[36] Yu J, Ge L, Huang J, Wang S and Ge S 2011 Microfluidic paper-based chemiluminescence biosensor for simultaneous determination of glucose and uric acid *Lab Chip* **11** 1286–91
[37] Delaney J L, Hogan C F, Tian J and Shen W 2011 Electrogenerated chemiluminescence detection in paper-based microfluidic sensors *Anal. Chem.* **83** 1300–6
[38] Zhao W and van den Berg A 2008 Lab on paper *Lab Chip* **8** 1988–91
[39] Mahato K, Purohit B, Kumar A and Chandra P 2020 Paper-based biosensors for clinical and biomedical applications: emerging engineering concepts and challenges *Comprehensive Analytical Chemistry* vol 89 (Amsterdam: Elsevier), pp 163–88
[40] Nie Z, Deiss F, Liu X, Akbulut O and Whitesides G M 2010 Integration of paper-based microfluidic devices with commercial electrochemical readers *Lab Chip* **10** 3163–9
[41] Hossain S Z, Luckham R E, McFadden M J and Brennan J D 2009 Reagentless bidirectional lateral flow bioactive paper sensors for detection of pesticides in beverage and food samples *Anal. Chem.* **81** 9055–64
[42] Apilux A, Dungchai W, Siangproh W, Praphairaksit N, Henry C S and Chailapakul O 2010 Lab-on-paper with dual electrochemical/colorimetric detection for simultaneous determination of gold and iron *Anal. Chem.* **82** 1727–32
[43] Li X, Ballerini D R and Shen W 2012 A perspective on paper-based microfluidics: current status and future trends *Biomicrofluidics* **6** 011301
[44] Chandra P 2016 *Nanobiosensors for Personalized and Onsite Biomedical Diagnosis* (London: The Institution of Engineering and Technology)
[45] Purohit B, Kumar A, Mahato K and Chandra P 2020 Smartphone-assisted personalized diagnostic devices and wearable sensors *Curr. Opin. Biomed. Eng.* **13** 42–50
[46] Li L, Wang T, Zhang Y, Xu C, Zhang L, Cheng X, Liu H, Chen X and Yu J 2018 Editable TiO_2 nanomaterial-modified paper *in situ* for highly efficient detection of carcinoembryonic antigen by photoelectrochemical method *ACS Appl. Mater. Interfaces* **10** 14594–601
[47] Li L., Wang T., Zhang Y., Xu C., Zhang L., Cheng X., Liu H., Chen X. and Yu J. 2018 Editable TiO_2 nanomaterial-modified paper in situ for highly efficient detection of carcinoembryonic antigen by photoelectrochemical method. *ACS Appl. Mater. Interfaces* **10** 14594–601
[48] Gao C, Su M, Wang Y, Ge S and Yu J 2015 A disposable paper-based electrochemiluminescence device for ultrasensitive monitoring of CEA based on $Ru(bpy)_3^{2+}$@Au nanocages. *Rsc Advances* **5** 28324–31

Chapter 3

Fabrication of paper-based immunochromatography assay

Jyoti Jain, Vaibhav Misra, Meenu Jain, Rishika khetan, Ruchira Chaudhary, Aditya Raj and Savita Bharat Jain

Paper-based immunochromatography assay includes devices made of paper or any porous membrane that works on the principal of capillary action. These devices are involved in the development of point-of-care (POC) diagnostic which does not need time-consuming and costly equipment-based procedures. These devices have several advantages, e.g., they are cost effective, easy to fabricate, easy to dispose, no need of any supporting equipment to operate. In this chapter we discuss the methods involved in the fabrication of paper-based devices their applications in different fields and briefly discuss their limitations and future challenges.

3.1 Introduction

Infectious disease is the second leading cause of death worldwide [1]. So, there is a need for rapid diagnosis of diseases. The developed countries have many medical tools and are rich in resources to conduct diagnostic tests but unfortunately the developing countries are suffering from a paucity of diagnostic resources [2–5], in such countries most death occur in the absence of early diagnosis. These deaths could be prevented if the disease could have been diagnosed earlier; the early diagnosis of disease reduces its chance of outbreak.

The WHO has given the ASSURED (affordable, sensitive, specific, user friendly rapid and robust, equipment free and deliverable to end users) criteria for plotting the diagnostic tool [3, 6].

Paper-based immunochromatography assays are developed as POC diagnostics that meet the ASSURED criteria [7, 8]. Paper has been exploited to design a paper-based diagnostic assay due to its low cost, its ability to handle small volumes of fluid by capillary action, ease of fabrication and ability to be operated without using computer controlled pumps.

doi:10.1088/978-0-7503-5820-0ch3 © IOP Publishing Ltd 2023

3.2 Paper as a platform for POC diagnosis

3.2.1 Paper as a substrate and other alternatives

Paper is a flexible sheet usually constructed of an interwoven network of pressed cellulose fibres. A wide range of paper materials has been created in recent years. Diagnostic instruments for POC testing have traditionally been made from two types of material [9]. One is a cellulose fibre-based material, filter paper and chromatography paper, for example, are key substrates for dipsticks and microfluidic paper-based analytical equipment [10]. The nitrocellulose membrane, which is used in lateral flow assays (LFAs), is the other [11, 12]. Cellulose is a fibrous, hydrophilic, biodegradable macromolecule made up of hundreds of glucose units [13] that are insoluble in water and most organic solvents. Nitrocellulose is made when cellulose is partially nitrated. Nitration increases cellulose porosity and converts it from hydrophilic to hydrophobic. Porous materials include cellulose fibres and nitrocellulose membranes. As a medium for developing a POC diagnostic device, paper has several distinct advantages. It is low cost, readily available, and works with a variety of printing and processing methods. Because paper has a high surface-to-volume ratio, it can be used to dry and store chemicals and samples for subsequent analysis. Finally, because paper wicks fluids by capillary action, a paper-based device may transport fluids and run assays without the use of pumps or external power sources [14–17].

3.3 Paper-based immunoassay

The paper strips used to identify the presence of a biomarker in a sample are known as paper-based assays. The majority of paper-based tests are immunoassays, meaning that antibodies are used to bind to the biomarker of interest in the sample. Because of the presence of a gold nanoparticle (NP)–antibody combination that creates a bright colour signal during the assay, these assays may be read with the eyes.

A nitrocellulose membrane serves as the substrate for the paper-based tests, which also include NPs coupled with antibodies or immunoprobes and a capture antibody printed on the substrate. As a result, they have a small number of components and use a small amount of reagent. A single assay is inexpensive and easy to mass generate.

As a result, paper-based assays are seen as a point-of-care device with lower costs and shorter testing times, allowing physicians to make more timely treatment decisions and therefore benefiting the healthcare system. Different types of paper-based immunoassay formats are given below.

3.3.1 Dipstick examination

Dipstick assays, such as pH strips and urine test strips, are simple to develop, inexpensive to produce, and easy to use. Dipsticks or test strips are made up of paper pads that are glued to plastic strips and contain dried chemicals. The strip is dipped into the liquid sample to perform the dipstick assay. The colour change occurs when analytes in the sample react with reagents on the pad. The results are then compared to a standard chart depending on the colour intensity produced. Dipstick assays are used to assess the analyte in a semi-quantitative manner.

3.3.2 Lateral flow assay

In POC diagnostics, LFAs are the most often used technology. LFA is exemplified by a home pregnancy test. These are POC devices that work in a strip format. The device is built on a plastic backing. A sample application pad, a conjugate pad, a nitrocellulose membrane, and an adsorption pad make up the device. The test and control lines are separated on the nitrocellulose membrane. LFA is based on chromatographic principles: a liquid sample containing the desired analyte passes through several zones of polymeric strips where the molecule can interact with the analyte without any external force. User-friendliness, excellent specificity, enhanced sensitivity, long-term stability under varied environmental circumstances, and device portability are the advantages of LFAs [18, 19].

LFAs are simple, quick, and inexpensive. Furthermore, the LFA architecture can accommodate multiplex testing. As a result, it represents an appropriate solution to the ongoing requirement for POC multiplexing analysis in theory. Multiplexed LFAs are promising POC candidates that precisely meet the ASSURED criteria [20–23], unlike other multiplex testing procedures like as PCR and ELISA, which require expensive instrumentation, a long analysis time, and specialized staff.

LFAs offer a wide range of applications in medicine, including the diagnosis of tumours, infections, allergies, and neurological and cardiac issues [24, 25]. The LFAs also suffer from some limitations such as difficulty in obtaining multiplex system and in quantitative analysis.

3.3.3 Microfluidic paper-based analytical devices (μPADs)

The drawbacks of LFA can be overcome by μPADs. μPADs are paper-based microfluidic devices that are constructed by fabricating hydrophilic channels in hydrophobic paper. Techniques such as photolithography, plotting, cutting, wax printing, inkjet etching, etc, are used to fabricate the paper and to generate μPADs. These microfluidic devices are used for multiplexing and in quantitative analysis. Table 3.1 depicts the benefits and limitations of different paper-based assays.

3.4 Components of LFA

Formats, biorecognition molecules, labels, and detection systems are some of the components of lateral flow assays.

3.4.1 Formats

LFA runs in a variety of formats. A membrane is made up of four primary parts. A quick description of each component follows before explaining the types of format.

Sample application pad The region where the sample is applied is known as the sample application pad. Its job is to disperse the sample evenly and convey it to the

Table 3.1. Different types of paper-based assays.

Method	Advantage	Disadvantage
Dipstick assay	1. Simple and cheap 2. Enhances workflow-saving labour and time 3. Fast optimization 4. A large number of samples can be processed in less time 5. Easy to scale up	1. Cannot be used with pressurized pumps 2. Visual indication only 3. High false positives rates 4. Some false negative 5. Subjected to observer error 6. Mostly no quantification
Lateral flow immunoassay	1. One step assay without washing step 2. Simple and user friendly 3. Low cost, need small volume of sample 4. Give result in short time 5. Long life span without precise storage 6. Good reproducibility 7. High sensitivity and specificity 8. High prospective for commercialization	1. Poor qualitative discrimination 2. Reproduciblity may vary from lot to lot 3. Low signal intensity 4. Pretreatment of sample is required for non-fluidic samples 5. Mostly qualitative or semi-quantitative
μPADs	1. Versatile 2. Cost effective 3. Fast reaction using low volume 4. Ability to drive and manipulate flow without equipment 5. Multianalysis 6. High capillary flow	1. It is very complex to pattern the channels on paper 2. Long optimization time

conjugate pad in a smooth, continuous, and uniform way. The sample pad is treated with buffers, salts, surfactants, proteins, and other liquids to control the flow rate and make it acceptable for the detecting system. Sample application pads serve as filters, removing unnecessary material from the sample, such as red blood cells.

Labelled biorecognition molecules (such as antibodies, nanoparticles, enzymes, or oligonucleotides) are delivered in this area. These biorecognition molecules should be released promptly upon contact with the moving liquid sample during the assay. During the experiment, the labelled conjugate should stay stable. The conjugate buffer's composition, which includes carbohydrate (such as sucrose) ensures this. It acts as a preservative as well as a resolubilizer. Sugar forms a coating around the particles when they are dried in the presence of sugar, stabilizing them. The sugar molecules dissolve and transfer the particles into the fluid stream when the sample enters the conjugate pad.

Membrane The most important component of the LFA strip is the membrane. The most frequent materials used to make the strips are cellulose and nitrocellulose.

These come in a variety of pore diameters (from 0.05 to 12 mm). Capillary forces, as well as the ease of binding and immobilizing proteins required for subsequent reaction and detection systems, should all be present in a suitable membrane. The capillary time should be addressed while choosing a membrane material. The capillary flow time is the time it takes for the liquid to get to the membrane strip and completely fill it. Over this piece of membrane, test and control lines are drawn. Non-specific binding at the test and control lines may have a major impact on the results. As a result, a good membrane has less non-specific binding.

Absorbent pad Cellulose filters are used to make adsorbent pads. The adsorbent pad's job is to wick liquid through the membrane and collect the treated liquid. It acts as a sink at the end of the strip, maintaining the liquid flow rate over the membrane and preventing sample backflow.

All of these elements are adhered to a backdrop card. It is extremely adaptable and serves as a foundation for the proper assembly of all components. Figure 3.1 depicts the main components of a LFA.

The liquid sample containing the desired analyte of interest is placed on the sample pad at one end of the strip, it flows through the capillary action of the strip, passing through several zones where biomolecules that can interact with the analyte are attached. Finally, it arrives at the conjugation pad, which includes antibodies to the target analyte that have been coupled with coloured fluorescent nanoparticles [26–33]. The sample, together with the conjugated antibody attached to the analyte, is then passed through a nitrocellulose membrane, where specific biological components (antibodies or antigens) are immobilized in a zone known as the test line. In the control line, a control reagent is immobilized. The analyte is either collected at the test line and causes a colour shift that may be seen with the naked eye or with a specialized reader, or it continues to migrate through the absorbent pad, indicating that the assay has run successfully. Figure 3.2 describes the assay mechanism of LFA.

Two basic formats of LFAs have been developed, named the sandwich and the competitive format.

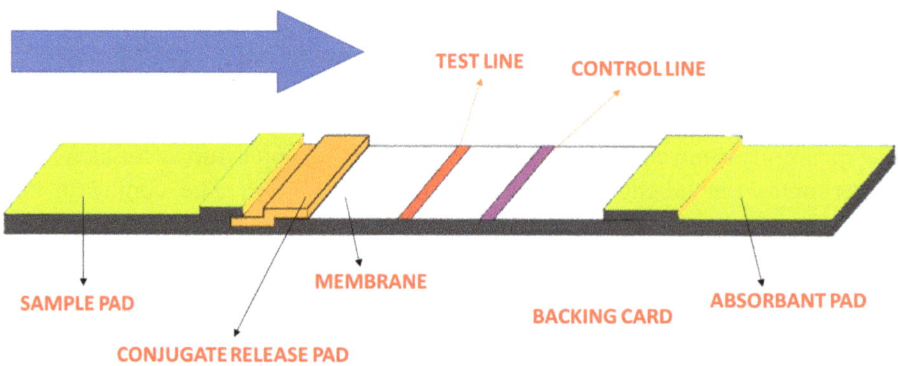

Figure 3.1. A lateral flow immunoassay test strip typical configuration.

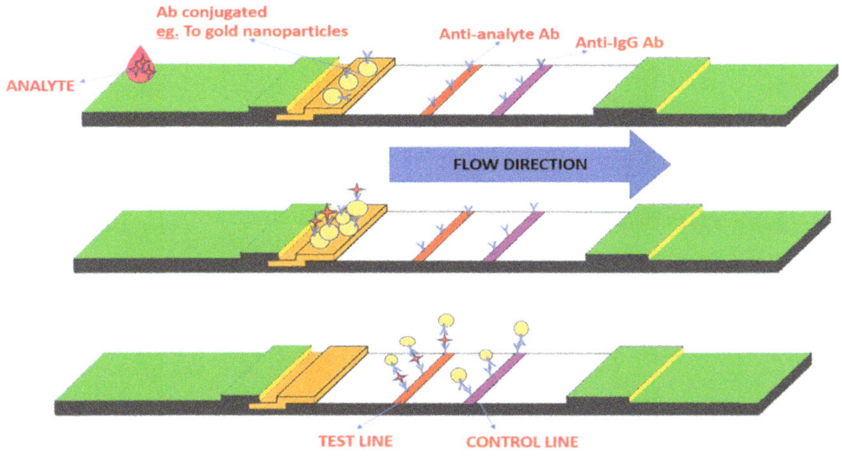

Figure 3.2. Assay's mechanism schematic representation. (1) Sample is poured on the sample pad and moves towards the conjugate pad. (2) Conjugate antibody binds to the target analyte. (3) Moved to test line where the bound target analyte is captured.

3.4.1.1 Sandwich format

A large analyte having more than two antigenic sites can be evaluated in this way. On the conjugate pad, tagged antibodies (enzymes, nanoparticles, fluorescent dyes) are immobilized. Over the test line, a primary antibody against the target analyte is immobilized. On the control line, a secondary antibody or probe against the labelled conjugate is immobilized.

When an analyte-containing sample is put on the sample pad, it migrates to the conjugation pad, where it is caught by the labelled antibody and forms a labelled antibody–analyte conjugate. This conjugate is now sandwiched between the labelled and primary antibodies on the nitrocellulose membrane, generating a labelled antibody conjugation/analyte/primary antibody complex. Secondary antibody buffers will catch excess labelled antibody conjugate at the control line, and surplus solution will flow to the adsorption pad. The signal strength at the test line is proportional to the amount of analyte in the sample and can be measured using an optical strip reader or visually assessed. The presence of colour on the control line indicates that the strip is operational. Figure 3.3 shows the schematic representation of the sandwich format.

3.4.1.2 Competitive format

This format is ideal for detecting small analytes that cannot bind two antibodies at the same time as shown in figure 3.4. This format has two different layouts. A solution containing the target analyte is applied to the sample pad in the first configuration, and the pre-immobilized labelled antibody conjugate is hydrated and begins to flow with moving liquid. The test line comprises antigen that has been pre-immobilized (the same analyte to be detected) and binds to the label conjugate precisely. The control line comprises secondary antibodies that have been pre-immobilized and can bind to labelled antibody conjugates. If the target analyte in

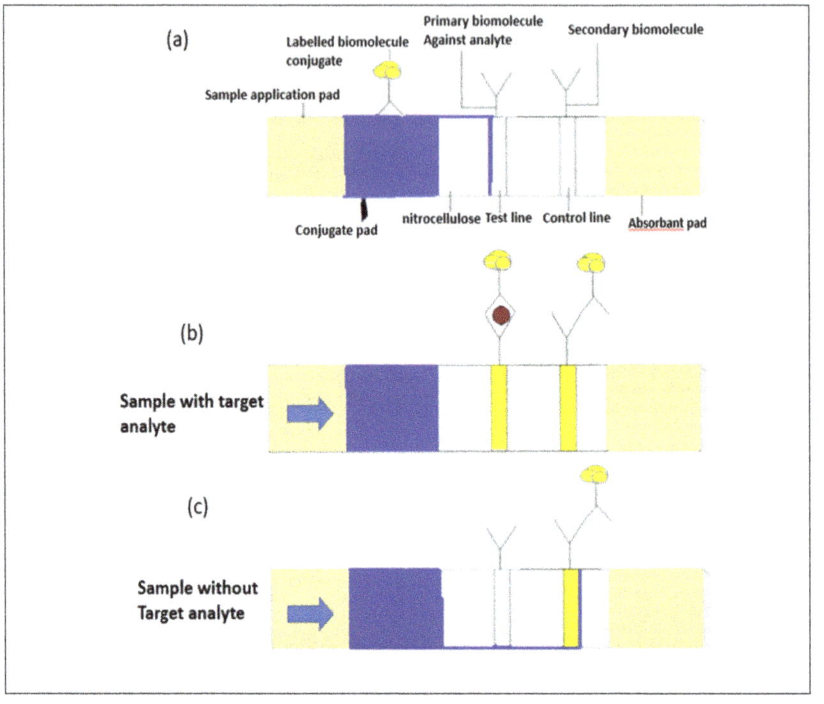

Figure 3.3. Schematic representation of the sandwich format (a) labelled lateral flow assay (LFA) strip. (b) When a sample with analyte is applied on the sample application pad, it flows over the strip under capillary action and colour appears at the test and control line. (c) When a sample without target analyte is applied, it flows and a colour only appears on the test line.

the sample solution is absent or present in such a low quantity that some sites of the labelled antibody conjugate remain unoccupied when the liquid sample reaches the test line, pre-immobilized antigen will attach to the labelled conjugation. The antigen in the sample solution and the antigen immobilized at the test line of the strip compete for the labelled conjugate's attention. A tagged analyte conjugate is dispensed at the conjugation pad, while a primary anti-analyte antibody is dispensed at the test line in another pattern. Following the administration of an analyte solution, the analyte and the labelled analyte compete for binding with the primary antibody at the test line.

In summary, in the sandwich and competitive forms, the presence or absence of a visual signal at the test line indicates a positive outcome.

3.4.1.3 Multiplex detection

For the detection of several analytes, different detection formats are used. Multiple test lines of antibodies unique to the target species are immobilized in an array format on a strip and analysed under the same set of circumstances in this format [34] Miniaturized versions of LFA based on microarrays for multiplex detection of DNA sequences have been reported to have various benefits, including lower test reagent usage, a smaller sample volume requirement, and improved sensitivity [35].

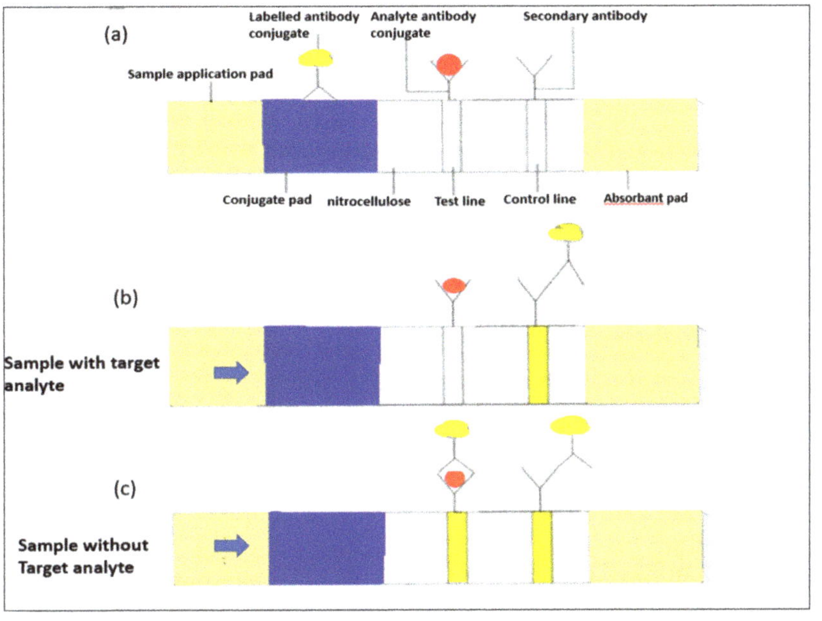

Figure 3.4. Schematic representation of the competitive format. (a) Labelled lateral flow assay strip. (b) When a sample with target analyte is applied on sample application pad, it flows through the strip and a colour appears on a test line. (c) When a sample without target analyte is applied, it flows on the strip and colour appears on both lines.

3.4.1.3.1 COVID-19 antibody rapid test kit

Because the COVID-19 pandemic has altered people's lifestyles in every country, stringent testing has become necessary. As a result, LFA has been hailed as the most promising method for identifying new coronaviruses. LFA detects antibodies produced by the body when it is exposed to SARSCOV-2, the virus that causes COVID-19.

After around five days of a fresh infection, the human immune system develops 'IgM' antibodies, which have an instant binding strength to coronavirus. The 'IgG' antibodies, on the other hand, have a significant binding affinity for COVID-19 after 8–10 days. Hence, the COVID-19 IgM/IgG test kit detects the presence of IgM/IgG antibodies together or separately in a qualitative manner. As a result, COVID-19 lFA cannot identify SARSCOV-2 in an infected person. In fact, it is utilized to work out how immune responses behave.

3.4.2 Molecules of biorecognition

3.4.2.1 Antibodies

The presence of viruses or bacteria in a patient can be recognized using genetic information, pathogen envelope proteins, or the patient's immune response, which detects antibodies produced in reaction to the infection [36, 37].

Although the physical components of the test strip, fabrication techniques, and buffers all play a part in optimizing the test, the antibodies, which must be carefully developed and properly purified, are at the heart of the process.

The antibodies are immobilized on the test and control lines of the lateral flow strip as biorecognition molecules and attach to the analyte, involving immunochemical interaction between antigen and antibody. The lateral flow immunochromatographic assay (LFIA) is the product of this process.

The following considerations should be considered when choosing an antibody:

1. To ensure that antibodies are available at all times.
2. Antigen specificity must be determined. The variable region of the antibody determines antigen specificity; if this area recognizes a common molecular motif, the antibody may bind to the same epitope on different targets. Because non-specific binding can cause data to be misinterpreted, using an antibody that recognizes a single target is preferred.
3. The antibody's binding affinity must also be determined. An antibody with a high binding affinity is required for a sample with a high analyte concentration.
4. Monoclonal antibodies are favored over polyclonal antibodies because they can be generated in high quantities and recognize a single antigenic epitope. Although polyclonals can yield satisfactory findings, they are subject to variation between animals and over time, and their supply cannot be guaranteed for the duration of the lateral flow immunoassay.

3.4.2.2 Aptamer

Aptamers are made up of natural DNA or RNA nucleotide sequences and are produced *in vitro* using the SELEX (systematic evolution of ligands by exponential enrichment) procedure [38] Importantly, the SELEX process can assist in the development of aptamers that bind to low-molecular-weight molecules that are not favorable to generate antibodies. Aptamers have high association constants and can bind to a range of analytes selectively. Aptamers are chosen over antibodies because they are easier to manufacture, smaller in size, need a simple labelling method, have a high affinity for the target, are easier to modify and immobilize, have higher reproducibility, and are more stable [39]

3.4.3 Labels

To increase antibody detectability, many labelling compounds are used [40]. Gold nanoparticles, magnetic particles, coloured cellulose particles, coloured latex particles, carbon nanoparticles, quantum dots, fluorophores, and enzymes are some of the materials. A label should be detectable at a very low concentration. A good labelling material should be stable and not alter the biorecognition molecule's characteristics. When the label concentration is reduced to $10^{-9.}$ optical detection is possible [41]. Some labels generate direct signals after a test is completed.

Gold colloidal generates colours, whereas enzymes require a further step to provide a signal, which is measured after a reaction with a suitable substrate. Labels that produce direct signals are preferable in the LFA assay because they take less time and reduce the number of procedures required for POC diagnosis. Some of the labels are briefly discussed.

3.4.3.1 Nanoparticles of gold

Gold nanoparticles are the most commonly employed nanoparticles in LFA due to their chemical and optical characteristics. Because gold is chemically inert, gold nanoparticles have extraordinary resilience against degradation over long periods of time. Because gold nanoparticles have a high affinity for biomolecules, they can be conjugated to antibodies and aptamers quickly and reliably. Shape and size have a big impact on the optical characteristics of spherical gold nanoparticles. Smaller nanoparticles absorb light more efficiently, with maxima about 520 nm. Larger nanoparticles, on the other hand, scatter more and have peaks at longer wavelengths. Gold nanoparticles have many other unique qualities, such as large specific areas, ease of synthesis, low cost, and simple preparation methods, which save analysis time and provide reliable analysis on-site.

3.4.3.2 Megnetic particles

A new generation of magnetic lateral flow immunoassays is proving to be a valuable diagnostic tool. Magnetic nanoparticles are used as a detection label. Magnetic particle labels can be seen with the naked eye [42, 43], or magnetic characteristics can be identified with magnetic sensors [44]. They can generate magnetic signals that are more stable over time than optical signals and boost LFA sensitivity by 10–1000 times [45] Magnetic particles can be quantified by detecting their magnetic characteristics, albeit this requires a specialized reader. Using 111 nm superparamagnetic nanoparticles and a magnetic assay reader, Xu *et al* established a very sensitive lateral flow assay with a detection limit of 0.01 ng ml^{-1} cardiac troponin I, compared to 10 ng ml^{-1} detected by enzyme-linked immunosorbent assay (ELISA) [45].

3.4.3.3 Materials which are fluorescent or luminous

LFA uses fluorescent compounds as labels. Fluorescent labelling will increase sensitivity. A fluorescent label absorbs a specific colour or wavelength of light, and a slightly different colour of light is released after a very brief time. Filters can be used to block the detection of the original light, allowing only the emitted light to be viewed against a reduced background. Fluorescein isothiocyanate or fluorescently labelled latex particles were used as direct labels. Fluorescence systems are generally costly due to the high cost of the light source needed to illuminate the fluorescent reporters, the interference filters and detection systems used to analyse and collect the produced light, and the data processing required to obtain the result. Several papers [46–48] have documented the use of fluorescence in lateral flow systems, but the results do not provide a sufficient benefit of fluorescence over gold in terms of sensitivity or dynamic range to justify the additional expense and complexity.

3.4.3.4 Quantum dots for labeling

QDs are fluorescent semiconductor nanocrystals with distinct optical and electrical features. Quantum dots have a particle size range of 1.5–10 nm [49]. Depending on the functional group on the quantum dots' surface, carbodiimide-mediated approaches can be used to label antibodies utilizing quantum dots. For conjugation, antibody elements (Fv and Fc) are preferred. When compared to organic dyes used for fluorescent labelling, QDs have better photostability, high fluorescence, and broad absorption spectra with particular emission spectra [50]. A fluorometric technique can be used to read a QD-based LFA in the test zone.

3.4.3.5 Enzymes

In LFAs, enzymes are also utilized as labels. In the case of enzymes, the assay requires the selection of an appropriate enzyme substrate combination. Horseradish peroxidase (HRP) is the most extensively utilized enzyme, which catalyses the oxidation of organic substrates in the presence of hydrogen peroxide. HRP is coupled to detection molecules in LFAs, which are labelled and caught in the test region. A wash step is conducted after a sample has been processed on the LFA to remove any excess labels from the membrane. Finally, HRP substrate and H_2O_2 solutions are pumped through the LFA to achieve enzymatic amplification and a high colour enhancement or chemiluminescence in the test area. The enzyme substrate combination determines the procedure's sensitivity [51].

3.4.3.6 Carbon colloidal

Carbon black or colloidal carbon nanoparticles (CNPs) are the cheapest labels, and suspensions of them are exceedingly stable and simple to make. Furthermore, no activation is required. They come in a variety of commercial formats [52, 53]. They are used in two ways in LFA: nanostrings and nanotubes [54, 55]. The antibody is conjugated to the probe by simple incubation (physical adsorption). The results can be analysed via a colorimetric method or by visual observation as black provides a stronger contrast to the nitrocellulose's white background. Despite the numerous advantages of carbon nanoparticles, black chemicals and black matrixes should not be utilized on strips made from these nanoparticles.

3.4.4 Detection system

Paper-based lateral flow tests have a lot of commercial success, and they are now widely utilized in medical diagnostics and environmental monitoring. Traditional LFAs are identified visually by inspecting the colour shift in the test band. This read-out method, on the other hand, is insufficiently sensitive and not trustworthy for the identification of key biomarkers in clinical samples that are present in extremely minute levels. A variety of technologies for detecting high-sensitivity LFA have been developed, and commercialization attempts are now underway.

The label used in the analysis plays a big role in deciding which detection method to use.

Visual assessment of the colours at the test and control lines provides quantitative or semi-quantitative analysis of the gold nanoparticles or other colour-producing labels. Optical strip readers are used to evaluate the intensity of colours produced at the test line and control line for the quantification of nano gold immunochromatography test strips [56, 57]. Fluorescent dyes and paramagnetic particles cannot be seen with the naked eye, therefore quantitative analysis requires specialized readers. Instruments that can generate high-intensity light of a specific wavelength or colour, filters that can prevent stray light from that light source, and a light detecting system to collect the emitted light are all required for fluorescence reading [58]. A specific instrument is required to detect magnetic particles' minute magnetic fields. Carbon nanoparticles are not as visible as gold nanoparticles, and can only be detected with high-intensity infrared light and specialized detection devices. A smartphone-based dual-modality imaging system [59] that can quantitatively detect colour or fluorescence lateral flow test strips was recently created and may be used anywhere at any time.

Furthermore, automated detection systems outperform manual imaging and processing in terms of time consumption, interpretation, and variable modification.

3.5 Lateral flow in immunoassay application

3.5.1 Clinical applications

The diagnostic tests carried out in hospitals can take several hours or even days to give the results. Most of the time, timely actions can have an impact on the clinical result. LFAs can help in diagnosis, prognosis, monitoring, and surveillance of diseases. LFIA tests help to minimize workload, improve clinical care, improve workflow, and reduce costs. Aside from that, there are long-term advantages to the LFIA. It aids in the differentiation of bacterial and viral illnesses, hence preventing antibiotic misuse. LFIA can be utilized in hospital wards, health centers, clinics, or even at home for self-testing [60]. HCG hormone was tested using the first lateral flow immunochromatographic method. This technology is commonly used in pregnancy testing. The HCG lateral flow test, often known as a pregnancy kit, is used to measure HCG levels in urine samples. POCT uses immunochromatographic technology extensively in clinical diagnostics. Myoglobin (Mb) [61], CK-MB [62], troponin I (cTnI) [63], troponin T (cTnT) [64], and other cardiac markers are frequently used by doctors to help detect acute myocardial infarction (AMI). In the experimental comparison, the detection sensitivity was determined to be higher than the classic ELISA detection approach.

The increasing number of infectious diseases threatens human life globally. There is, therefore, a need for the establishment of accurate and accessible point-of care testing technology which allows the rapid checking of disease at home. This will reduce the spread of infectious disease in hospitals or public places.

The immunochromatography test technology is being used to detect pathogens such as adenovirus, hepatitis B surface antigen [65], vibrio cholerae, *Helicobacter pylori* [66], HIV-1 etc. The secreted protein antigen of mycobacterium can also be utilized to detect the serum and pleura effusions TB antibody [67].

Recently the lateral flow immunochromatography technique has been used in the testing of novel coronavirus [68] and in the detection of neutralizing antibodies in COVID-19 patients for the development of vaccine [69].

This technique can detect the microbial indicator of various diseases for patients easily, quickly and with low cost. This technology can readily, rapidly, and economically detect the microbiological signs of a variety of questionable patients.

3.5.2 Applications for food safety

Because it is well recognized that hazardous food can cause more than 200 diseases, the food sector tries to produce and market food products that do not harm the consumer. Furthermore, tainted food kills around 420 000 individuals each year and causes sickness to over 600 million people [70]. To avoid the presence of harmful substances such as veterinary medications, pesticides, heavy metals, toxic fertilizers, and pathogens, food safety procedures should be implemented throughout the food chain [71–73]. Following appropriate agricultural and manufacturing practises can help to reach this goal [74].

LFIA can be used to manage the risk of foodborne illness. LFIA enhances the number of analyses and makes the entire process from manufacture to ready-to-eat food simple, quick, and economical. All of these characteristics combine to make the LFIA an excellent tool for hazard analysis and critical control points (HACCP) processes [75].

In comparison to the LFIA used in clinical diagnostics, the LFIA for food safety must cope with the difficulty of food matrices [76] that can be extremely diverse, requiring a different LFIA apparatus to analyse different food items such as cereals, meat, spices, milk, and alcoholic drinks.

One of the most generally accepted uses of LFIA in this sector is the detection of poisons, antibiotics or other medications, pesticides, pathogens, food adulterants, and allergies.

3.5.3 Environmental application

Today the major subject of concern is environmental pollution. Environmental monitoring is the activity that safeguards the environment and protects living organisms from exposure to toxic pollutants, contamination sources, and pathogens.

LFIAs are used for the detection of heavy metals in soil, pesticides, algae, pathogens, toxins, and other compounds. They are mainly used for the detection of soil and water contaminants

3.5.4 Veterinary applications

Veterinary services are mandatory to assure the health of animal, to control and prevent animal diseases and diseases which are transmitted to humans through animals (zoonotic diseases), to ensure the safety of animal products and to improve the welfare of animals worldwide [77]. World Organisation for Animal Health (OIE, historic acronym of the Office International des Epizooties) works to control animal diseases and in improving the welfare of animals. Effective surveillance, early detection and rapid response mechanisms are the key to prevent and control outbreaks of disease.

The use of POCT in the veterinary field has increased in the last decade which helps in the identification and prevention of infectious diseases. Considering the fact that 60% of human pathogens are of animal origin [78, 79], it is important to understand the crucial role of rapid detection. LFIA have been developed for the detection of African swine fever [80, 81]

3.6 New challenges

LFIA is the ideal device for POC testing having low cost, operational reliability, no need for transportation and storage of samples, works in poor or non-laboratory environment. LFIAs are used for used for qualitative screening. Their use is limited when highly quantitative and reproducible results are demanded. So there is a need to develop existing LFIA systems and to overcome their weakness. The sensitivity of LFIA can be enhanced by the use of dedicated strip readers [82].

The external readers allow the quantitative analysis of LFIA strips by measuring the intensities of signals generated at two lines. Thus, these readers on one hand increase the cost of analysis, but on the other hand ensure the testing quality by allowing the digitalization of data track, stores the data and reduces the interpretation and transmission errors. In this sense, there is an increasing use of smartphone technology to be used in LFIA readers [83].

The use of strip readers provides an alternative detection method (fluorescence, chemiluminescence). The use of the fluorescence method has increased from 3.8% to 15.8% and the use of surface-enhanced Raman spectroscopy (SERS) has increased from 0% to 3.6% but the colorimetric method of detection still predominates all the methods.

3.7 Future developing directions

The commercial application of any device includes the reproducibility of test, ease in sample addition, recording and processing of data. As already discussed the applications of multiplex LFIAs in various fields, there is an exponential growth in the use of multiplexing LFIAs as various analytes can be detected at the same time in a particular condition. But multiplex LFIAs have certain limitations regarding the number of analytes to be detected. This can be overcome by the use of microarray LFIAs with reading devices which improves the multiplex capability [84, 85]. The use of new labels such as fluorescence labels in place of traditional colloidal gold particles improves the sensitivity of the assay. Fluorescence labels are much more sensitive, qualitative and can be prepared in a multiplex way through the selection of different dyes. The use of quantum dots provides the additional advantage of stability, wide range excitation, narrow range emission, and large absorption coefficients. Quantum dots can be applied as reporters in fluorescence LFIAs. Surface-enhanced Raman scattering based LFIAs provide a novel direction to build a better assay with better sensitivity and specificity [86].

References

[1] Yager P, Edwards T, Fu E, Helton K, Nelson K and Tam M R 2006 Microfluidic diagnostic technologies for global public health *Nature* **442** 412–8

[2] Weigl B, Domingo G, Labarre P and Gerlach J 2008 Towards non- and minimally instrumented, microfluidics-based diagnostic devices *Lab Chip* **12** 1999–2014

[3] Tomazelli Coltro W K, Cheng C M, Carrilho E and de Jesus D P 2014 Recent advances in low-cost microfluidic platforms for diagnostic applications *Electrophoresis* **8** 2309–24

[4] Lei R, Huo R and Mohan C 2019 Current and emerging trends in point-of-care urinalysis tests *Expert Rev. Mol. Diagn.* **20** 69–84

[5] Li F, You M, Li S, Hu J, Liu C, Gong Y, Yang H and Xu F 2020 Paper-based point-of-care immunoassays: recent advances and emerging trends *Biotechnol. Adv.* **39** 107442

[6] Cate D M, Adkins J A, Mettakoonpitak J and Henry C S 2015 Recent developments in paper-based microfluidic devices *Anal. Chem.* **87** 19–41

[7] Hu J, Wang S, Wang L, Li F, Pingguan-Murphy B, Lu T J and Xu F 2014 Advances in paper-based point-of-care diagnostics *Biosens. Bioelectron.* **54** 585–97

[8] Yetisen A K, Akram M S and Lowe C R 2013 Paper-based microfluidic point-of-care diagnostic devices *Lab Chip* **13** 2210–51

[9] Ballerini DR, Li X and Shen W 2012 Nov Patterned paper and alternative materials as substrates for low-cost microfluidic diagnostics. *Microfluidics and nanofluidics.* **13** 769–87

[10] Pelton R 2009 Sep 1 Bioactive paper provides a low-cost platform for diagnostics. *TrAC Trends in Analytical Chemistry.* **28** 925–42

[11] Millipore 2009 Rapid lateral flow test strips: consideration for product development. http://millipore.com/techpublications/tech1/tb500en00 (accessed 15 December 2012)

[12] Wang J 2008 Electrochemical glucose biosensors *Chem. Rev.* **108** 814–25

[13] O'Sullivan A C 1997 *Cellulose: The Structure Slowly Unravels* vol 4 (Berlin: Springer), 173–207

[14] Hu J, Wang S, Wang L, Li F, Pingguan-Murphy B, Lu T J and Xu F 2014 Advances in paper-based point-of-care diagnostics *Biosens. Bioelectron.* **54** 585–97

[15] Costa MN, Veigas B, Jacob JM, Santos DS, Gomes J, Baptista PV, Martins R, Inácio J and Fortunato E 2014 Feb 12 A low cost, safe, disposable, rapid and self-sustainable paper-based platform for diagnostic testing: lab-on-paper. *Nanotechnology.* **25** 094006

[16] Martinez A W, Phillips S T, Whitesides G M and Carrilho E 2010 Diagnostics for the developing world:microfluidic paper-based analytical devices *Anal. Chem.* **82** 3–10

[17] Martinez A W, Phillips S T and Whitesides G M 2008 Three-dimensional microfluidic devices fabricated in layered paper and tape *Proc. Natl Acad. Sci. USA* **105** 19606–11

[18] Li Z, Wang Y, Wang J, Tang Z, Pounds J G and Lin Y 2010 Rapid and sensitive detection of protein biomarker using a portable fluorescence biosensor based on quantum dots and a lateral flow test strip *Anal. Chem.* **82** 7008–14

[19] Anon 2008 *Rapid Lateral Flow Test Strips: Considerations for Product Development* (Billerica, MA: Merck Millipore)

[20] Anfossi L, Di Nardo F, Cavalera S, Giovannoli C and Baggiani C 2018 Multiplex lateral flow immunoassay: an overview of strategies towards high-throughput point-of-need testing *Biosensors (Basel)* **9** 2

[21] Li J and Macdonald J 2016 Multiplexed lateral flow biosensors: technological advances for radically improving point-of-care diagnoses *Biosens. Bioelectron.* **83** 177–92

[22] Yen C W, Puig H, Tam J, Gomez-Marquez J, Bosch I, Schifferli K H and Gehrke L 2015 Multicolored silver nanoparticles for multiplexed disease diagnostics. Distinguishing dengue, yellow fever, and Ebola viruses *Lab Chip* **15** 1638–41

[23] Xu Y, Liu Y, Wu Y, Xia X, Liao Y and Li Q 2014 Fluorescent probe-based lateral flow assay for multiplex nucleic acid detection *Anal. Chem.* **86** 5611–4

[24] Eyad H, Hawamdeh G, Jarrad N A, Yasin O, Al-Gharabli S I and Shad Fan R 2018 Detection of human chorionic gonadotropin (hCG) hormone using digital lateral flow immunoassay *40th Annual Int. Conf. of the IEEE Engineering in Medicine and Biology Society (EMBC) (July)* pp 3845–8

[25] Andryukov B G 2020 Six decades of lateral flow immunoassay: from determining metabolic markers to diagnosing COVID-19 *AIMS Microbiol* **6** 280–304

[26] Yadavalli T and Shukla D 2017 Role of metal and metal oxide nanoparticles as diagnostic and therapeutic tools for highly prevalent viral infections *Nanomed. Nanotechnol. Biol. Med.* **13** 219–30

[27] Posthuma-Trumpie G A, Korf J and van Amerongen A 2009 Lateral flow (immuno)assay: its strengths, weaknesses, opportunities and threats. A literature survey *Anal. Bioanal. Chem.* **393** 569–82

[28] Jiuchuan G, Chen S, Guo J and Ma X 2021 Nanomaterial labels in lateral flow immunoassays for point-of-care-testing *J. Mater. Sci. Technol.* **60** 90–104

[29] Parolo C, de la Escosura-Muñiz A and Merkoçi A 2013 Enhanced lateral flow immunoassay using gold nanoparticles loaded with enzymes *Biosens. Bioelectron.* **40** 412–6

[30] Eden M N, Naghdi T, Zor E and Merkoçi A 2015 Photoluminescent lateral-flow immunoassay revealed by graphene oxide: highly sensitive paper-based pathogen detection *Anal. Chem.* **87** 8573–7

[31] Parolo C, Sena-Torralba A, Bergua JF, Calucho E, Fuentes-Chust C, Hu L, Rivas L, Álvarez-Diduk R, Nguyen EP, Cinti S and Quesada-González D. 2020 Dec Tutorial: Design and fabrication of nanoparticle-based lateral-flow immunoassays. *Nature Protoc.* **15** 3788–816

[32] Zhan L, Guo S Z and Song F 2017 The role of nanoparticle design in determining analytical performance of lateral flow immunoassays *Nano Lett.* **17** 7207–12

[33] Wild D 2013 *The Immunoassay Handbook: Theory and Applications of Ligand Binding, ELISA, and Related Techniques* 4th edn (Oxford/Waltham, MA: Elsevier)

[34] Panhotra B, Hassan Z, Joshi C and Bahrani A 2005 Visual detection of multiple viral amplicons by dipstick assay. Its application in screening of blood donors a welcome tool for the limited resource settings *J. Clin. Microbiol.* **43** 6218

[35] Carter D J and Cary R B 2007 Lateral flow microarrays: a novel platform for rapid nucleic acid detection based on miniaturized lateral flow chromatography *Nucleic Acids Res.* **35** e74

[36] Lee S, Mehta S and Erickson D 2016 Two-color lateral flow assay for multiplex detection of causative agents behind acute febrile illnesses *Anal. Chem.* **88** 8359–63

[37] Peeling R W *et al* 2010 Evaluation of diagnostic tests: dengue *Nat. Rev. Microbiol.* **8** S30–8

[38] Tuerk C and Gold L 1990 Systematic evolution of ligands by exponential enrichment: RNA ligands to bacteriophage T4 DNA polymerase *Science* **249** 505–10

[39] Ellington A D and Szostak J W 1990 In vitro selection of RNA molecules that bind specific ligands *Nature* **346** 818–22

[40] Sajid M, Kawde A and Daud M 2015 Design, formats and applications of lateral flow assays *J. Saudi Chem. Soc.* **19** 689–705

[41] Gubala V, Harris L F, Ricco A J, Tan M X and Williams D E 2012 Point of care diagnostics: status and future *Anal. Chem.* **84** 487–515

[42] Liu C, Jia Q, Yang C, Qiao R, Jing L and Wang L *et al* 2011 Lateral flow immunochromatographic assay for sensitive pesticide detection by using Fe_3O_4 nanoparticle aggregates as color reagents *Anal. Chem.* **83** 6778–84

[43] Wang D B, Tian B, Zhang Z P, Wang X Y, Fleming J and Bi L J *et al* 2015 Detection of Bacillus anthracis spores by super-paramagnetic lateral-flow immunoassays based on 'Road Closure' *Biosens. Bioelectron.* **67** 608–14

[44] Wang Y, Xu H, Wei M, Gu H, Xu Q and Zhu W 2009 Study of superparamagnetic nanoparticles as labels in the quantitative lateral flow immunoassay *Mater. Sci. Eng.* C **29** 714–8

[45] Xu Q, Xu H, Gu H, Li J, Wang Y and Wei M 2009 Development of lateral flow immunoassay system based on superparamagnetic nanobeads as labels for rapid quantitative detection of cardiac troponin I *Mater. Sci. Eng.* C **29** 702

[46] Wang L, Lu D and Wang J *et al* 2011 A novel immunochromatographic electrochemical biosensor for highly sensitive and selective detection of trichloropyridinol, a biomarker of exposure to chlorpyrifos *Biosens. Bioelectron.* **26** 2835–40

[47] Khreich N, Lamourette P, Lagoutte B, Ronco C, Franck X, Créminon C and Volland H 2010 A fluorescent immunochromatographic test using immunoliposomes for detecting microcystins and nodularins *Anal. Bioanal. Chem.* **397** 1733–42

[48] Li Z, Wang Y, Wang J, Tang Z, Pounds J G and Lin Y 2010 Rapid and sensitive detection of protein biomarker using a portable fluorescence biosensor based on quantum dots and a lateral flow test strip *Anal. Chem.* **82** 7008–14

[49] Maxwell T, Nogueira Campos M G, Smith S, Doomra M, Thwin Z and Santra S 2019 Quantum dots *Nanoparticles for Biomedical Applications: Fundamental Concepts, Biological Interactions and Clinical Applications* (Amsterdam: Elsevier), 243–65

[50] Resch-Genger U, Grabolle M, Cavaliere-Jaricot S, Nitschke R and Nann T 2008 Quantum dots versus organic dyes as fluorescent labels *Nat. Methods* **5** 763–75

[51] Parolo C, de la Escosura-Muñiz A and Merkoçi A 2013 Enhanced lateral flow immunoassay using gold nanoparticles loaded with enzymes *Biosens. Bioelectron.* **40** 412–6

[52] Kaviani D, Pirmohamadi P, Saghi M, Padidaran B and Bigtan M H 2015 Synthesis of carbon nanoparticles from polystyrene wastes *Int. J. Sci.* **4** 53–7

[53] Muhsan M S, Nadeem S, Hassan A U, Din A M U, Shahid S and Ali S 2019 Synthesis of carbon nanoparticles by using seed oils *Pakistan J. Sci. Ind. Res. Ser. A: Phys. Sci.* **62** 1–7

[54] Kalogianni D P, Boutsika L M, Kouremenou P G, Christopoulos T K and Ioannou P C 2011 Carbon nano-strings as reporters in lateral flow devices for DNA sensing by hybridization *Anal. Bioanal. Chem.* **400** 1145–52

[55] Qiu W, Baryeh K, Takalkar S, Chen W and Liu G 2019 Carbon nanotube-based lateral flow immunoassay for ultrasensitive detection of proteins: application to the determination of IgG *Mikrochim. Acta* **186** 436

[56] Shen G, Zhang S and Hu X 2013 Signal enhancement in a lateral flow immunoassay based on dual gold nanoparticle conjugates *Clin. Biochem.* **46** 1734–8

[57] Xu H, Mao X, Zeng Q, Wang S, Kawde A N and Liu G 2009 Aptamer-functionalized gold nanoparticles as probes in a dry-reagent strip biosensor for protein analysis *Anal. Chem.* **81** 669–75

[58] Li Z, Wang Y, Wang J, Tang Z, Pounds J G and Lin Y 2010 Rapid and sensitive detection of protein biomarker using a portable fluorescence biosensor based on quantum dots and a lateral flow test strip *Anal. Chem.* **82** 7008–14
[59] Hou Y, Wang K and Xiao K 2017 Smartphone-based dual-modality imaging system for quantitative detection of color or fluorescent lateral flow immunochromatographic strips *Nanoscale Res. Lett.* **12** 291
[60] Urusov A E, Zherdev A V and Dzantiev B B 2019 Towards lateral flow quantitative assays: detection approaches *Biosensors (Basel)* **9** 89
[61] Ecollan P *et al* 2007 Pre-hospital detection of acute myocardial infarction with ultra-rapid human fatty acid-binding protein (H-FABP) immunoassay *Int. J. Cardiol.* **119** 349–54
[62] Hampl J, Hall M, Mufti N A, Yao Y M, MacQueen D B, Wright W H and Cooper D E 2001 Upconverting phosphor reporters in immunochromatographic assays *Anal. Biochem.* **288** 176–87
[63] Xu Q, Xu H, Gu H, Li J, Wang Y and Wei M 2009 Development of lateral flow immunoassay system based on superparamagnetic nanobeads as labels for rapid quantitative detection of cardiac troponin I *Mater. Sci. Eng.* **29** 702–7
[64] Xu Q, Xu H, Gu H, Li J, Wang Y and Wei M 2009 Development of lateral flow immunoassay system based on superparamagnetic nanobeads as labels for rapid quantitative detection of cardiac troponin I *Mater. Sci. Eng.* **29** 702–7
[65] Lin S and Zhang Y 2008 Optimization of production process of diagnostic reagent of colloidal gold for HBsAb *Prog. Modern Biomed.* **8** 289–92
[66] Chen T S, Chang F Y and Lee S D 1997 Serodiagnosis of *Helicobacter pylori* infection: comparison and correlation between enzyme-linked immunosorbent assay and rapid serological test results *J. Clin. Microbiol.* **35** 184–6
[67] Yang Y 2009 Application of gold immunochromatographic assay in rapid diagnosis of tuberculosis *Gansu Sci. Technol.* **24** 173–4
[68] Li Z *et al* 2020 Development and clinical application of a rapid IgM–IgG combined antibody test for SARS-CoV-2 infection diagnosis *J. Med. Virol.* **10** 1–7
[69] Lake D F, Roeder A J, Kaleta E, Jasbi P, Pfeffer K and Koelbela C *et al* 2021 Development of a rapid point-of-care test that measures neutralizing antibodies to SARS-CoV-2 *J. Clin. Virol.* **145** 105024
[70] WHO Estimates of the Global Burden of Foodborne Diseases: Foodborne Disease Burden Epidemiology Reference Group 2007–2015 http://apps.who.int/iris/bitstream/10665/199350/1/9789241565165_eng.pdf (accessed 17 May 2021)
[71] Choi J R, Yong K W, Choi J Y and Cowie A C 2019 Emerging point-of-care technologies for food safety analysis *Sensors (Basel)* **19** 817
[72] Eltzov E, Guttel S, Kei A L Y, Sinawang P D, Ionescu R E and Marks R S 2015 Lateral flow immunoassays—from paper strip to smartphone technology *Electroanalysis* **27** 2116–30
[73] Anfossi L 2019 Immunoassays: food applications *Encyclopedia of Analytical Science* 3rd edn (Amsterdam: Elsevier)
[74] Fetzer J C, Worsfold P, Townshend A and Poole C 2006 Encyclopedia of analytical science *Anal. Bioanal. Chem.* **385** 1035–6
[75] General Standard for Contaminants and Toxins in Food and Feed (CODEX STAN 193-1995) http://fao.org/faowhocodexalimentarius/shproxy/en/?lnk=1&url=https%253A%252F%2Fworkspace.fao.org%252Fsites%252Fcodex%252FStandards%252FCXS%2B193–1995%252FCXS_193e.pdf (accessed 27 July 2021)

[76] DiNardo F and Anfossi L 2020 Commercial biosensors for detection of food additives, contaminants, and pathogens ed M K Sezgintürk *Commercial Biosensors and Their Applications. Clinical, Food, and Beyond* 1st edn (Amsterdam: Elsevier), ch 8, pp 183–215
[77] Anfossi L 2019 Immunoassays| food applications *Encyclopedia of Analytical Science* ed J C Fetzer, P Worsfold, A Townshend and C Poole 3rd edn (Amsterdam: Elsevier), 25–30
[78] Veterinary Services https://oie.int/fileadmin/Home/eng/Media_Center/docs/pdf/VS-FINAL-EN.pdf (accessed 17 May 2021)
[79] Taylor L H, Latham S M and Woolhouse M E J 2001 Risk factors for human disease emergence *Phil. Trans. R. Soc.* B **356** 983–9
[80] Sastre P, Gallardo C, Monedero A, Ruiz T, Arias M, Sanz A and Rueda P 2016 Dec Development of a novel lateral flow assay for detection of African swine fever in blood. *BMC Vet. Res.* **12** 1–8
[81] Mak W C, Beni V and Turner A P F 2016 Lateral-flow technology: from visual to instrumental *TrAC Trends Anal. Chem.* **79** 297–305
[82] Bishop J D, Hsieh H V, Gasperino J D J and Weigl B H 2019 Sensitivity enhancement in lateral flow assays: a systems perspective *Lab Chip* **19** 2486–99
[83] Nguyen V, Song S, Park S and Joo C 2020 Recent advances in high-sensitivity detection methods for paper-based lateral-low assay *Biosens. Bioelectron.* **152** 112015
[84] Mahmoudi T, de la Guardia M, Shirde B, Mokhtarzadeh A and Baradan B 2019 Recent advancements in structural improvements of lateral flow assays towards point-of-care testing *TrAC Trends Anal. Chem.* **116** 13–30
[85] Thakur R, Akram F, Rastogi V, Mitra A, Nawani R, Av V, Dubey S K and Shakher C 2020 Development of smartphone-based lateral flow device for the quantification of LH and E3G hormones *IEEE Sens. J.* **20** 14491–500
[86] Wang R, Kim K, Choi N, Wang X, Lee J and Jeon J H *et al* 2018 Highly sensitive detection of high-risk bacterial pathogens using SERS-based lateral flow assay strips *Sensors Actuators* B **270** 72–9

Chapter 4

Fabrication of surface-enhanced Raman scattering based lateral flow assay for disease diagnosis

Nidhi Puranik and Shiv Kumar Yadav

Surface-enhanced Raman scattering (SERS) based technologies such as dipstick and lateral flow formats have been gaining interest in the consumer market over the last three decades due to their compactness, facile interpretation, and portability without the use of any external instrumentations. SERS tags development has taken a major step forward for spectroscopic analysis of biological/biomedical samples because of its numerous advantagous properties. Several reviews demonstrate the potency of SERS for therapeutic drug monitoring in the detection of cancer cells and tumour for *in vivo* situations and DNA bio-sensing. The reported studies also explained the potential of SERS in numerous applications in the field of biomedical. SERS has become a powerful tool in chemical, material, and life sciences. The SERS tag consists of easy colloidal gold so can be used in lateral flow immunoassay (LFIA) designs due to similar properties and also having an optical point of view so has numerous advantages. SERS tags have specificity and are used for the quantitative detection of a wide range of samples. The structure of SERS tags could be designed to improve the performance of assays. The SERS-based LFIA methods are suitable due to their guidance for treatment as a fast, accurate, ultrasensitive, and efficient method to detect pathogens. SERS-LFIA based devices are capable of reducing the limit of the detection (LOD) and possibilities of quantitative and multiplex detection in a wider range of analytes such as proteins, nucleic acids, heavy metals, antibiotics, distinct pathogens, virus bacteria, etc.

4.1 Introduction

The surface-enhanced Raman scattering (SERS) method has gained attention in numerous analytical roles due to its straightforward properties. It provides ultra-sensitive detection and structural information at a singular molecular level and is

doi:10.1088/978-0-7503-5820-0ch4

© IOP Publishing Ltd 2023

capable of detecting via unique Raman fingerprints, SERS related lateral flow immunoassay (LFIA) by targeting analytes for detection. The SERS-based LFIA system exhibits promising results as it overcomes the lower sensitivity issues of conventional LFIA and the deficient precision character of signal measurement via optical or fluorescence signal reader [1, 2].

The application of SERS that is most interesting is in the field of imaging, analytical, and disease diagnosis. The SERS tags have more optical efficiency than the fluorescent labels and have the same efficiency as organic dyes and quantum dots. These consist of gold (Au) nanoparticles (NPs) belonging to the plasmonic core, Raman active molecules adsorbed in nanoparticles, and the protective polymers or inorganic layers. Zhang and his group develop a single T line SERS lateral flow assay in his study for the detection of distinct cardio markers [3, 4].

On the other hand, SERS tags have numerous advantages including their optical method use. Firstly this enhances the intensity of Raman scattering that makes it capable of detecting a single SERS tag by the use of the general optical procedure. Secondly, its intensity is proportional to the tag number for a wider range of concentrations. Finally, the small spectral band of Raman scattering makes it suitable for multiplexing. There are numerous types of SERS tag preparations including nanostars, nanoflowers, nanoprobes, etc. The gap-enhanced Raman tags (GERTs), a type of SERS nanoprobe, is attractive in showing the Raman enhancement, photostability and reproducibility. These types of particles were recently used for the detection of cardiac troponin I by the SERS-LFIA method [5–7]. The general scheme of SERS is shown in figure 4.1 [8].

Now point of care technology (POCT) is one of the focused methods for current health monitoring due to its aim of providing rapid and facile health information in a cost reduced manner. This includes all points from variability in genes,

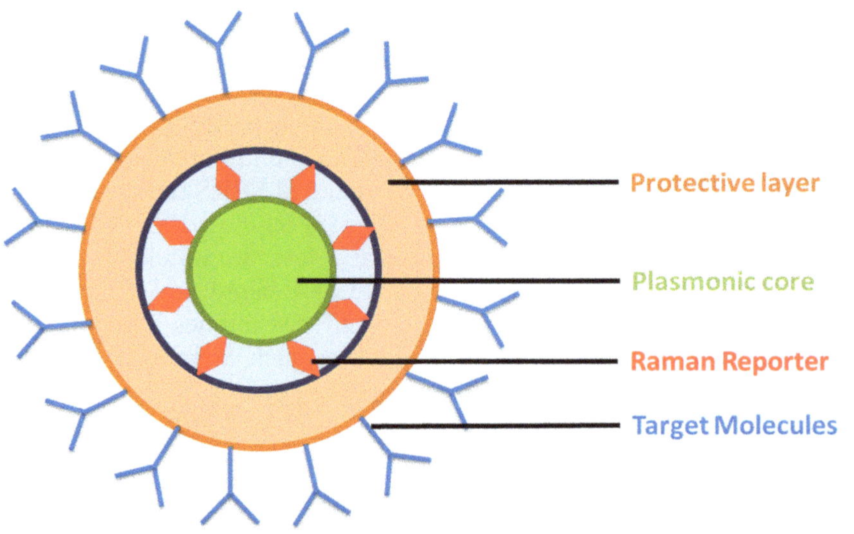

Figure 4.1. General scheme of SERS tag composition.

environment, and style of living, and also the precision medicine (PM) modernizes disorder prevention and treatment. This reported study has collected data from millions of patients and confirms that PM is highly dependent upon the health condition status of the individual. This results in the new POCT method, known to have higher accuracy, becoming one of the important pathways for future development [9, 10]. Examples of SERS-based technologies that are gaining interest in the consumer market over the last three decades are dipstick and lateral flow formats due to their compactness, facile interpretation, and portability without the use of any external instrumentations. Viewing all scenarios the current demand of present assay formats is a lack of quantitation in measurement [11, 12]. The lateral flow assay depends upon the immuno-strips used and the gold colloids like nanoparticles used mostly in the POCT techniques to govern their simple operation, fast detection method, and robustness in numerous applications such as detection of cardio markers, high sensitivity for myoglobin by using LFIA assay [13], the multiplex LFIA for detection of mycotoxin [14], Disease detection causes due to infection from distinct pathogens like dengue, chikungunya virus [15], diagnostics associated with a distinct type of chemical and biological targets [16] and their LFA associated with SERS nanotags for determination of multiplex and quantitation cardiac biomarkers, which helps in early detection of acute myocardial infarction. The recently used technologies for quantitative LFA detection are fluorescence and Raman/magnetic labels rather than gold colloids [3, 16, 17].

The preparation of SERS tags is done by attachment of intrinsically strong Raman reporters (i.e., Raman scattering molecules) to the plasmon-resonance surface (Ag (silver) or Au NPs), that are capable of creating the SERS spectrum of Raman reporters. SERS tag development has taken a major step forward for spectroscopic analysis of biological/biomedical samples due to its numerous advantageous properties which are given in table 4.1.

SERS is used widely as a spectroscopic method because of its property of giving structural information at the single-molecule level [20, 21]. The technique is gaining traction due to features such as non-invasiveness, obliviousness to water, which is ubiquitous in biological samples, and the ability to analyse conformational changes as well as offering vibrational information on the analytes of interest [22]. Several reviews exhibit the potency of SERS for therapeutic drug monitoring in the

Table 4.1. Basic properties of SERS tags [18, 19].

S. No.	Characteristics/properties	SERS tags
1	Based on physical principal	Raman scattering
2	Structural information	Fingerprint
3	Photostability	Anti-photo bleaching
4	Core composition	Au and Ag based NPs
5	Size bandwidth	Less than 2 nm
6	Multiplexing capacity	10–100
7	Toxicity	Non-toxic

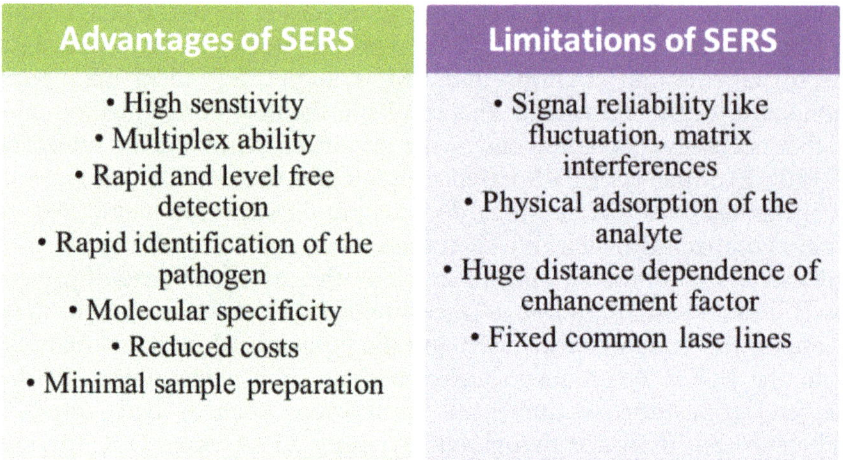

Figure 4.2. Advantages and limitation of SERS.

detection of cancer cells and tumour for *in vivo* situations and DNA bio-sensing as well. The reported studies also explained the SERS potential in numerous applications in the field of biomedical [23, 24]. Various advantages and limitations of SERS are shown in figure 4.2 as reported earlier [25].

More analytes were also used for detection using LFIA and multiple assays on a single immune strip that enhances the complete information, reduces the time and is cheap to use, and improves accuracy in health monitoring. Numerous cardiac biomarkers are detected in this way such as myoglobin, cardiac troponin I, and creatine kinase-MB isoenzymes also known as Myo, cTnI and CK-MB respectively, which it is required to rapidly diagnose to have early knowledge of acute myocardial infarction, which is a major cause of death and is a life-threatening issue throughout the world. Recently the SERS nanotags gained attention due to their properties that proved to be excellent where the signal of Raman dyes with Raman scattering cross-sections are used and enhanced by the use of plasmonic gold/silver nanoparticles. When compared to fluorescence, SERS signals come from the dye molecule via vibration and rotation movements and are more stable than the single nano-tag detected through the higher enhancement factor of rationally planned plasmonic nanostructures [26–28].

4.2 Surface-enhanced Raman scattering

The Raman effect was first discovered by C V Raman in 1928 using simple optical materials and instruments [29]. Further described as a particular optical readout platform that involves the scattering of irradiation light followed by interaction of polarizable molecule under interrogation to monochromatic laser sources. The scattered photon's larger proportion has similar energy to the incident light; this is termed Rayleigh scattering. So, this does not have any specific chemical information. The common requirement of Raman spectra is a good signal-to-noise ratio, high power density, long collection time, and clinically unrealistic concentration.

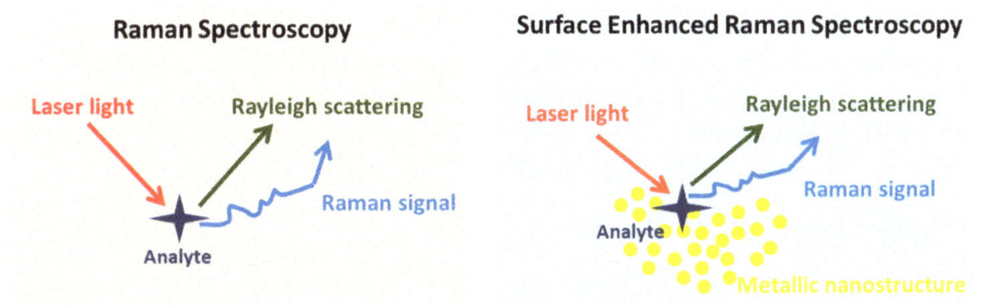

Figure 4.3. Differentiation between the Raman spectroscopy and SERS.

These measuring parameters enhance the fluorescence and photo-degradation that commonly mask Raman spectral lines. This might become a limitation of disorder diagnosis for Raman spectroscopy in the field of biofluids and cells. It is interesting that major consideration has now shifted to SERS to overcome the quantum incompetence of conventional Raman spectroscopy [30–32]. The basic differences in SERS and Raman spectroscopy is shown in figure 4.3.

Fleischmann and colleagues at the University of Southampton in the United Kingdom discovered the SERS effect accidentally in 1974. Where the Raman signals of monolayer pyridine adsorbed into electrochemically roughened Ag electrodes showed a significant increase. For nanoscale rough metallic particles with a smaller diameter than the wavelength of excitation radiation, the SERS involves interactions between electromagnetic radiation and molecules adsorbed into close proximity [33, 34].

SERS is a well-known spectroscopic technique with extremely high spatial resolution that outperforms traditional techniques like fluorescence: it has narrow bands of 0.1 nm in contrast to fluorescence's 20–80 nm bandwidth, making it ideal for multiplexing detection in the same sample, allowing multiple targets to be identified in simple assays [35]. Due to its inherent features (i.e., fingerprint recognition capabilities and high sensitivity) and technical advances that have reduced the cost of the instruments while improving their sensitivity and user-friendliness, SERS has become a powerful tool in chemical, material, and life sciences [36–38]. SERS has gained popularity in the last decade for the study of biological samples ranging from environmental studies to diagnostics [2]. SERS-based nanometric probes with intrinsic quantitative molecular specificity are attractive candidates for all-optical environmental, biological, and technical sensing applications [39]. In the fabrication of SERS-based diagnostic systems various components are involved having different properties such as plasmonic nanoparticle (gold or silver nanoparticles) [40–42] with different shapes (spheres [43], pillar [44, 45], stars [46–48], boot shaped [49] and road [50, 51]) [52, 53], reporter molecule (fluorescent dyes) [54, 55], stabilizer (ethylene glycol [56, 57], poly(methyl meth-acrylate) [50, 58], silica [59, 60], graphene [60–62] and bovine serum albumin [63]), and various conjugation molecules [64, 65].

4.2.1 Fabrication of SERS tags for use in the field of medical science

Fabrication of SERS tags used in the medical field is basically completed in four steps as shown in figure 4.4 and discussed in research papers [36]. These steps include (i) design of SRRS substrate, (ii) adsorption of reporter, (iii) surface coating, and (iv) conjugation of various ligands on surface coated tags.

4.3 Fabrication of SERS-based LFIA

The design consists of:

Step I—LFIA preparation
Step II—SERS tags preparation
Step III—sandwich of these two to precede further diagnosis

4.3.1 Step I—LFIA preparation

LFIA was found to be the simplest and cheapest technique for diagnosis at the POCT in the early 1990s. The system is a paper-based system consisting of signal readout time and less sample preparation. The LFIA preparation consists of five important constituents that are:

- backing card,
- nitrocellulose membrane,
- sample pad,
- conjugate pad, and
- absorbent pad.

The widely used labels for this are gold nanoparticles due to their easy fabrication, potent light extinction, and functionalization [36–38].

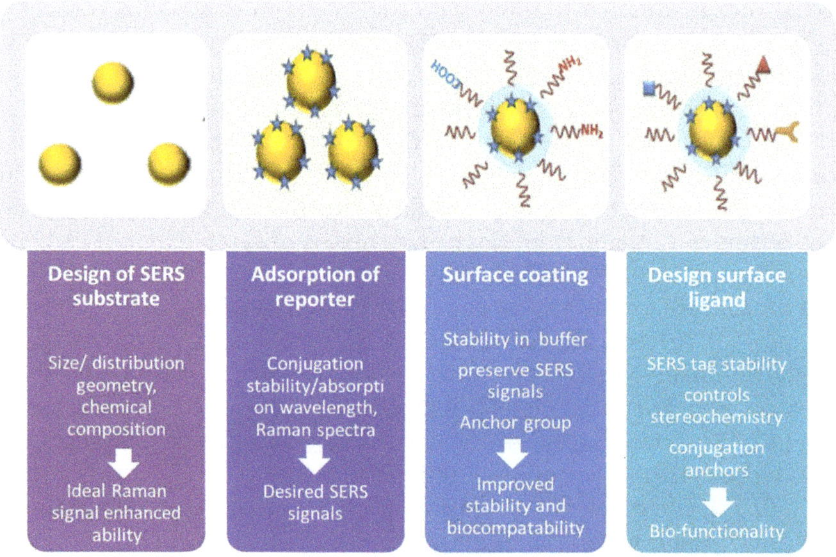

Figure 4.4. General steps in designing of SERS tags for use in field of medical science.

4.3.2 Step II—SERS tags preparation

The SERS tag consists of four parts:

- Metal nano-substrate: like Au nanoparticles, that serve as a plasmonic core.
- Organic Raman reporter molecule: these are Raman active molecules that are absorbed or embedded in nanoparticles. The reporters are larger cross-sections and various Raman peaks ranging from 400 to 1600 cm^{-1}.
- Protection shell: consisting of polymer or inorganic layer for protection that functions for the identification of antibodies [3].
- Targeting molecules.

The conjugation of Raman reporters is often carried out by simple physical adsorption of the dye to the particle's surface for longer periods of incubation. The most common type of paper used for Raman reporters is Nile blue dyed paper (as Raman reporter). Because the adsorption of dye molecules on the surface of nanoparticles does not completely block it, additional conjugation has been done with antibodies that are simply adsorbable.

Because of the high affinity of the thiol group for Au or Ag and the recognized Raman peaks of benzene ring vibration, thiol-based aromatic compounds are important for Raman reporters. Mercaptobenzoic acid and di-thionitro benzoic acid are two more known reporters. This reporter molecule has a carboxyl group that enables conjugation to antibodies utilizing the EDC/NHS cross-linking method. Aminothiophenol benzene dithiol naphthalenethiol and nitrobenzene thiol are some examples of thiolated aromatic compounds that can be used as Raman reporters and improve the colloidal stability of SERS tags. Various Raman reporters used in fabrication of SERS tags for LFIA are given in table 4.2.

Table 4.2. Types of Raman reporters used in designing of SERS tags for LFIA [66–68].

Type	Examples	Benefits	Limitation
Sulfur-containing dyes (dye molecules)	3,3′diethylthiadicarbocy-anineiodide, malachite green isothiocyanate, tetramethylrhodamine-5-isothiocyanate	Large Raman cross section, high binding affinity to metal, suitable for further tag coating and modification, ready for SERRS	Expensive, limited type, hard to form SAM
Nitrogen-containing cationicdye (dye molecules)	Crystal violet, rhodamine B rhodamine 6G, Nile blue	Cheap, high Raman cross section, ready for SERRS	Weak affinity to metal, weak signal stability, hard for further tag surface coating,
Thiolated aromatic molecules	4-aminothiophenol, 4-methylbenzenethiol, 2-naphthalenethiol, benzenethiol	Inexpensive, durable binding affinity to metal	Small Raman cross section, not ready for surface-enhanced resonance Raman scattering (SERRS)

4.3.3 Step III—sandwich of these two to precede diagnosis

The SERS tag consists of easy colloidal gold so it can be used in LFIA designs due to similar properties and also having an optical point of view so has numerous advantages. The intensity of SERS allows it to detect single SERS tags by using the general optical technique. Further, the SERS intensity of SERS signals is proportional to tag numbers in a wider range for concentrations and its narrow spectral band makes it appropriate for multiplexing. From numerous reported studies it was observed that this property stated the enhancement in sensitivity and dynamic range of using the SERS readout. The example is SERS tags for LFIA using Au core@ satellite nanoparticles, nanoparticles consisting of interior nanogaps used in numerous published reports. The use of the SERS tag in LFIA has many advantages, including specificity determination and quantitative detection of sample; however, its structure could also be differently designed for enhancing the performance of assays. Figure 4.5 explains the processing of SERS-based LFIA for diagnosis purposes [5].

4.4 SERS-based LFIA approaches

The example of SERS tags for LFIA consists of nanoformulations that are like nanostars, which are used in the detection of the pathogen causing dengue and Zika disorders [69], nanoflowers [70], raspberry similar particles [70], and composite Au/PT nano-rods. The nanoparticles for this technique have been gaining attention due to their properties like enhancing the surface to volume ratios permitting more Raman reporters for attachment on their surface. On the other hand, these types of particles have a larger size of about 70–100 nm. This, together with their rough surfaces, reduces the colloidal stability and prepares a uniform pathway via a membrane under lateral flow [71]. Various SERS-based LFIAs used for diagnosis of different biomolecules are listed in table 4.3.

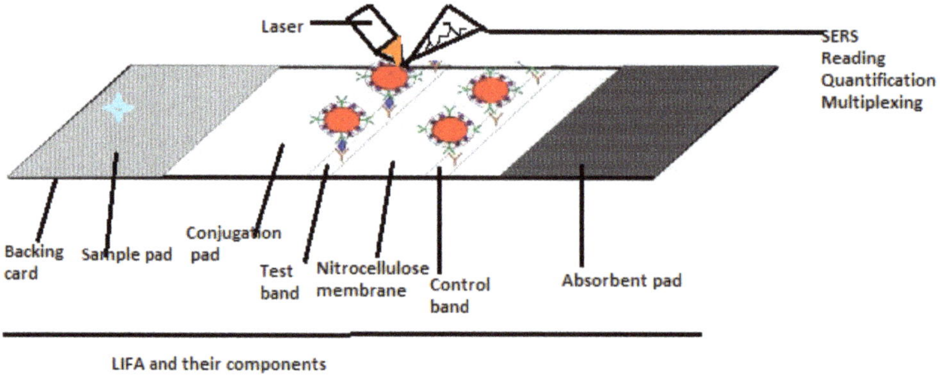

Figure 4.5. Illustrating SERS-based LFIA for diagnosis purpose.

Table 4.3. SERS LFIA used for diagnosis purpose.

Examples	Application	Advantage	References
Simple spherical Au nanoparticle	Used for detection and the quantification of Staphylococcal Enterotoxin B	Enhances the performance of assays sensitivity, chemical and physical stability, and also their multiplexing ability	[72]
Single T line SERS-LFA	Fast detection of distinct cardio markers	Permit more Raman reporters to attach on their surfaces.	[4]
Au nanostar	Neuron-specific enolase (NSE) and the S100-b protein	Enhances performance of assays sensitivity	[73, 74]
AuNP	Detection of pathogen in disease diagnosis (thyroid-stimulating hormone)	—	[75]
Gap-enhanced Raman tags (GERTs)	Quantitative detection of cardiac troponin I and hCG	Raman enhancement, reproducibility, and photostability	[6, 7]
Multi-branched gold nanostars (AuNS)	Immuno-chromatographic assay for sensitive influenza detection	Ultra-high detection sensitivity, which enhances a sensitive POCT for diagnosis in disorders	[76]
Au–Ag@MBA SERS tags	Detection of *Listeria monocytogenes* and Salmonella enteric	—	[77]

4.4.1 SERS-based pathogen detection methods

Pathogen detection is one of the most important problems faced by humanity, and most of them spread widely so need quick detection. The SERS-based LFIA methods are suitable due to their guidance for treatment as a fast, accurate, ultrasensitive, and efficient method to detect the pathogen. This reduces the diagnosis time and enhances the accuracy of testing results, which helps in the reduction of infection-associated morbidity and mortality rates [78]. The SERS related LFA method for point-of-care diagnostics of infectious diseases has been reported in various research papers [79]. The basic diagrammatic presentation of LFA is shown in figure 4.6.

4.4.2 Cancer detection

Recently, SERS-based LFIA gains special attention in this field and has been serving as non-invasive photothermal therapy based on specificity for treating the tumour cells.

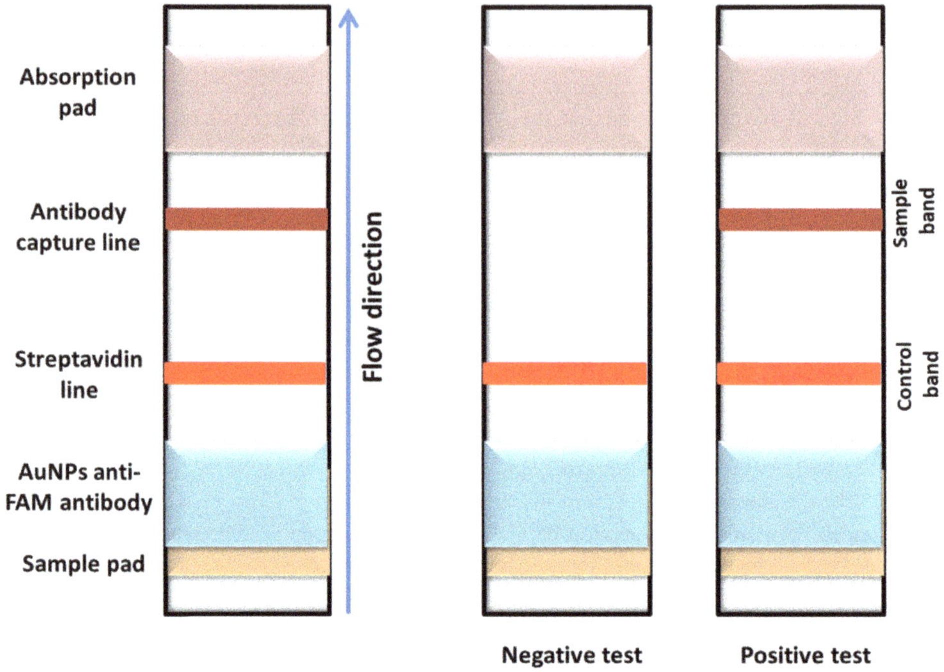

Figure 4.6. SERS related lateral flow assay method for point-of-care diagnostics of infectious diseases.

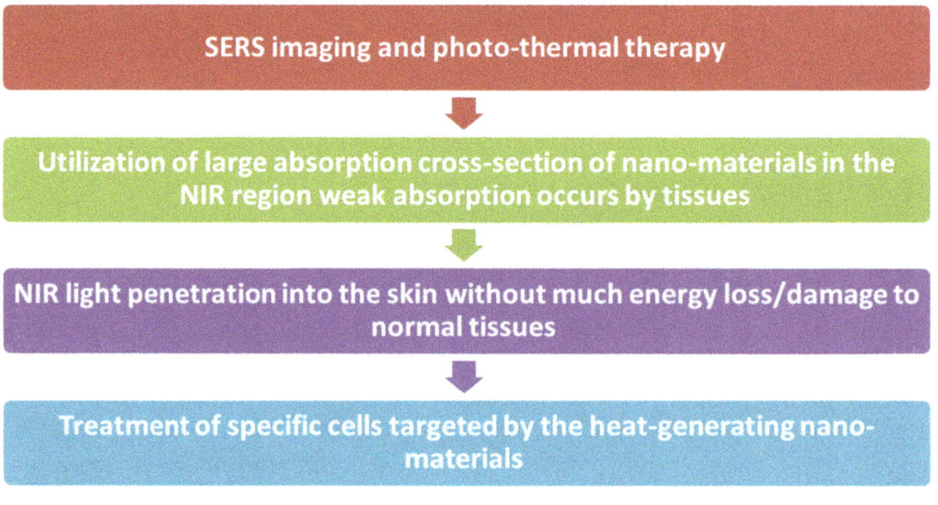

Nano platforms based on SERS imaging and photothermal therapy is a major advantage for NIR light absorption purpose for specific SERS-active noble metals NPs. The targeted cell such as tumour location can also be detected *in vivo* via spectrophotometric Raman analysis between the specific and non-specific bindings [80–82]. An example is Maltzahn's group which developed in their studies a bifunctional Au NR-based SERS tag used for *in vivo* imaging and also controlled by the use of the remote, used for treating cancer by photothermal heating mechanism [83].

4.4.3 Detection of respiratory disorders

The respiratory disorders consist of the breath patterns and type of air that is inhaled and exhaled. The term used breathomics is known as 'metabolomics of exhaled air'. The human exhaled breath consists of various constituents including water, oxygen (O_2), nitrogen (N_2), nitric oxide (NO_2), and carbon dioxide (CO_2). Additionally, it contains minor gaseous volatile organic components (VOC) that are formed from numerous highly regulated metabolic reactions in distinct metabolic ways. Recent studies and research have been done on GC–MS gold-standard techniques for global profiling of exhaled volatile organic components associated with abnormal metabolisms that are the reason for the origin of diabetes and cancer. The VOC is present in trace amounts/concentration in breath exhaled. With the help of SERS, it can be detected down to the single-molecule level by using the nanomaterial base, so SERS-associated methods show exciting vision in this field [84–86]. An example is GSP coating with ZIF-8, known as GSP@ZIF-8, it makes a 3D core–shell that behaves as a SERS-active substrate and metal–organic framework that is an interesting one. It is a biosensor that is more attractive and practical for analysis purposes, specifically clinical and for the detection of lung cancer volatile organic biomarkers at the time of need [86].

4.4.4 Protein analysis for Alzheimer disease biomarkers

SERS-associated analysis for proteins is attracting interest because of its simple fabrication, ease of use and rapid results with minimum cost. The other capabilities is its revelation of structural changes and concentration belonging to targeted components. These are all factors that are important for early-stage diagnosis and in clinical therapy usage. Park and his group state the development of 'carboxylic-acid-functionalized, graphitic nanolayer-coated three-dimensional SERS substrate' prepared from gold nano-wires that are used for diagnosis of biomarkers of Alzheimer's disease (AD), i.e., tau protein, and amyloid β. The researchers looked at tau protein and amyloid, both of which are linked to AD, which is the cause of dementia. These proteins are already present in body fluids and can be used as biomarkers for AD, thus their concentration is a useful indicator [87].

4.5 Conclusion

It has been found from reported studies that the SERS-associated platform shows higher sensitivity and promising application in the field of bioanalysis of analytes and disease diagnosis. The major advantages are that SERS-LFIA based devices are capable of reducing the LOD and possibilities of quantitative and multiplex detection wider range of analytes like proteins, nucleic acids, heavy metals, antibiotics, distinct pathogens, virus bacteria, etc. The benefits were obtained due to the presence of higher optical efficiency SERS tags and slower Raman readings and signal isolation. The SERS-LFIA has become the most interesting equipment for point of care testing in immunological testing due to its simple use and lower cost campared to the expensive equipment with longer signal acquisition time. These types of device are highly sensitive, non-invasive, have no requirement for sample preparation, and also particularly belong to small structural changes with higher spatial resolution. The variety of SERS-associated assays on the paper-based substrate offer a number of choices in the biomedical and clinical fields for diagnosis of various disorders. The combination of detection via SERS multiplex and *in vivo* endoscopic methods shows more interesting uses in assays performed, and surgical treatments. SERS is an important factor and plays a major role in target-based detection of particular biomarkers in cells/human biofluids/tissues and further use is being investigated for several disorders urgently.

References

[1] Baniukevic J, Hakki Boyaci I, Goktug Bozkurt A, Tamer U, Ramanavicius A and Ramanaviciene A 2013 Magnetic gold nanoparticles in SERS-based sandwich immunoassay for antigen detection by well oriented antibodies *Biosens. Bioelectron.* **43** 281–8

[2] Wang Y, Yan B and Chen L 2013 SERS tags: novel optical nanoprobes for bioanalysis *Chem. Rev.* **113** 1391–428

[3] Wang Z, Zong S, Wu L, Zhu D and Cui Y 2017 SERS-activated platforms for immunoassay: probes, encoding methods, and applications *Chem. Rev.* **117** 7910–63

[4] Zhang D, Huang L, Liu B, Ni H, Sun L and Su E *et al* 2018 Quantitative and ultrasensitive detection of multiplex cardiac biomarkers in lateral flow assay with core–shell SERS nanotags *Biosens. Bioelectron.* **106** 204–11

[5] Khlebtsov B N, Burov A M, Bratashov D N, Tumskiy R S and Khlebtsov N G 2020 Petal-like gap-enhanced Raman tags with controllable structures for high-speed Raman imaging *Langmuir* **36** 5546–53

[6] Khlebtsov B N, Bratashov D N, Byzova N A, Dzantiev B B and Khlebtsov N G 2018 SERS-based lateral flow immunoassay of troponin I by using gap-enhanced Raman tags *Nano Res.* **12** 413–20

[7] Ye Z, Lin L, Tan Z, Zeng Y J, Ruan S and Ye J 2019 Sub-100 nm multi-shell bimetallic gap-enhanced Raman tags *Appl. Surf. Sci.* **487** 1058–67

[8] Khlebtsov B and Khlebtsov N 2020 Surface-enhanced Raman scattering-based lateral-flow immunoassay *Nanomater* **10** 2228

[9] Parolo C and Merkoçi A 2012 Paper-based nanobiosensors for diagnostics *Chem. Soc. Rev.* **42** 450–7

[10] Xia Y, Si J and Li Z 2016 Fabrication techniques for microfluidic paper-based analytical devices and their applications for biological testing: a review *Biosens. Bioelectron.* **77** 774–89

[11] Yetisen A K, Akram M S and Lowe C R 2013 Paper-based microfluidic point-of-care diagnostic devices *Lab Chip* **13** 2210–51

[12] Jung W, Han J, Choi J W and Ahn C H 2015 Point-of-care testing (POCT) diagnostic systems using microfluidic lab-on-a-chip technologies *Microelectron. Eng.* **132** 46–57

[13] Zhu J, Zou N, Zhu D, Wang J, Jin Q and Zhao J *et al* 2011 Simultaneous detection of high-sensitivity cardiac troponin i and myoglobin by modified sandwich lateral flow immunoassay: proof of principle *Clin. Chem.* **57** 1732–8

[14] Song S, Liu N, Zhao Z, Njumbe Ediage E, Wu S and Sun C *et al* 2014 Multiplex lateral flow immunoassay for mycotoxin determination *Anal. Chem.* **86** 4995–5001

[15] Lee S, Mehta S and Erickson D 2016 Two-color lateral flow assay for multiplex detection of causative agents behind acute febrile illnesses *Anal. Chem.* **88** 8359–63
[16] Zarei M 2017 Advances in point-of-care technologies for molecular diagnostics *Biosens. Bioelectron.* **98** 494–506
[17] Hu J, Zhang Z L, Wen C Y, Tang M, Wu L L and Liu C *et al* 2016 Sensitive and quantitative detection of C-reaction protein based on immunofluorescent nanospheres coupled with lateral flow test strip *Anal. Chem.* **88** 6577–84
[18] Wang R, Yu C, Yu F, Chen L and Yu C 2010 Molecular fluorescent probes for monitoring pH changes in living cells *TrAC Trends Anal. Chem.* **29** 1004–13
[19] Wang Y and Chen L 2011 Quantum dots, lighting up the research and development of nanomedicine *Nanomed. Nanotechnol. Biol. Med.* **7** 385–402
[20] Kneipp K, Wang Y, Kneipp H, Perelman L T, Itzkan I and Dasari R R *et al* 1997 Single molecule detection using surface-enhanced Raman scattering (SERS) *Phys. Rev. Lett.* **78** 1667
[21] Blackie E J, Le Ru E C and Etchegoin P G 2009 Single-molecule surface-enhanced Raman spectroscopy of nonresonant molecules *J. Am. Chem. Soc.* **131** 14466–72
[22] Jaworska A, Fornasaro S, Sergo V and Bonifacio A 2016 Potential of surface enhanced Raman spectroscopy (SERS) in therapeutic drug monitoring (TDM). A critical review *Biosensors* **6** 47
[23] Tuma R 2005 Raman spectroscopy of proteins: from peptides to large assemblies *J. Raman Spectrosc.* **36** 307–19
[24] Pyrak E, Krajczewski J, Kowalik A, Kudelski A and Jaworska A 2019 Surface enhanced Raman spectroscopy for DNA biosensors—how far are we? *Molecules* **24** 4423
[25] Tahir M A, Dina N E, Cheng H, Valev V K and Zhang L 2021 Surface-enhanced Raman spectroscopy for bioanalysis and diagnosis *Nanoscale* **13** 11593–634
[26] Wang X, Choi N, Cheng Z, Ko J, Chen L and Choo J 2017 Simultaneous detection of dual nucleic acids using a SERS-based lateral flow assay biosensor *Anal. Chem.* **89** 1163–9
[27] Wall M A, Shaffer T M, Harmsen S, Tschaharganeh D F, Huang C H and Lowe S W *et al* 2017 Chelator-free radiolabeling of SERRS nanoparticles for whole-body PET and intra-operative Raman imaging *Theranostics* **7** 3068
[28] Yang K, Hu Y, Dong N, Zhu G, Zhu T and Jiang N 2017 A novel SERS-based magnetic aptasensor for prostate specific antigen assay with high sensitivity *Biosens. Bioelectron.* **94** 286–91
[29] Raman C V and Krishnan K S 1928 A new type of secondary radiation *Natrue* **121** 501–2
[30] Laing S, Jamieson L E, Faulds K and Graham D 2017 Surface-enhanced Raman spectroscopy for *in vivo* biosensing *Nat. Rev. Chem.* **1** 1–19
[31] Ellis D I and Goodacre R 2006 Metabolic fingerprinting in disease diagnosis: biomedical applications of infrared and Raman spectroscopy *Analyst* **131** 875–85
[32] Zhao X, Li M and Xu Z 2018 Detection of foodborne pathogens by surface enhanced Raman spectroscopy *Front. Microbiol.* **9** 1236
[33] Fleischmann M, Hendra P J and McQuillan A J 1974 Raman spectra of pyridine adsorbed at a silver electrode *Chem. Phys. Lett.* **26** 163–6
[34] Sharma B, Frontiera R R, Henry A I, Ringe E and Van Duyne R P 2012 SERS: materials, applications, and the future *Mater. Today* **15** 16–25
[35] Blanco-Formoso M and Alvarez-Puebla R A 2020 Cancer diagnosis through SERS and other related techniques *Int. J. Mol. Sci.* **21** 2253–72

[36] Dykman L and Khlebtsov N 2012 Gold nanoparticles in biomedical applications: recent advances and perspectives *Chem. Soc. Rev.* **41** 2256–82

[37] Wang P, Lin Z, Su X and Tang Z 2017 Application of Au based nanomaterials in analytical science *Nano Today* **12** 64–97

[38] Verheijen R, Stouten P, Cazemier G and Haasnoot W 1998 Development of a one step strip test for the detection of sulfadimidine residues *Analyst* **123** 2437–41

[39] Liebel M, Pazos-Perez N, Hulst N F and Van Alvarez-Puebla R A 2020 Surface-enhanced Raman scattering holography *Nat. Nanotechnol.* **15** 1005–11

[40] Hong S and Li X 2013 Optimal size of gold nanoparticles for surface-enhanced Raman spectroscopy under different conditions *J. Nanomater.* **2013** 49

[41] Foti A, D'Andrea C, Villari V, Micali N, Donato M G and Fazio B *et al* 2018 Optical aggregation of gold nanoparticles for SERS detection of proteins and toxins in liquid environment: towards ultrasensitive and selective detection *Materials (Basel)* **11** 440–63

[42] Hu X, Zhang Y, Ding T, Liu J and Zhao H 2020 Multifunctional gold nanoparticles: a novel nanomaterial for various medical applications and biological activities *Front. Bioeng. Biotechnol.* **8** 990

[43] Lloyd J A, Liu Y, Ng S H, Thai T, Gómez D E and Widmer-Cooper A *et al* 2019 Self-assembly of spherical and rod-shaped nanoparticles with full positional control *Nanoscale* **11** 22841–8

[44] Chen J, Li Y, Huang K, Wang P, He L and Carter K R *et al* 2015 Nanoimprinted patterned pillar substrates for surface-enhanced Raman scattering applications *ACS Appl. Mater. Interfaces* **7** 22106–13

[45] Polemi A, Wells S M, Lavrik N V, Sepaniak M J and Shuford K L 2010 Local field enhancement of pillar nanosurfaces for SERS *J. Phys. Chem.* C **114** 18096–102

[46] Costa J C S and Corio P 2010 Star-shaped silver nanoparticles as SERS substrates for trace analysis of polycyclic aromatic hydrocarbons *AIP Conf. Proc.* **1267** 940–1

[47] Barveen N R, Wang T J and Chang Y H 2020 Synergistic action of star-shaped Au/Ag nanoparticles decorated on $AgFeO_2$ for ultrasensitive SERS detection of a chemical warfare agent on real samples *Anal. Methods* **12** 1342–52

[48] Lai C H, Wang G A, Ling T K, Wang T J, Chiu P K and Chou Chau Y F *et al* 2017 Near infrared surface-enhanced Raman scattering based on star-shaped gold/silver nanoparticles and hyperbolic metamaterial *Sci. Rep.* **7** 1–8

[49] Hu J, Wang Z and Li J 2007 Gold nanoparticles with special shapes: controlled synthesis, surface-enhanced Raman scattering, and the application in biodetection *Sensors* **7** 3299–311

[50] Yang N, You T, Gao Y, Zhang C and Yin P 2018 Rapid fabrication of flexible and transparent gold nanorods/poly (methyl methacrylate) membrane substrate for SERS nanosensor application *Spectrochim. Acta* A

[51] Rekha C R, Nayar V U and Gopchandran K G 2018 Synthesis of highly stable silver nanorods and their application as SERS substrates *J. Sci. Adv. Mater. Devices* **3** 196–205

[52] Wei C, Li M and Zhao X 2018 Surface-enhanced Raman scattering (SERS) with silver nano substrates synthesized by microwave for rapid detection of foodborne pathogens *Front. Microbiol.* **9** 2857–66

[53] Novikov S M, Popok V N, Evlyukhin A B, Hanif M, Morgen P and Fiutowski J *et al* 2018 Highly stable silver nanoparticles for SERS applications *J. Phys. Conf. Ser.* **1092** 12098

[54] Bartolowits M D, Xin M, Petrov D P, Tague T J and Davisson V J 2019 Multimeric rhodamine dye-induced aggregation of silver nanoparticles for surface-enhanced Raman scattering *ACS Omega* **4** 140–5

[55] Sánchez-Purrà M, Roig-Solvas B, Rodriguez-Quijada C, Leonardo B M and Hamad-Schifferli K 2018 Reporter selection for nanotags in multiplexed surface enhanced Raman spectroscopy assays *ACS Omega* **3** 10733–42
[56] Shkilnyy A, Soucé M, Dubois P, Warmont F, Saboungi M L and Chourpa I 2009 Poly (ethylene glycol)-stabilized silver nanoparticles for bioanalytical applications of SERS spectroscopy *Analyst* **134** 1868–72
[57] Šimáková P, Gautier J, Procházka M, Hervé-Aubert K and Chourpa I 2014 Polyethylene-glycol-stabilized ag nanoparticles for surface-enhanced Raman scattering spectroscopy: Ag surface accessibility studied using metalation of free-base porphyrins *J. Phys. Chem.* C **118** 7690–7
[58] Gushiken N K, Paganoto G T, Temperini M L A, Teixeira F S and Salvadori M C 2020 Substrate for surface-enhanced Raman spectroscopy formed by gold nanoparticles buried in poly(methyl methacrylate) *ACS Omega* **5** 10366–73
[59] Lupa D, Oćwieja M, Piergies N, Baliś A, Paluszkiewicz C and Adamczyk Z 2019 Gold nanoparticles deposited on silica microparticles—electrokinetic characteristics and application in SERS *Colloids Interface Sci. Commun.* **33** 100219
[60] Zhang Y, Li X, Xue B, Kong X, Liu X and Tu L *et al* 2015 A facile and general route to synthesize silica-coated SERS tags with the enhanced signal intensity *Sci. Rep.* **5** 14934
[61] Lee J, Shin S, Kang S, Lee S, Seo J and Lee T 2015 Highly stable surface-enhanced Raman spectroscopy substrates using few-layer graphene on silver nanoparticles *J. Nanomater.* 2015
[62] Jabłońska A, Jaworska A, Kasztelan M, Berbeć S and Pałys B 2018 Graphene and graphene oxide applications for SERS sensing and imaging *Curr. Med. Chem.* **26** 6878–95
[63] Zheng X S, Hu P, Cui Y, Zong C, Feng J M and Wang X *et al* 2014 BSA-coated nanoparticles for improved SERS-based intracellular pH sensing *Anal. Chem.* **86** 12250–7
[64] Salehi M and Hamann-Steinmeier A 2017 Bioconjugation of SERS nanotags and increasing the reproducibility of results *BioNanoMaterials* **18** 20160011
[65] Langer J, de Aberasturi D J, Aizpurua J, Alvarez-Puebla R A, Auguié B and Baumberg J J *et al* 2020 Present and future of surface-enhanced Raman scattering *ACS Nano* **14** 28–117
[66] Mcnay G, Eustace D, Smith W E, Faulds K and Graham D 2011 Surface-enhanced Raman scattering (SERS) and surface-enhanced resonance Raman scattering (SERRS): a review of applications *Appl. Spectrosc.* **65** 825–37
[67] Maiti K K, Dinish U S, Fu C Y, Lee J J, Soh K S and Yun S W *et al* 2010 Development of biocompatible SERS nanotag with increased stability by chemisorption of reporter molecule for *in vivo* cancer detection *Biosens. Bioelectron.* **26** 398–403
[68] Maiti K K, Dinish U S, Samanta A, Vendrell M, Soh K S and Park S J *et al* 2012 Multiplex targeted *in vivo* cancer detection using sensitive near-infrared SERS nanotags *Nano Today* **7** 85–93
[69] Sánchez-Purrà M, Carré-Camps M, De Puig H, Bosch I, Gehrke L and Hamad-Schifferli K 2017 Surface-enhanced Raman spectroscopy-based sandwich immunoassays for multiplexed detection of Zika and Dengue viral biomarkers *ACS Infect. Dis.* **3** 767–76
[70] Fu X, Chu Y, Zhao K, Li J and Deng A 2017 Ultrasensitive detection of the β-adrenergic agonist brombuterol by a SERS-based lateral flow immunochromatographic assay using flower-like gold-silver core–shell nanoparticles *Microchim. Acta* **184** 1711–9
[71] He D, Wu Z, Cui B, Xu E and Jin Z 2019 Establishment of a dual mode immunochromatographic assay for *Campylobacter jejuni* detection *Food Chem.* **289** 708–13
[72] Hwang J, Lee S and Choo J 2016 Application of a SERS-based lateral flow immunoassay strip for the rapid and sensitive detection of staphylococcal enterotoxin B *Nanoscale* **8** 11418–25

[73] Sun J, Zhao Y, Hou Y, Li H, Yang M and Wang Y *et al* 2019 Multiplexed electrochemical and SERS dual-mode detection of stroke biomarkers: rapid screening with high sensitivity *New J. Chem.* **43** 13381–7

[74] Gao X, Zheng P, Kasani S, Wu S, Yang F and Lewis S *et al* 2017 Paper-based surface-enhanced Raman scattering lateral flow strip for detection of neuron-specific enolase in blood plasma *Anal. Chem.* **89** 10104–10

[75] Choi S, Hwang J, Lee S, Lim D W, Joo H and Choo J 2017 Quantitative analysis of thyroid-stimulating hormone (TSH) using SERS-based lateral flow immunoassay *Sensors Actuators* B **240** 358–64

[76] Maneeprakorn W, Bamrungsap S, Apiwat C and Wiriyachaiporn N 2016 Surface-enhanced Raman scattering based lateral flow immunochromatographic assay for sensitive influenza detection *RSC Adv.* **6** 112079–85

[77] Bin L H, Du X J, Zang Y X, Li P and Wang S 2017 SERS-based lateral flow strip biosensor for simultaneous detection of *Listeria monocytogenes* and *Salmonella enterica* serotype enteritidis *J. Agric. Food Chem.* **65** 10290–9

[78] Yoo S M and Lee S Y 2016 Optical biosensors for the detection of pathogenic micro-organisms *Trends Biotechnol.* **34** 7–25

[79] Kim K, Kashefi-Kheyrabadi L, Joung Y, Kim K, Dang H and Chavan S G *et al* 2021 Recent advances in sensitive surface-enhanced Raman scattering-based lateral flow assay platforms for point-of-care diagnostics of infectious diseases *Sensors. Actuators* B **329** 129214

[80] Kim J, Park S, Lee J E, Jin S M, Lee J H and Lee I S *et al* 2006 Designed fabrication of multifunctional magnetic gold nanoshells and their application to magnetic resonance imaging and photothermal therapy *Angew. Chem.* **118** 7918–22

[81] Maiti K K, Samanta A, Vendrell M, Soh K S, Olivo M and Chang Y T 2011 Multiplex cancer cell detection by SERS nanotags with cyanine and triphenylmethine Raman reporters *Chem. Commun.* **47** 3514–6

[82] Kim J, Piao Y and Hyeon T 2009 Multifunctional nanostructured materials for multimodal imaging, and simultaneous imaging and therapy *Chem. Soc. Rev.* **38** 372–90

[83] Von Maltzahn G, Centrone A, Park J H, Ramanathan R, Sailor M J and Alan Hatton T *et al* 2009 SERS-coded gold nanorods as a multifunctional platform for densely multiplexed near-infrared imaging and photothermal heating *Adv. Mater.* **21** 3175–80

[84] Neerincx A H, Vijverberg S J H, Bos L D J, Brinkman P, van der Schee M P and de Vries R *et al* 2017 Breathomics from exhaled volatile organic compounds in pediatric asthma *Pediatr. Pulmonol.* **52** 1616–27

[85] Aizpurua J, Arnolds H, Baumberg J, Bruzas I, Chikkaraddy R and Chisanga M *et al* 2017 Ultrasensitive and towards single molecule SERS: general discussion *Faraday Discuss.* **205** 291–330

[86] Qiao X, Su B, Liu C, Song Q, Luo D and Mo G *et al* 2018 Selective surface enhanced Raman scattering for quantitative detection of lung cancer biomarkers in superparticle@MOF structure *Adv. Mater.* **30** 1702275

[87] Park H J, Cho S, Kim M and Jung Y S 2020 Carboxylic acid-functionalized, graphitic layer-coated three-dimensional sers substrate for label-free analysis of Alzheimer's disease biomarkers *Nano Lett.* **20** 2576–84

Chapter 5

Design and fabrication of tag/probe-based and label-free paper-based devices

Nidhi Puranik and Shiv Kumar Yadav

Paper-based devices are useful because they are an inexpensive technology which is easy to manufacture and portable for diagnosis of disorders. Testing can be undertaken where resources are limited, for example in developing countries and non-favourable conditions/environments where there is a lack of trained staff and facilities do not have full equipment. Their use varies from medical diagnosis to detection of environmental pollutants, agricultural analysis from pesticides to crop quality, and also in sensing of cell cultures and various others. Distinct physical and chemical properties are needed for biosensors and the other properties of paper are also being explored depending upon the target use. The wide use of label-free devices was facilitated up to a maximum extent due to the use of biological and chemical receptors for direct detection of samples and their moleculare analysis without using any specific enzymes and fluorescent labels. There are distinct papers used for the preparation of paper-based devices such as sensors depending upon the type of fabrication and application of the sensor. Some examples are bioactive paper, Whatman brand chromatography paper, Whatman filter paper No. 4, nitrocellulose membranes, glossy paper, etc. The paper-based devices are easy for diagnosis of disorders; these are equipment free, simple to operate, sensitive, user-friendly, affordable, and suitable for robust assays from care point, so can be categorized as lifesavers under limited resources and conditions and WHO also assured paper-based devices, ideal for the rapid test.

5.1 Introduction

Paper-based devices are commonly used for the detection of biomarkers, and toxins, monitoring of food quality and safety, checking the environmental factor, sun exposure, and also for detecting the pathogens like bacteria and fungi [1]. Papers are flexible, environment-friendly, porous, and are utilized for the fabrication of inexpensive devices and biosensors for fast detection of analytes. Paper-based devices have numerous

doi:10.1088/978-0-7503-5820-0ch5 © IOP Publishing Ltd 2023

advantages and are simple to fabricate in less expenditure with excellent action for detection of disorders, monitoring of food quality and safety, environment factor check, sun exposure, and also for detecting the pathogens like bacteria and fungi [2, 3].

Paper-based devices are useful because are inexpensive technology with easy to manufacture and portable for diagnosis of disorders, tests, where there is a limitation of resources like in developing countries and non-favourable conditions/environments where there is a lack of trained staff and facilities of full equipment [4, 5]. Overall from all published research it can be said that paper-based approaches like sensors, devices, and microfluidics all are capable of providing the best approach to diagnosis [6].

There are various types of detection methods for such devices like the electrochemical method that uses biological/chemical incident to an electronic signal, electro-chemiluminescence, optical, immunoassay, colorimetric, fluorescence methods. Paper-based sensors give the assured criteria and fulfil requirements and also have various advantages related to surface volume ratio, bio-compatibility, costing (low), light (weight), flexibility, biodegradability, and porosity [7]. These are developed by delimiting the lipophobic zones of cellulose substrate along with lipophilic reagents. These designs perform easy detection and their fabrication and patterning can be done with the help of methods such as wax printing, screen printing, inkjet printing, photolithography, etc to obtain high resolution [8–11].

The paper biosensors are simply made by the use of patterning on lipophilic and phobic papers and are useful in biological testing, for example, blood, urine, saliva, sweat, and tears and can also be used for environmental reagent testing of heavy metal ions and hydrogen sulfide gas that consist of the analyte of interest. The simple procedure used is to apply the sample to the device and wick to find the zone with the help of capillary action without using an external pump [12]. The detection of analyte from sample uses the mechanism of facilitating chemical reaction that enhances a change in colour, their electrochemical property, and light emission/absorption. Among all methods, the colorimetric procedure is used widely for such detection, due to the simple evaluation of results by the colour produced, formed from ligand–analyte binding like in antibody–antigen that is a quantified method and low in cost [13]. Benefits and limitations of paper-based detection system are given in table 5.1.

Paper-based devices have vast applications and are a suitable approach for all laboratories either fully equipped or with limited resources. Their use varies from medical diagnosis to detection of environmental pollutants, agricultural analysis from pesticides to crop quality, and also in sensing of cell cultures and various others. The recent research also shows that paper-based sensors are capable of detecting analytes if present in low concentration and are low cost and portable also easy to maintain and use. Paper is natural and is biodegradable, compatible, disposable, chemically and biologically inert so is found to be suitable and important for reagent immobilization [16].

5.2 Paper types

Paper has recently been widely used in the preparation for microfluidic uses and is an attractive and promising substitute not only because of its ubiquity and lower cost

Table 5.1. Important benefits and limitation of including paper [10, 14, 15].

Benefits	Limitation
• Great surface-to-volume ratio • Adsorption characteristics • Have capillary activity • Compatibility with various biological samples • Compatible with various chemical changes and addition of different molecules • Direct sterilization possible • Easy disposal through incineration • Store and transportation is easy • Lightweight and accessible globally • Low cost	• Related to sensitivity • Accuracy measures • Multiple analytes at the same time • Shows disadvantages related with cost • Delicate equipment • Unstable on heating sometimes • Low resolution in some procedures

Table 5.2. Types of paper used in biosensor and their applications [18–20].

Type of paper	Application	References
Bioactive paper	Biosensors, immobilization of biomolecules	[21]
Whatman brand chromatography paper	Higher wicking ability, uniform thickness	[22]
Whatman filter paper No. 4	Have some extra qualities including having greater adsorption power and strong holding of reagents	[23]
Nitrocellulose membranes	Covalent immobilization of biomolecules, high protein binding	[24]
Glossy paper	Used for detection of ethanol	[25]
Conventional printing paper	High flexibility and foldability	[26]

but also because of its numerous properties like flexibility, light weight, minimal thickness, and other mechanical functions. For its development, the general method used is the preparation of a dilute aqueous suspension of cellulose fibres. Paper is drained via a sieve, pressed and dried, providing a sheet formed by a network of randomly interwoven fibre [17]. There are distinct papers used for the preparation of paper-based devices like sensors depending upon the type of fabrication and application of the sensor. Some examples are given in table 5.2.

The paper-based analytical device brings a new platform and technology into the field of analysis and has a vast range of applications that give low cost, easy fabrication, and operations, and is also simple to use. The widely used paper is Whatman brand chromatography paper and this has superior wicking capability [26]. This specific type of paper has a moderate type of retention and flow rate that is due to the thickness and pore size of the paper, i.e., around 180 and 11 μm respectively. Other paper types like Whatman filter paper No. 4 are used because of their bigger pore size, approximately 20–25 μm, and have a higher retention rate [24]. Recently filter paper has been used as a paper-based sensor, also manufactured using Whatman filter paper. These technologies are widely used for uniformity of thickness and wicking characteristics and also having superior adsorption and retention of reagents compared to the same type of papers [27]. The nature and characteristics of the paper is given in table 5.3, and the historical aspect of paper-based devices is mentioned in table 5.4.

Distinct physical and chemical properties needed for biosensors and the other properties of paper are also being explored depending upon the target use.

Table 5.3. Nature and characteristics of paper and their impact in preparation.

Properties of paper	Advantages	Application/use	References
Mechanical	Flexibility, high specific stiffness, lightness	Used for preparation of 3D structure, that will not tear on bending	[28]
	Thickness	Important for device preparation (should be in 10/100 μm)	[29]
	Soft texture	Helps in maintaining direct contact with the solid objects and collection of traces of analytes by swabbing	[30]
Fibrous and porous	Absorbency	Increases storage and delivery of a specific volume of reagents inside the paper matrix Enriches the sample through numerous addition/desiccating steps	[31]
	Air permeability	Free diffusion of gas in complete material that removes problems mostly associated with microfluidic system like air bubbles.	[32]
	Network structure	Helps the filtration of samples that are contaminated with solids and also separation of analytes by means of chromatography	[33]
	High surface-to-volume ratio	Increase the number of enzyme molecules or colorimetric probes that can be immobilized	[34]
	Capillary action	Increase the number of enzyme molecules or colorimetric probes that can be immobilized	[35]
Natural source	Compatible with biological samples	Enhance thermal stability of immobilized molecules, including enzymes and gold nanoparticles	[36]
	Easy to sterilize	Decrease the problem of contamination with biological material	[37]
	Chemically and biologically inert	Thermal stability of immobilized molecules	[38]
	Disposability and biodegradability	Recyclable, fast degradation by microorganisms, and easy to disposed of by incineration	[39]

Table 5.4. Historical aspect of paper-based devices/sensors.

Year	Application	References
79–79	Process for determining the quality of Tyrian purple dye using a method similar to papyrus chromatography and a papyrus-associated ferrous sulphate spot test	[65]
Early 1800s	Testing of acid by litmus paper test	[66, 67]
19th century	Developing the dry chemistry test papers and dipsticks	[66]
1906	Chromatography-related spot test for bilirubin from urine	[68]
1937	Spot test with defined walls made by paraffin embossing	[69]
1950	Electrophoresis on paper become a breakthrough in the separation of proteins	[70]
1952	Martin and Synge get the Nobel Prize in chemistry for the invention of paper chromatography	[71]
1957	The first use of reported earlier urine glucose test strips with blood samples	[73]
2007	A scientific journal publishing multichannel system with photoresist walls by Whitesides' group	[48]

5.2.1 Nitrocellulose membrane

The nitrocellulose membrane is being used because of the chemical functional group that is capable of covalent immobilization of biomolecules. Nitrocellulose allows for the charge to charge interactions, Vander Waals interaction along with the protein-related substrate, and weak hydrogen bonds. Resulting from the paper-based devices with high protein binding capabilities widely used for ELISA and assay associated with gold nanoparticles [40]. These types of membrane are also used as they prevent diffusion and leaching of samples via a membrane that allows a higher degree of retention and then a longer reaction time within the sensor. These types of membrane are smoother and have pore size uniformity (0.45 μm). Such membranes can be customized through the wax printing method of fabrication that is followed by heating. The penetration of wax into nitrocellulose membranes is slow compared to filter paper.

5.2.2 Bioactive paper

The other type of paper used is bioactive paper for the preparation of paper-based sensors, where the modification of the matrix is done with biomolecules, if no modification is made then it is only used for adsorption of cationic molecules on their wet surface. On the other hand, proteins are adsorbed on cellulose, but the rate and extent of this method is not as effective as other hydrophilic surfaces, so cellulose fibres are modified in such a way that they can absorb biomolecules, which is achieved by activating paper surfaces with aldehyde and amide, and then covalently conjugating biomolecules [41–43]. Piezoelectric inkjet printing of enzymes within biocompatible sol–gel silica layers is the approach utilized to create bioactive paper-based devices. When making paper-based devices, cellulose filter paper is used. Biomolecules can be immobilized by graft copolymerization of glycidyl methacrylate, which is employed in dot ELISA and gold nanoparticle assays.

5.2.3 Glossy paper

Another form of paper used to make paper-based sensors is glossy paper, which is made up of cellulose fibres and inorganic fillers that are mixed and blended into the paper matrix. Arena *et al* in their study use glossy paper for developing a flexible device for sensing used in the detection of ethanol. This particular paper is widely used for preparing numerous sensing devices due to its properties of easily accepting surface alteration. There are distinct types of papers used for developing paper-based sensors like convectional printing paper also being used. The paper is used for wearable devices that are meant to fold and be flexible. Carbon black modified electrodes are printed on paper towels as well. Due to their excellent features such as low cost and high porosity, this is also employed as a wicking layer for filter paper-based biosensor devices, making them appropriate for measurement of a wide range of analytes [44–46].

5.3 Tags based paper devices

This type of device is used widely in the food industry, security, and environmental monitoring applications. The method gains attention because of its properties such as being non-invasive, oblivious to water which is omnipresent in the biological samples and having investigational conformational changes that provide vibrational information on the targeted analytes [22].

5.4 Non-labels/non-tag-based paper devices

The employment of biological and chemical receptors for direct detection of samples and their molecular analysis without the use of specialized enzymes or fluorescent labels aided the widespread usage of label-free devices to the greatest extent possible. These devices only require single-element recognition, simplifying pattern analysis and reducing analysis time and reagent costs. This type also offers real-time quantification products for biomolecular reactions, enabling for continuous data recording and kinetic monitoring of parameters in the ligand–receptor interaction remodelling procedure. The detection of target analytes in their natural form without tagging or chemical modification, allowing them to be used for further analysis, is one of the major advantages of this type of technology. The benefits of such devices are simplifying pattern of analysis, reduction in analysis time by the rapid response time which lowers the analysis cost, lowers the organic solvent consumption cost, detection of smaller molecules, and detection of targeted analytes in natural form and also does not require a qualified medical person. The general classification of paper-based devices based on strategies for detection purpose is shown in figure 5.1.

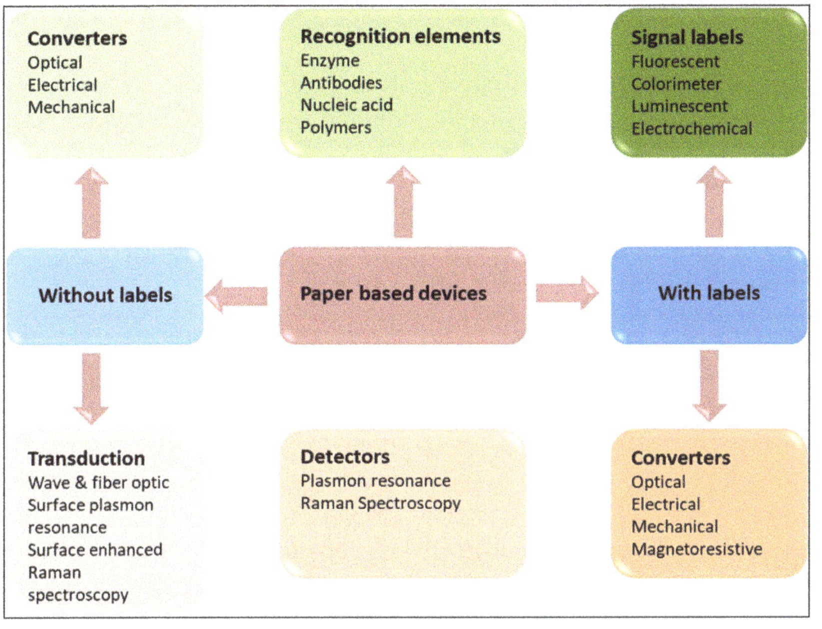

Figure 5.1. Classification of paper-based devices based on strategies for detection purpose.

5.5 Fabrication and patterning

In 1949, Muller and Clegg invented a paraffin-based paper, which was the first time a fluidic channel was created on paper, as well as the first paper-related assay. Whitesides Group at Harvard University was the first to introduce paper-related microfluidics, which is a protein glucose test created by the lithography technique in paper. Following that, a variety of fabrication techniques were developed. Paper-based microfluidic device fabrication can be split into two kinds [47–49]:

- two-dimensional shaping/cutting of paper and
- patterning hydrophilic/hydrophobic contrasts on paper.

5.5.1 Two-dimensional shaping/cutting of paper

Paper channels are often obtained in this class by cutting paper with a cutter plotter capable of regulating the X–Y-axis with CO_2 laser cutting equipment. The next step is to apply adhesive tape as a backing to the cut channels, which will provide specific microfluidics such as structure and strength to the entire device. The disadvantage of this technology is that it cannot be used for mass production since it requires a unique instrument that is not economically possible, as well as energy power constraints in fixed resource locations or fields [50].

5.5.2 Patterning hydrophilic/hydrophobic contrasts on paper

To receive a lipophilic/lipophobic combination on paper numerous patterning methods are categorized into three sub-categories, depending upon the binding form of lipophilic agents to paper:

- physical blocking of the pores: using agents like photoresist and polydimethylsiloxane (PDMS)
- physical deposition of a hydro-phobising agent on the paper fibre surfaces: polystyrene, wax or commercial ink, any chemical reaction between the agents and the paper fibres
- chemical modification of the paper fibre surface.

These types of lipophilic agents change the wetting characteristics of paper by filling the paper pores or adsorbing on the fibre surface [5].

5.5.1.1 Wax printing

This type of fabrication method is used widely because of its simple fabrication method and low cost. The process is performed for the development of paper-associated microfluidics devices because of the low cost of wax printers. The wax patterns are directly printed on the paper in this approach, which is then utilized to control the flow of fluid, which includes samples and reagents. Lu *et al* introduced the processes of wax printing in 2009 [51] as shown in figure 5.2:

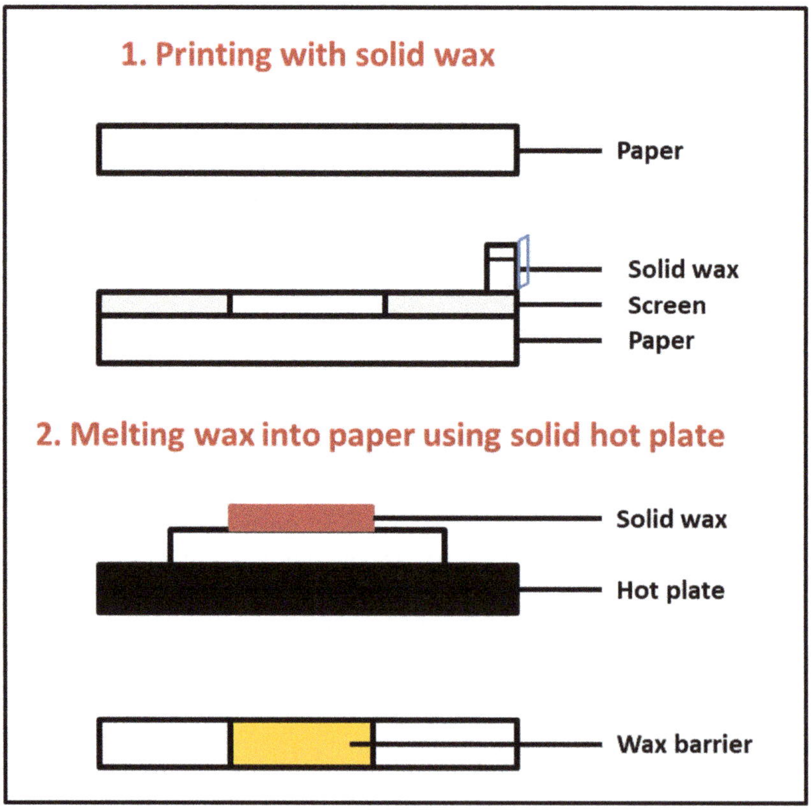

Figure 5.2. Wax printing fabrication (cross sectional) step wise.

Step I—Printing
Step II—Heating

This method is also suitable for mass production due to the availability of wax commercially and is also cheap and easy to operate [51, 52].

5.5.1.2 Ink stamping method

Curto *et al* explained this method, and details about the double-side stamping procedure developed by Akyazi *et al* became alternatives to traditional wax printing because they are a quick and inexpensive prototyping method associated with forming lipophilic ink channels on paper using a PDMS stamp and indelible inks [53, 54].

5.5.1.3 Origami and kirigami

Using origami principles, a unique device was created in this approach, which consists of two zones divided by a crease. The detector zone is the I zone, while the enzymatic immobilization zone is the II zone. The reported design by researchers using this method is the preparation of an analytical device for detecting glucose. The method is widely used and favourable due to its simplicity, affordability, reliable characteristics. This method was also favourable for the development of 2D and 3D vertical flow paper-based devices [55, 56].

5.5.1.4 Photolithography

This method is used for the fabrication of paper-associated sensors that have high resolution and are good for large-scale production as well. Paper-related microfluidic devices that can detect multiple biomarkers were generated using this method [57].

5.5.1.5 Hot embossing

The roll-to-roll technique of hot embossing allows for great throughput due to short cycle periods, making this technology efficient. The laminated paper was made by pressing it at 450 °C for 3 min, while the infused paper was pressed at a higher temperature for longer [15, 58, 59].

5.5.1.6 PDMS

This method is widely used due to its low cost of fabrication and is used for developing flexible sensor-based devices through PDMS patterns on paper. These methods allow the sensor-based devices to bend/fold and are flexible without harming the microfluidics channels, PDMS along with hexanes was used in ratio 3:1 and loaded in the plotter and then finally printed on paper [60].

Fabrication of paper-based biosensors and advantages and disadvantages of various paper-based biosensors [61, 62] are shown in figures 5.3 and 5.4, respectively.

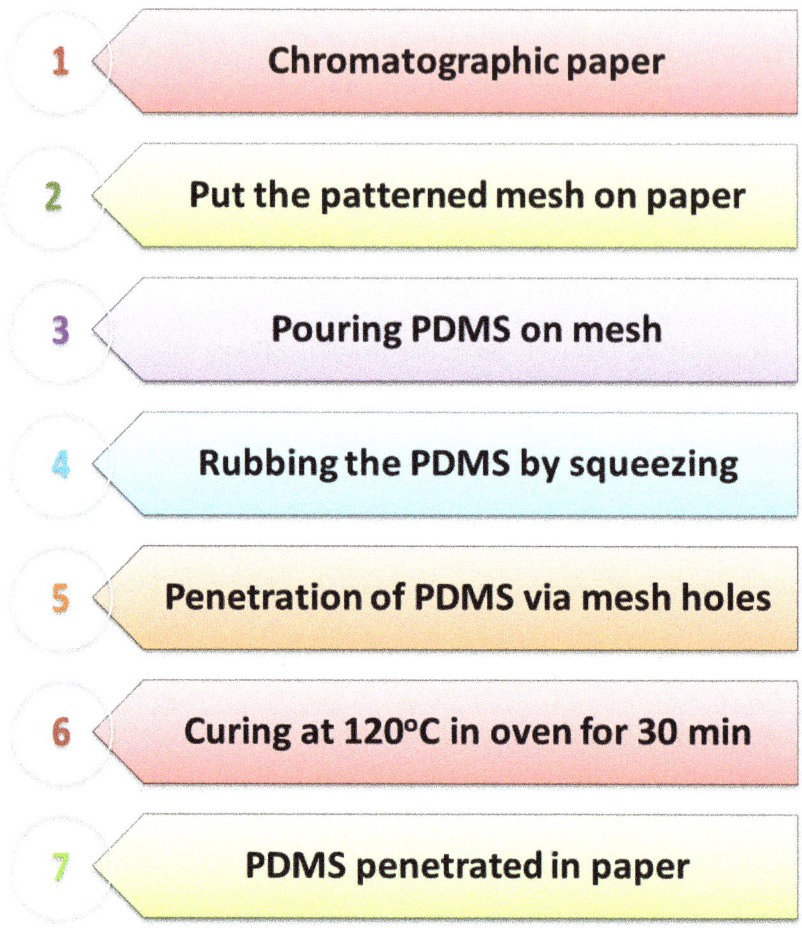

Figure 5.3. Fabrication methods for paper-based sensors.

5.6 Applications of paper-based devices

Paper-based devices are easy to use for the diagnosis of disorders; these are equipment free, simple to operate, sensitive, user-friendly, affordable, and suitable for robust assays from care point, so can be categorized as lifesavers under limited resources and conditions and WHO also assured paper-based devices, ideal for the rapid test. The uses of such devices are very wide from health diagnostic fields to environment and food beverages industries as well. Used for the detection of cancer and biomolecules for liver function like glucose uric acid etc. Able to detect water quality with limited resources and in all conditions seems to be one of the beneficial points of such devices. Checking the quality of food and beverages will help farmers at a minimal cost [4, 63, 64]. Various applications of paper-based biosensors reported in research papers [7, 62] are summarized in figure 5.5.

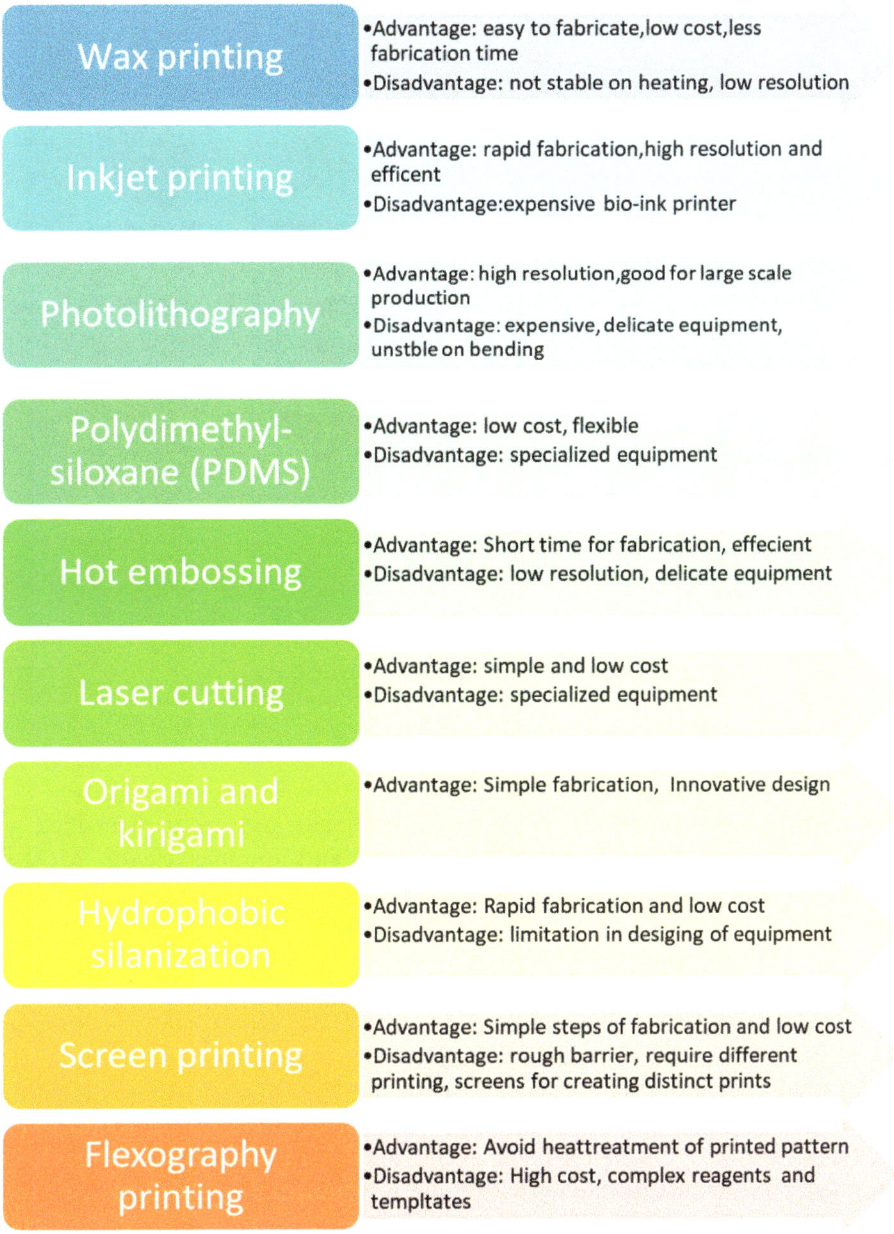

Figure 5.4. Advantages and disadvantages of various paper-based sensors.

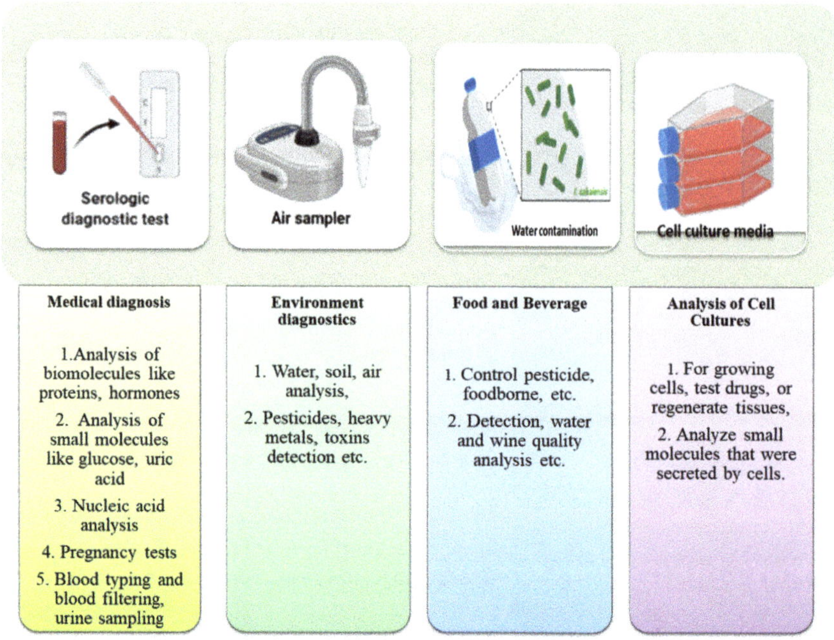

Figure 5.5. Application of paper-based devices.

5.7 Conclusions

Paper-based devices like sensors have vast advantages and are a diversified group consisting of optical, electrochemical, piezoelectric, and immune sensors. Most often these devices help in cost reduction and provide unique applications that are not possible to obtain in other ways. The great benefits of paper-based devices are in the field of rapid testing, still, there are some parameters that need further studies and improvements in analytical performance in the field of detection to improve specificity. These have various advantages such as, they are inexpensive, user-friendly, quick detection, simple to use, portable device and because of these benefits, they are not only useful in fully equipped industries but also in the field where there is a limitation of resources. In numerous disorders they used for easy diagnosis of biomarkers, e.g., diabetes, liver and kidney function as well. These are also useful in the field of food and beverages to check and monitor food quality and in agricultural, environmental applications.

References

[1] Nie J, Zhang Y, Lin L, Zhou C, Li S and Zhang L *et al* 2012 Low-cost fabrication of paper-based microfluidic devices by one-step plotting *Anal. Chem.* **84** 6331–5

[2] Gong M M and Sinton D 2017 Turning the page: advancing paper-based microfluidics for broad diagnostic application *Chem. Rev.* **117** 8447–80

[3] Katis L, He P, Eason R and Sones C 2017 *Bacterial Pathogen Detection Using Laser-Structured Paper-Based Diagnostic Sensors* (Southampton: ePrints Soton)

[4] Hu J, Wang S Q, Wang L, Li F, Pingguan-Murphy B and Lu T J *et al* 2014 Advances in paper-based point-of-care diagnostics *Biosens. Bioelectron.* **54** 585–97
[5] Li X, Ballerini D R and Shen W 2012 A perspective on paper-based microfluidics: current status and future trends *Biomicrofluidics* **6** 011301
[6] Nilghaz A, Guan L, Tan W and Shen W 2016 Advances of paper-based microfluidics for diagnostics—the original motivation and current status *ACS Sens.* **1** 1382–93
[7] Akyazi T, Basabe-Desmonts L and Benito-Lopez F 2018 Review on microfluidic paper-based analytical devices towards commercialisation *Anal. Chim. Acta* **1001** 1–17
[8] Zhang Y, Zhou C, Nie J, Le S, Qin Q and Liu F *et al* 2014 Equipment-free quantitative measurement for microfluidic paper-based analytical devices fabricated using the principles of movable-type printing *Anal. Chem.* **86** 2005–12
[9] Ahmed S, Bui M P N and Abbas A 2016 Paper-based chemical and biological sensors: Engineering aspects *Biosens. Bioelectron.* **77** 249–63
[10] Nery E W and Kubota L T 2013 Sensing approaches on paper-based devices: a review *Anal. Bioanal. Chem.* **405** 7573–95
[11] He Y, Wu Y, Fu J Z and Bin W W 2015 Fabrication of paper-based microfluidic analysis devices: a review *RSC Adv.* **5** 78109–27
[12] Costa M N, Veigas B, Jacob J M, Santos D S, Gomes J and Baptista P V *et al* 2014 A low cost, safe, disposable, rapid and self-sustainable paper-based platform for diagnostic testing: lab-on-paper *Nanotechnology* **25** 094006
[13] Park T S, Li W, McCracken K E and Yoon J Y 2013 Smartphone quantifies *Salmonella* from paper microfluidics *Lab Chip* **13** 4832–40
[14] Pelton R 2009 Bioactive paper provides a low-cost platform for diagnostics *TrAC Trends Anal. Chem.* **28** 925–42
[15] Liana D D, Raguse B, Justin Gooding J and Chow E 2012 Recent advances in paper-based sensors *Sensors* **12** 11505–26
[16] Cate D M, Adkins J A, Mettakoonpitak J and Henry C S 2015 Recent developments in paper-based microfluidic devices *Anal. Chem.* **87** 19–41
[17] Credou J and Berthelot T 2014 Cellulose: from biocompatible to bioactive material *J. Mater. Chem.* B **2** 4767–88
[18] Martinez A W, Phillips S T, Whitesides G M and Carrilho E 2010 Diagnostics for the developing world: microfluidic paper-based analytical devices *Anal. Chem.* **82** 3–10
[19] Cretich M, Sedini V, Damin F, Pelliccia M, Sola L and Chiari M 2010 Coating of nitrocellulose for colorimetric DNA microarrays *Anal. Biochem.* **397** 84–8
[20] Gao B, Chi J, Liu H and Gu Z 2017 Vertical paper analytical devices fabricated using the principles of quilling and kirigami *Sci. Rep.* **7** 1–8
[21] Tyagi C, Tomar L K and Singh H 2009 Surface modification of cellulose filter paper by glycidyl methacrylate grafting for biomolecule immobilization: influence of grafting parameters and urease immobilization *J. Appl. Polym. Sci.* **111** 1381–90
[22] Ellerbee A K, Phillips S T, Siegel A C, Mirica K A, Martinez A W and Striehl P *et al* 2009 Quantifying colorimetric assays in paper-based microfluidic devices by measuring the transmission of light through paper *Anal. Chem.* **81** 8447–52
[23] Ali M M, Brown C L, Jahanshahi-Anbuhi S, Kannan B, Li Y and Filipe C D M *et al* 2017 A Printed multicomponent paper sensor for bacterial detection *Sci. Rep.* **7** 1–10
[24] Lu Y, Shi W, Qin J and Lin B 2010 Fabrication and characterization of paper-based microfluidics prepared in nitrocellulose membrane by wax printing *Anal. Chem.* **82** 329–35

[25] Arena A, Donato N, Saitta G, Bonavita A, Rizzo G and Neri G 2010 Flexible ethanol sensors on glossy paper substrates operating at room temperature *Sensors Actuators* B **145** 488–94

[26] Santhiago M, Corrêa C C, Bernardes J S, Pereira M P, Oliveira L J M and Strauss M *et al* 2017 Flexible and foldable fully-printed carbon black conductive nanostructures on paper for high-performance electronic, electrochemical, and wearable devices *ACS Appl. Mater. Interfaces* **9** 24365–72

[27] Cassano C L and Fan Z H 2013 Laminated paper-based analytical devices (LPAD): fabrication, characterization, and assays *Microfluid. Nanofluidics* **15** 173–81

[28] Werner O, Quan C, Turner C, Pettersson B and Wågberg L 2009 Properties of superhydrophobic paper treated with rapid expansion of supercritical CO_2 containing a crystallizing wax *Cellulose* **17** 187–98

[29] Tseng S C, Yu C C, Wan D, Chen H L, Wang L A and Wu M C *et al* 2012 Eco-friendly plasmonic sensors: using the photothermal effect to prepare metal nanoparticle-containing test papers for highly sensitive colorimetric detection *Anal. Chem.* **84** 5140–5

[30] Prikhozhdenko E S, Bratashov D N, Gorin D A and Yashchenok A M 2018 Flexible surface-enhanced Raman scattering-active substrates based on nanofibrous membranes *Nano Res.* **11** 4468–88

[31] Gu Z, Zhao M, Sheng Y, Bentolila L A and Tang Y 2011 Detection of mercury ion by infrared fluorescent protein and its hydrogel-based paper assay *Anal. Chem.* **83** 2324–9

[32] Xu M, Bunes B R and Zang L 2011 Paper-based vapor detection of hydrogen peroxide: Colorimetric sensing with tunable interface *ACS Appl. Mater. Interfaces* **3** 642–7

[33] Martinez A W, Phillips S T, Carrilho E, Thomas S W, Sindi H and Whitesides G M 2008 Simple telemedicine for developing regions: camera phones and paper-based microfluidic devices for real-time, off-site diagnosis *Anal. Chem.* **80** 3699–707

[34] Osborn J L, Lutz B, Fu E, Kauffman P, Stevens D Y and Yager P 2010 Microfluidics without pumps: reinventing the T-sensor and H-filter in paper networks *Lab Chip* **10** 2659–65

[35] Hossain S M Z, Luckham R E, McFadden M J and Brennan J D 2009 Reagentless bidirectional lateral flow bioactive paper sensors for detection of pesticides in beverage and food samples *Anal. Chem.* **81** 9055–64

[36] Zhang Y and Rochefort D 2011 Activity, conformation and thermal stability of laccase and glucose oxidase in poly(ethyleneimine) microcapsules for immobilization in paper *Process Biochem.* **46** 993–1000

[37] Martinez A W 2011 Microfluidic paper-based analytical devices: from POCKET to paper-based ELISA *Bioanalysis* **3** 2589–92

[38] Zhao W, Ali M M, Aguirre S D, Brook M A and Li Y 2008 Paper-based bioassays using gold nanoparticle colorimetric probes *Anal. Chem.* **80** 8431–7

[39] Noh H and Phillips S T 2010 Fluidic timers for time-dependent, point-of-care assays on paper *Anal. Chem.* **82** 8071–8

[40] Barr M C, Rowehl J A, Lunt R R, Xu J, Wang A, Boyce C M, Im S G, Bulović V and Gleason K K 2011 Paper Electronics: Direct Monolithic Integration of Organic Photovoltaic Circuits on Unmodified Paper *Adv. Mater.* **31** 3499

[41] Li L, Xiang H, Zhou X, Li M and Wu D 2012 Detection of Fe^{3+} and Al^{3+} by test paper *J. Chem. Educ.* **89** 559–60

[42] Zhao W and Van Den Berg A 2008 Lab on paper *Lab Chip* **8** 1988–91

[43] Luckham R E and Brennan J D 2010 Bioactive paper dipstick sensors for acetylcholinesterase inhibitors based on sol–gel/enzyme/gold nanoparticle composites *Analyst* **135** 2028–35
[44] Apilux A, Siangproh W, Praphairaksit N and Chailapakul O 2012 Simple and rapid colorimetric detection of Hg(II) by a paper-based device using silver nanoplates *Talanta* **97** 388–94
[45] Songjaroen T, Dungchai W, Chailapakul O, Henry C S and Laiwattanapaisal W 2012 Blood separation on microfluidic paper-based analytical devices *Lab Chip* **12** 3392–8
[46] Tao H, Chieffo L R, Brenckle M A, Siebert S M, Liu M and Strikwerda A C *et al* 2011 Metamaterials on paper as a sensing platform *Adv. Mater.* **23** 3197–201
[47] Müller R H and Clegg D L 1949 Automatic paper chromatography *Anal. Chem.* **21** 1123–5
[48] Martinez A W, Phillips S T, Butte M J and Whitesides G M 2007 Patterned paper as a platform for inexpensive, low-volume, portable bioassays *Angew. Chem.* **119** 1340–2
[49] Cheng C-M, Martinez A W, Gong J, Mace C R, Phillips S T and Carrilho E *et al* 2010 Paper-based ELISA *Angew Chem.* **122** 4881–4
[50] Yetisen A K, Akram M S and Lowe C R 2013 Paper-based microfluidic point-of-care diagnostic devices *Lab Chip* **13** 2210–51
[51] Lu R, Shi W, Jiang L, Qin J and Lin B 2009 Rapid prototyping of paper-based microfluidics with wax for low-cost, portable bioassay *Electrophoresis* **30** 1497–500
[52] Dungchai W, Chailapakul O and Henry C S 2010 A low-cost, simple, and rapid fabrication method for paper-based microfluidics using wax screen-printing *Analyst* **136** 77–82
[53] Curto V F, Lopez-Ruiz N, Capitan-Vallvey L F, Palma A J, Benito-Lopez F and Diamond D 2013 Fast prototyping of paper-based microfluidic devices by contact stamping using indelible ink *RSC Adv.* **3** 18811–6
[54] Akyazi T, Saez J, Elizalde J and Benito-Lopez F 2016 Fluidic flow delay by ionogel passive pumps in microfluidic paper-based analytical devices *Sensors Actuators* B **233** 402–8
[55] Mohammadifar M, Zhang J, Yazgan I, Sadik O and Choi S 2018 Power-on-paper: origami-inspired fabrication of 3-D microbial fuel cells *Renew. Energy* **118** 695–700
[56] Li W, Qian D, Wang Q, Li Y, Bao N and Gu H *et al* 2016 Fully-drawn origami paper analytical device for electrochemical detection of glucose *Sensors Actuators* B **231** 230–8
[57] Dungchai W, Chailapakul O and Henry C S 2010 Use of multiple colorimetric indicators for paper-based microfluidic devices *Anal. Chim. Acta* **674** 227–33
[58] Gosselin D, Belgacem M N, Joyard-Pitiot B, Baumlin J M, Navarro F and Chaussy D *et al* 2017 Low-cost embossed-paper micro-channels for spontaneous capillary flow *Sensors Actuators* B **248** 395–401
[59] Ng S H, Wang Z F, Tjeung R T and De Rooij N F 2007 Development of a multi-layer microelectrofluidic platform *Microsyst. Technol.* **13** 1509–15
[60] Bruzewicz D A, Reches M and Whitesides G M 2008 Low-cost printing of poly(dimethylsiloxane) barriers to define microchannels in paper *Anal. Chem.* **80** 3387–92
[61] Mohammadi S, Maeki M, Mohamadi R M, Ishida A, Tani H and Tokeshi M 2015 An instrument-free, screen-printed paper microfluidic device that enables bio and chemical sensing *Analyst* **140** 6493–9
[62] Singh A T, Lantigua D, Meka A, Taing S, Pandher M and Camci-Unal G 2018 Paper-based sensors: emerging themes and applications *Sensors* **18** 2838
[63] Yager P, Edwards T, Fu E, Helton K, Nelson K and Tam M R *et al* 2006 Microfluidic diagnostic technologies for global public health *Nature* **442** 412–8

[64] Rozand C 2013 Paper-based analytical devices for point-of-care infectious disease testing *Eur. J. Clin. Microbiol. Infect. Dis.* **33** 147–56

[65] Gudger E W n.d. *Pliny's Historia Naturalis* 3

[66] Rocco R M 2006 *Landmark Papers in Clinical Chemistry* 504

[67] Crosland M 2004 *Gay–Lussac: Scientist and Bourgeois* (Google Books)

[68] Morgan E D and Wilson I D 2004 An early description of paper chromatography? *Chromatography* **60** 135–6

[69] Yagoda H 1937 Applications of confined spot tests in analytical chemistry: preliminary paper *Ind. Eng. Chem.—Anal. Ed.* **9** 79–82

[70] Kunkel H G and Tiselius A 1951 Electrophoresis of proteins on filter paper *J. Gen. Physiol.* **35** 89–118

[71] Ettre L S 2001 The birth of partition chromatography *LC-GC North Am.* **19** 506

IOP Publishing

Paper-Based Diagnostic Devices for Infectious Diseases

Nidhi Puranik, Arpana Parihar and Raju Khan

Chapter 6

Development of aptamer-based lateral flow assays

Meerambika Mishra and Nidhi Puranik

The advantages of lateral flow assays (LFAs) as point-of-care (POC) devices are that they are inexpensive, easy to use by non-technical users, and require low sample amounts. Because of these benefits, LFAs are excellent tools for detecting analytes on-site with qualitative or semi-quantitative results in a very short time. Nuclei acid-based LFAs are in demand for the detection and diagnosis of diseases caused by bacterial and viral infection. Aptamers are DNA or RNA based single-stranded nucleic acid (ssNA) oligomers with different conformational forms that may molecularly recognise and bind their appropriate targets. Aptamers appear to be appropriate biological recognition elements due to their unique qualities such as efficient chemical synthesis, prolonged shelf life, and ease of modification. Furthermore, they allow for the creation of intelligent detection techniques that are not possible with antibodies (Abs). This chapter focuses on LFAs that use aptamers as a molecular recognition component for LFAs. A brief summary of LFAs and aptamers, including their generation and properties, will be provided in the first section of the chapter and a review of newly published research on this topic will be presented in the second part, demonstrating the wide range of applications and analytes detectable using aptamer-based LFAs.

DNA	deoxyribonucleic acid
NA	nucleic acid
LFA	lateral flow assay
POCT	point-of-care testing
RNA	ribonucleic acid
siRNA	small-interfering RNA

doi:10.1088/978-0-7503-5820-0ch6

© IOP Publishing Ltd 2023

6.1 Introduction

In medical analysis, point-of-care testing (POCT) is a widely applicable approach for early detection and diagnosis of any entities in biological samples. POCT, unlike centralized laboratories, reduces the time between sample gathering and therapeutic intervention (turnaround time) by delivering quicker results. The dipstick pregnancy kit, which was initially introduced in 1991, is the most widely used POCT. The lateral flow assay (LFA), in which the analyte is moved along with the test platform via capillary forces, is the basis for this low-cost test. As POCT may be accomplished not only at medical facilities and exercises, but also in patients' homes, specimen transportation is not necessary, which reduces the risk of unstable analytes and is especially beneficial for patients with chronic conditions [1]. To assess and reduce risks to human health, effective detection of pollutants in food and toxins, hormones, proteins, and other biological substances is critical. The lack of infrastructure, a dearth of skilled personnel, and an increase in healthcare-associated infections, particularly in developing countries, remain the fundamental hurdles to monitoring and controlling these parameters. LFAs are part of the POC device category and can address all of these issues by combining properties such as ease of use, rapid response, resilience, and low cost. During the development phase, false negative results due to the hook effect, where a high concentration of target precludes proper signal creation, or false positive results due to non-specific binding to the LFA, might cause problems [2].

For a long time, nucleic acids (NAs) were thought to be molecules whose primary tasks were to store genetic information in the form of DNA and transport it from gene to protein via RNA. Although, investigations have shown that NAs fulfil various tasks as the enzymatic catalysis also the transcription control over time. The finding of these supplementary NA functions has caused the academic group to re-evaluate its initial perspective on NA functions. The scientific community has proposed the 'RNA world theory' as a result of this transition. This theory claims that NAs can perform a variety of jobs and have aided all of the catalytic reactions that have occurred since the beginning of time on Earth. Recent finding of aptamers has been significantly involved in the realistic fortitude of the multifunctional aspect of NAs.

6.2 Aptamers

These are single-stranded DNA (ssDNA) or RNA oligonucleotides which may connect with target molecules not only with great specificity but also with high affinity [3]. They are typically 25–80 nucleotides long [4]. Aptamers have been accessible for about three decades because of the methodical progression of ligands by the exponential enrichment (SELEX) technique. Craig Tuerk and Larry Gold's work in 1990, in particular, is credited with the invention of aptamers [5]. Aptamers are ssNA sequences that transform into a complicated 3D form, allowing them to connect tightly to a specific target in the strictest sense (figure 6.1). Aptamers can be made of DNA (deoxyribonucleic acid) or RNA (ribonucleic acid). Peptide aptamers exist as well, however they will not be discussed here because they do not fulfil the technical definition of an aptamer as a nucleic acid-based molecule. Aptamer is

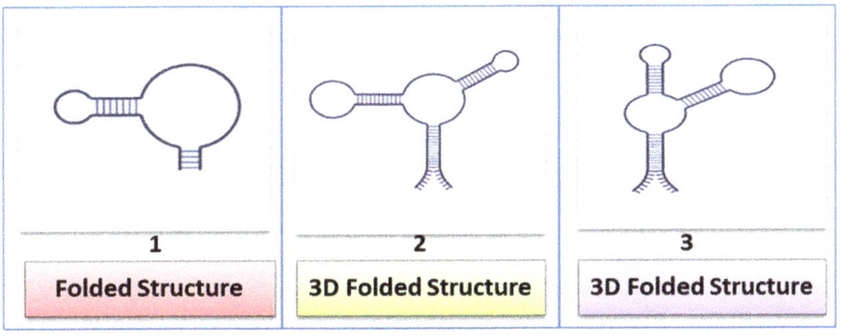

Figure 6.1. Different forms of aptamer.

derived from the Latin word 'aptus', which means 'suited to,' and the Greek word 'meros', which refers to 'part', and refers to the smallest unit of a repeating pattern [6]. Antibody (Ab)-antigen (Ag) tests are used to trap and choose target molecules because of their superior affinity and specificity aptamers. Because the functional groups of aptamers are physically similar to Abs, they can duplicate and expand many of Abs capabilities. As a result, these synthetic oligonucleotides have been dubbed 'chemical Abs'. Aptamers have a wide range and can be used to create a wide spectrum of analytes, including ions, tiny compounds, proteins, viruses, small biomolecules, bacteria, and even complete cells [7–9].

Aptamers have a lot of advantages, including the fact that they are inert to the cells around them (figure 6.2). Specific aptamers are intended to have high precision when attaching to a target molecule, allowing for a wide range of the analytical and restorative applications without the possibility of non-specific attachment. Another benefit is that they have a superior binding affinity [10, 11]. In situations where many ligands can attach to the same receptor site, aptamers have exhibited superior binding affinity than other ligands. It is noteworthy that the higher the affinity range of a molecule that is used in molecular identification, the lesser amount is required for molecular recognition, potentially reducing the costs for molecular identification [5].

K-turn, stem-loop, and pseudoknot motifs are common nucleic acid secondary structural elements, however high ranking tertiary motifs like coaxial stacking and G-quadruplexes can be created as well. The k-turn motif is a 3-nucleotide projection surrounded by normal matching bases that gives the helical aptamer a tight twist. K-turn motifs are highly conserved and are known to be crucial protein recognition sites. The most common motifs in aptamer folding are loops, particularly tetraloops, which can be maintained by mismatch base pairing and base stacking during target binding. Because pseudoknot structures have two layered stem-loop elements, they are more complicated. A separate tertiary structure is formed when a half of one stem intercalates between the two halves of the other stem. Furthermore, guanine-rich aptamer sequences can form G-quadruplexes, which are higher-ordered structures. Four Hoogsteen-paired guanine bases form a planar guanine tetrad that can be stacked on top of one another. Monovalent or divalent cations can be introduced into the quadruplex motif's centre, which stabilize the three-dimensional (3D) structure via

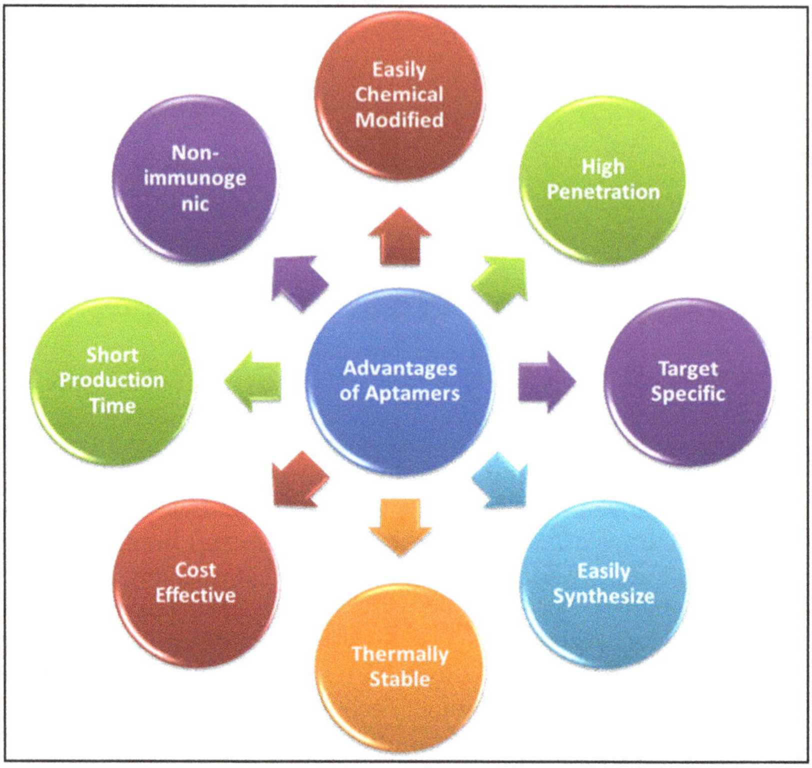

Figure 6.2. Advantages of aptamers.

electrostatic interactions. The effective quadruplex geometry is determined by the ion identity due to differing steric demands. All aptamer structures and associations are based on intramolecular and intermolecular hydrogen bonds, hydrophobic effects, and electrostatic interactions. Both match and mismatch base pairing can be induced via intramolecular hydrogen bonding. Apart from Watson–Crick base pairs that result in conventional helical forms, exceptional base pairing geometrics, base triples, and 'mismatch' all alter aptamer folding. In target recognition, all mismatch-paired or unpaired bases are crucial because they can form additional hydrogen bonds with target molecules, stabilizing the aptamer conformation. The hydroxyl groups on the ribose backbone can also assist in target binding [12]. The principle of the aptamer and its target molecular recognition are shown in figure 6.3. [14].

Understanding the binding interactions between an aptamer and its target is crucial since it will eventually assist in rationalizing and optimizing aptamer designs for downstream applications. The binding parameters includes affinity, avidity, specificity and selectivity [13].

6.3 Aptamer versus antibody

Aptamers have several distinct qualities or benefits over Abs, and they have sparked increased attention as a replacement for Abs in a variety of unique bioapplications,

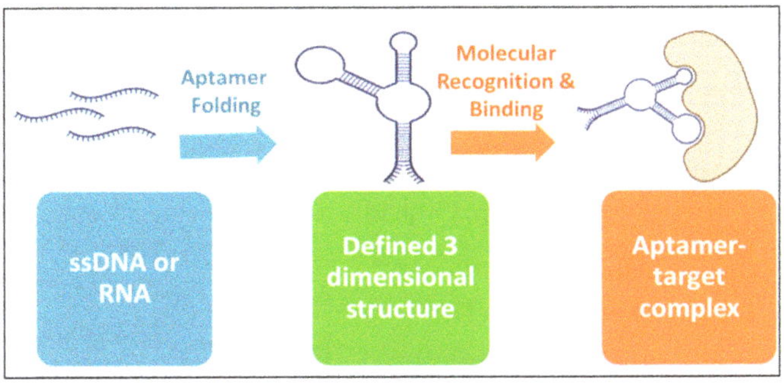

Figure 6.3. Principle of the aptamer molecular recognition.

including biosensing, diagnostic, therapeutic, and imaging studies (figure 6.2). Aptamers are used in an array of different uses besides clinical medicine, involving the recognition of bacterial and viral infections, tumour biomarkers, protein identification in Western blots, and *in vivo* imaging. These can be utilized as target-specific ligands in liquid chromatography and surface plasmon resonance (SPR) testing, besides biosensors (optical, electrochemical). Despite the fact that Abs are normally made *in vivo*, the synthesis of aptamers utilizing an *in vitro* election technique is easy and inexpensive, with good repeatability. This eliminates the requirement for animal use or for the animal models to be challenged in order to identify the target protein sites required for Ab synthesis. Aptamers are less immunogenic than Abs, are more selective, and have a greater affinity for the target. Refolding into distinct tertiary edifices, aptamers can recognise a wide range of targets, from small chemical compounds to large multidomain proteins or polysaccharides, including organic dyes, amino acids, drugs, Abs, and cancer cells and tissues; nevertheless, Abs can only bind to bigger molecules and only to immunogenic proteins. Aptamers have natural capacities to resist harsh circumstances such as heat, pH, ion concentration, and organic solvents, allowing them to be denatured and renatured several times without losing activity due to their capacity to restore their native conformation after chemical or thermal treatment. Aptamers also have a faster intracellular penetration than Abs because of their smaller size and molecular weight (1–2 nm, 5–15 kDa) as compared to Abs (10 nm, 155 kDa). Apart from their long-term stability, aptamers have a high surface density and low steric hindrance, no unwanted immunogenicity, and are non-toxic and non-proteinaceous. Furthermore, whereas site-specific modification of Abs is difficult, the chemical nature of aptamers allows for simple modification at different sites (5′ or 3′ end, aptamer backbone, or bases) by different functional moieties (such as nanomaterials, optical, electrochemical reporter, radioisotopes, and small-interfering RNA—siRNA), and they can be used for clinical, diagnostic, and healing tenacities in the same way as monoclonal Abs (mAbs) [15]. Comparative data of aptamers and Abs are given in table 6.1.

A selection cycle typically begins with the protein target being incubated with a combinatorial DNA or RNA library, which has roughly 10^{12}–10^{14} distinct

Table 6.1. Comparison between aptamers and antibodies.

Characteristics	Aptamer	Antibodies
Molecular weight	Approximately 15–30 kDa	Approximately 150–180 kDa
Production time	A few hours to months	Several months
Secondary structures	Hairpin, loop, G-quadruplex, etc	β-sheets
Variations in production batches	Less	High
Immunogenicity to individual	Less	High
Minimal target size	Targets small sizes ~60 Da	~600 Da
In vivo half-life	Around 20 min	Around one month
Shelf life	Long	Short
Nuclease degradation	Sensitive	Resistant
Targets	Wide range of targets	Antigen
Chemical alterations	Various alterations possible	Limited alterations possible
Stability *in vitro*	Highly stable	Delicate to temperature and pH changes
Production cost	Lower	Higher
Clearance rate	Fast circulation clearance	Small clearance rate
Conjugation of chemical group	Wide range of chemical conjugation from nanoparticles to drugs	Tough to conjugate
Clinical application	Immature	Mature

oligonucleotide sequences 20–80 bases in length. To construct the library for the next phase of selection, protein-bound aptamers are eluted and amplified. In the ensuing selection rounds, an enriched pool of candidate binders derived from PCR amplification is used. A negative selection step can be used to increase the selection stringency. Potential target-specific aptamers are developed after numerous rounds of selection. A negative selection phase can also be added to exclude sequences that bind to undesirable targets, enhancing the specificity of the selection [16].

6.4 Aptamer synthesis

As aptamers do not need to be extensively modified to improve their *in vivo* stability and pharmacokinetics in diagnostic assays, the development of diagnostics is even more common than clinical applications. The growing interest has fuelled technical advancements in *in vitro* selection technology (SELEX), which aims to improve the efficiency of producing aptamers for commercially valuable targets (figure 6.4) [17]. Individual aptamers from the subsequent extremely enhanced pool of aptamers can be further characterized using NGS methods. Indeed, by analysing population dynamics during SELEX, aptamer scientist's unravelled functional oligonucleotides from the past rounds as improved sequencing technology and bioinformatic software became accessible. However, producing more dependable and durable

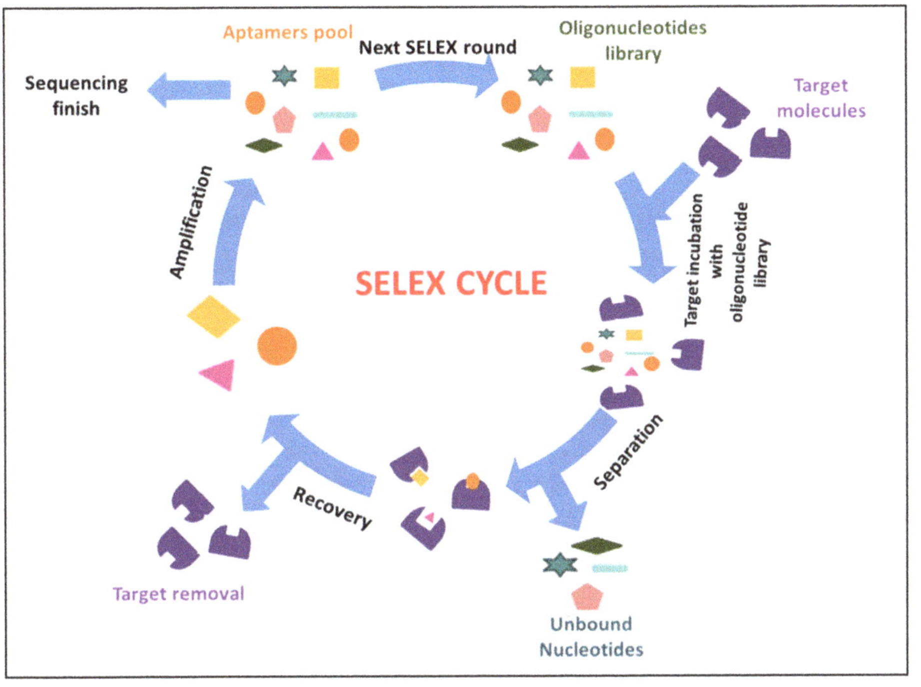

Figure 6.4. Diagrammatic representation of SELEX aptamer selection and enrichment cycle.

aptamers has been problematic due to the difficulties of producing extremely pure recombinant human proteins with native contour as SELEX-targets. Furthermore, SELEX is ineffective for proteins that are unknown, insoluble, and function in a multiprotein complex. As a result, scientists have been hard at work developing various aptamer choosing methodologies. Progress in classic SELEX permitted the creation of novel approaches that allow the assortment of aptamers compared to diverse targets, including living cells, microbes, and tissues, in addition to proteins. Among various new aptamer selection methods, the cell-based SELEX approach (cell-SELEX) stands out: the oligonucleotides selected with this technology can attach to not only cell surface molecules in original condition, but also undiscovered membrane receptors. As a result, cell-SELEX opens up new possibilities for dealing with aptamers that recognise proteins in their original state. Cell-SELEX based technology is employed for choosing particular aptamers for diagnostic and therapeutic applications over diverse cell surface targets, predominantly for tumour cells, during the past two decades. Using cell-SELEX, several studies projected the finding of novel significant biomarkers in various forms of cancer and further disorders. The SELEX approach can be tweaked in a variety of ways to improve aptamer specificity and SELEX efficiency including Cell-SELEX [18, 19], One-pot SELEX [20], Microfluidic SELEX [21], capillary electrophoresis (CE)-SELEX [22], counter-SELEX [18] and toggle-SELEX [23–25]. Cell, microfluidic and CE SELEX are the most common SELEX method for aptamer synthesis and selection and are described here in brief.

Morris and Jensen created cell-based SELEX methodology (cell-SELEX) in 1998 that established an *in vitro* procedure for quarantining highly affinitive aptamers especially against a complicated variety of possible targets. However, cell-SELEX chooses an aptamer that targets the entire cell as opposed to other SELEX methods, guaranteeing that cell surface molecular targets are in their natural state and have their usual folding conformation. Over the last 20 years, aptamers have been manufactured for diverse live cells and other complex systems, particularly for live cancer cells [26, 27]. Cell-SELEX techniques were developed to find aptamers that target proteins that persist in their natural habitat on the surface of the cell. Cell-SELEX can also be used to identify a specific cell type and find new biomarkers or cell membrane proteins that are unknown. The cell-SELEX procedure is similar to that of ordinary protein SELEX, however it is more complicated [28, 29].

Microfluidic technologies surpass managing tiny quantities of reagents, enhancing rigour while lowering costs [21]. Finally, one of the most significant disadvantages of SELEX is that every part of the cycle might be strenuous, onerous, and mandate specialized knowledge. Microfluidic approaches provide a significantly superior ability for automating and diversifying this process, thus reducing the time and the amount of energy spent on every new aptamer and streamlining the SELEX procedure. Many microfluidic SELEX separation techniques have resulted as a result of this, including capillary electrophoresis, microfluidic bead-based separations, and sol–gel encapsulation [30].

Due to great resolution of capillary electrophoresis (CE), CE has recently emerged as a more efficient separation approach for SELEX [22]. CE-based approaches can cut the entire SELEX process time in half; nevertheless, they still necessitate a significant amount of manual handling and a highly specialized set of skills, and they are not well suited to very big datasets [31]. CE was the original microfluidic procedure used to improve SELEX segmentation. CE isolates mixture elements built on electrophoretic mobility [32]. Liberated DNA or RNA travel simultaneously, whereas oligotarget complexes split from unbound sequences and are gathered due to their altered size and charge. Complexation causes a considerable and predictable decrease in mobility since DNA and RNA have a greater negative charge density than practically any desired target molecule [30]. CE has combined extraordinary resolving power with severe selection conditions to isolate aptamers. High-affinity aptamers can be created in substantially fewer rounds of selections using the much easier technique [22, 28, 33].

6.5 Aptamer modification and conjugation

Aptamers must be stabilized against nuclease degradation in order to be used *in vivo*, and the smaller sizes make it vulnerable to renal filtration. However, aptamers could be chemically changed to make them more stable in a variety of ways [34]. Furthermore, modifying nucleic acid libraries chemically increases aptamer binding and, as a result, the target range. Customized aptamers might have greater chemical variety than aptamers constructed exclusively of pure DNA or RNA nucleotides, allowing them to be used in a broader range of diagnostics, therapies, and

Table 6.2. Different approaches for aptamer modifications.

S. No.	Target	Different approaches for modification	References
1	Ribose modification	2′ and 4′ position replacement; 4′-oxygen replacement	[42]
2	Phosphate modification	Methylphosphonate or phosphorothioate	[43]
3	Base modification	Modification of 5th and 8th position of pyrimidine and purine, respectively through the addition of a hydrophobic, hydrophilic, charged or functional group	[42]
4	Modifications of the linkage	3′-capping with biotin–streptavidin and 5′-capping with amine, fatty acids, phosphate, PEG, cholesterol, and proteins	[42]

nanotechnology applications. Various approaches of aptamers modification are given in table 6.2.

Chemical alterations to oligonucleotides of aptamer are typically required to increase the nuclease resistance and reduce renal filtration. In rare cases, chemical modifications may boost the aptamer binding attraction. Several methods have been devised to improve the solidity of aptamers not including affecting their binding attraction and specificity for their targets. Some of the strategies employed include chemical phosphate backbone modification, sulphur substitution on the ribose unit and into the phosphodiester linkage, end capping at the 30 and/or 50 terminals, locked nucleic acids, and circular, multivalent, and dimerization of aptamers. The most common alteration is to the ribose sugar's 20-position [35].

Nanoparticles might be functionalized using a variety of aptamers as targeted ligands. The functionalization of nanoparticles can be performed in a variety of ways without impacting the 3D aptamer functioning. Chemical covalent bonding and physical coupling approaches were commonly employed through a spacer or a linker to maintain aptamer binding activity [35]. A range of coupling chemistry techniques, such as carbodiimide chemistry, thiol-maleimide chemistry, thiol-Aptamer gold coordination, direct conjugation, complementary base pairing, and electrostatic contact, have been employed for aptamer conjugation [36]. Applying the above conjugation chemistry a variety of synthetic macromolecules have been studied for aptamer conjugation, including gold nanorods [37], lipid-polymer nanoparticle [38], PEGylated liposomes [39], micelle [40] and dendrimers [41].

6.6 Aptamer-based LFAs

Hundreds of targets have been found thus far, ranging from tiny ions and small chemical compounds (e.g., neutral disaccharides, dyes, antibiotics etc) to large molecules such as glycoproteins (e.g., CD4) and even more complicated (e.g., whole living cells). For example, ethanolamine which contains only four non-hydrogen atoms and may induce a variety of disorders is probably the smallest aptamer target ever found [44]. In recent years, several research papers employing aptamers as probes in LFAs have been established. The most typical targets are proteins (thrombin) or whole organisms like bacteria and eukaryotic cells. However, there have been few publications on the detection of low molecular weight molecules such as metabolites or drugs utilizing aptamer-based LFAs [45]. Several critical difficulties must be considered while adapting LFAs for small-molecule detection, the most important of which being the working principle of LFAs. Similar to an enzyme-linked immunoassay (ELISA), they are usually set up in sandwich or in the competitive formats.

6.6.1 Competitive format

This format of LFA is often utilized in the recognition of molecules having only single epitope. The competition approach is as the target in the test matches for the opportunity to combine with the tagged aptamer with its corresponding DNA. An alternative option is for the target with regards to the sample to compete along with their hapten to blend with the tagged aptamer. In order to augment the specificity or sensitivity, various signal amplification methods are applied in the competitive format in the aptamer-based LFAs. Multiplexed recognition in this format of aptamer-based LFAs is currently of concern to researchers [46].

6.6.2 Sandwich format

For analyte detection various epitopes which attach to a pair of aptamers or a combination of aptamers and Abs, the sandwich format for these aptamer-based LFAs is the commonly used format. Various signal amplification approaches have been used to improve sensitivity. Employing the aptamer-based LFA sandwich design, researchers have made significant progress in multiplexed detection. For the detection of analytes having various epitopes that can attach to a pair of aptamers or their combination and Abs, the sandwich format for aptamer-based LFAs is the most used format. Various signal amplification approaches have been used to improve sensitivity. By employing the aptamer-based LFA sandwich design, researchers have made significant progress in multiplexed detection [46].

6.7 Developed aptamers for detection and diagnosis

Aptamer-based affinity tests have a great deal of potential as monitoring and diagnosis tools for bacteria. Various aptamers are synthesized to detect bacteria, virus and others [47]. Detection and diagnosis of various biomolecules and organism by aptamer-based different approaches are given in table 6.3. In a study a highly improved SELEX technique was used for selection of aptamers that could be beneficial for identifying *Streptococcus pyogenes*, obtaining M-type binding profiles, and developing new M-typing methods for non-specialized labs or POCT [48].

To test the potential of the aptamer against *S. aureus* enterotoxin C1 (SEC1) with a limit of detection of 6 ng ml^{-1}, a graphene oxide (GO)-based approach was used to quantify SEC1 in the food sample [56]. Aflatoxin B1 (AFB1) is detected by a swift and effortless dipstick assay that is based on an aptamer was developed, the

Table 6.3. Detection and diagnosis of various biomolecules and organism by aptamer-based different approaches.

Detection	Target	References
Salmonella Typhimurium	Whole bacteria	[49]
Aflatoxin B1	Aflatoxin B1	[50]
Aflatoxin B1	Aflatoxin B1	[51]
SARS coronavirus	Nucleocapsid protein	[52]
SARS-CoV-2	RBD domain of spike protein 1	[53]
Gram-negative bacteria	Outer membrane vesicles	[54]
Staphylococcus aureus	Enterotoxin A protein	[55]
	Enterotoxin C1 (SEC1)	[56]
	Enterotoxin Type A, B, C1	[57]
Campylobacter jenuni	Whole bacteria	[58]
Mycobacterium tuberculosis	Protein MPT64	[59]
Salmonella enteritidis	16s rRNA	[60]
Listeria monocytogenes	Internalin A protein	[61]
Lactobacillus acidophilus	Whole bacteria	[62]
Streptococcus pyrogenes	Whole bacteria	[48]

detection limit is 0.1 ng ml^{-1} in buffer [63]. Aptamers can also identify a variety of cancer metabolites, differentiating cells, chemicals that influence tumour activity, and cancer biomarkers. The conjugates of aptamer-nanoparticle (Apt-NP) are frequently utilized as cancer detection techniques. Cancer cells can be detected using these conjugates in complex bodily fluids like serum and blood [64]. Aptamer-based LFA for detection and identification of biomolecule and organism with detection limit is given in table 6.4.

6.8 Other applications of aptamers

Aptamers can be used for a variety of diagnostic and also medicinal objectives, including biosensors and target inhibitors. Aptamers have been employed in a variety of molecular biology, biotechnology, and biomedical applications due to their ease of synthesis, modification, and stability.

6.8.1 Therapeutic application

Aptamers are used as small-molecule medicinal medicines, which is an important application. DNA aptamers have been created as promising therapeutic agents in competition with Abs because they have significant therapeutic advantages. In general, DNA aptamers utilized for therapeutic purposes work in one of two ways. Firstly, DNA aptamers can behave as antagonists by attaching to the target protein and inhibiting protein–protein interactions. Second, when DNA aptamers attach to the target protein, they can act as agonists, promoting the target protein's function. Although DNA aptamers have comparable functions to Abs, their non-immunogenicity makes them

Table 6.4. Aptamer-based LFA for detection and identification of biomolecule and organism.

Target	Format	Aptamer conjugation with	Test and control line Ab	Detection limit	References
Aflatoxin B1	Competitive LFAs	Biotin modified aptamer	Streptavidin and anti-cy5 Ab	0.3 ng g^{-1}AFB	[63]
Escherichia coli	Sandwich LFAs	Aptamer-AuNP conjugates	Amino end-labelled capture aptamers and Anti-digoxigenin Ab	3000–6000 *E. coli* cells,	[65]
Ampicillin	Competitive LFAs	Aptamer-mFc-AuNP conjugates	Streptavidin and goat—anti-mouse Ab	260 mg l^{-1} ampicillin in milk sample	[45]
Ochratoxin	Competitive LFAs	Aptamer-AuNP conjugates	Streptavidin-biotin cDNA and Streptavidin-biotin-PolyT	1 ng ml^{-1} 0.18 ng ml^{-1}	[66]
Thrombin	Sandwich LFAs	Aptamer-AuNP conjugates	Ab and Streptavidin-biotin-cDNA to primary aptamer	0.25 nM	[67]
HCV core antigen	Competitive LFAs	Aptamer-AuNP conjugates	Streptavidin-biotin cDNA and Streptavidin-biotin-PolyT	100 pg ml^{-1}; 10 pg ml^{-1}	[68]
Salmonella typhimurium, *Escherichia coli* O157:H7 and *Staphylococcus aureus*	Sandwich LFAs	AuNP conjugated aptamer conjugates and	Streptavidin–aptamer conjugates	10^3 CFU ml^{-1}, 10^4 CFU ml^{-1}, and 10^4 CFU ml^{-1}, respectively	[69]

more useful in treatments. Because of their tiny size, DNA aptamers are easier to absorb than Abs. Aptamers are capable of recognising diverse targets, such as small molecules, proteins, and whole cells. Furthermore, aptamers are less expensive to generate than Abs since they may be produced and chosen *in vitro*. DNA aptamers have the traits and advantages listed above, making them a promising therapeutic tool [70].

6.8.2 Drug delivery system

Cell-specific drug delivery can help improve a therapy's efficacy while lowering side effects. Because of their high specificity and affinity, small size, minimal immunogenicity, low cost of production, and convenience of storage, aptamers are one of the best possibilities for particular ligands for nanoparticle functionalization [71]. Drug delivery system (DNA) aptamers are used as shuttles for tiny oligonucleotides such as small interference RNA (siRNA) and microRNA (miRNA), in addition to acting as therapeutic agents. Aptamers can recognise a specific target and can be altered quickly, making them a possible targeted delivery mechanism. DNA aptamers employed in two different methods for targeted drug delivery: either completely coupled to the drug molecules or combined with nanoparticles. Directly conjugating drug molecules to certain DNA aptamers could enable medications to be delivered more precisely, lowering the risk of non-specific consequences. Attaching DNA aptamers to pharmaceuticals or packaging the drug into an aptamer-folded formation, DNA aptamers–drug couples (ApDCs) transports medications to target cells with improved selectivity. *In vitro* and *in vivo*, many DNA aptamers have been chosen to economically deliver chemotherapeutic drugs such as doxorubicin (DOX), fluorouracil, and epirubicin [72]. ApDCs are promising tailored drug delivery systems for decreasing chemotherapy toxicity while enhancing efficacy [73].

6.8.3 Environmental pollution monitoring

Aptamers monitor and reduce environmental contaminants, as well as the illnesses that come from them. Antibiotics, heavy metals, poisons, and viruses are all potentially harmful to the neurological, endocrine, and reproductive systems. Antibiotics used on farm animals may accrue in the tissues of the animals and be passed on to humans eating them. Aptamers against antibiotics like chloramphenicol and tetracycline have been developed to address this problem [74].

6.8.4 Biosensors applications

Aptamers are commonly employed in biosensors because many aptamer structures can be created, as well as their competency to attach to specific targets by forming established tertiary structures. To date various aptamer-based biosensors have been developed such as aptamer-based biosensors for uncovering of platelet-derived growth factor BB (PDGF-BB), a cancer-biomarker, biosensors for antifungal medicines in the azole class, with applications in therapeutic medication observing of patients with hostile fungal infections, milk allergen identification using biosensors with DNA aptamers targeting B-lactoglobulin, high-sensitivity biosensors for detecting human epidermal growth factor receptor 2 (EGFR2) for identification of breast cancer cells and in bisphenol A detection [75–77].

6.9 Summary

The ability to effectively treat and manage animal diseases requires early diagnosis of the condition. Symptoms and biochemical, microbiological, and serological testing of biological samples are used to detect and differentiate animal diseases in the majority of instances. ELISA, DNA chips, real time PCR, and chromatographic procedures are a few examples of additional confirmatory tests that need sophisticated instruments, trained operators, and expensive reagents. Innovative POC biosensors have been developed as new diagnostic instruments in recent years; several have lower sensitivity, specificity, and dependability. Biosensors are quickly gaining traction as a new cutting-edge tool for the detection and treatment of illness. Biosensors are analytical instruments that generate signals from biological substances in order to detect a specific illness. Selectivity and sensitivity are two critical characteristics of biosensors. Various aptamers and aptasensors were analysed for the detection of a variety of infectious species, microbes and their toxins.

Aptamers are ssNAs with molecular identification properties like Abs. They are typically 22–100 nucleobases long and have a variable region surrounded by continuous sections, allowing for sequence amplification and identification. Aptamers, like mAbs, have a variety of uses, including biomarker discovery, therapies, diagnostics, and high-throughput screening. Aptamers, on the other hand, compete with Abs in numerous ways due to their physicochemical features [78].

Aptamer-based biosensors are gaining popularity as a result of their numerous benefits over other biosensors. The creation of biosensors for the detection of various diseases, on the other hand, remains a major issue for scientists and researchers. In the development of aptamer biosensors, the purpose of nanomaterials and the integration of modern multidisciplinary approaches will improve the sensitivity of the devices and allow them to be more economical for the initial recognition of illness, which is a pressing necessity. To summarize, while there are currently some limitations in the production of aptamers to be used in clinical applications in veterinary medicine, with the improvement of relevant technologies, aptamers will become broadly employed in the early and precise detection of sickness.

Despite the obvious advantages of aptamers, viable aptamer-based LFA applications have yet to be created. As a result, a number of hurdles to the commercialization of aptamer-based LFAs must be overcome. Only a few aptamers have been effectively used in LFAs, and their use in LFAs is usually considered proof-of-concept for innovative on-the-spot biosensors. Research has to be directed towards analytes that are in high demand in the market to tackle this problem. Coronavirus disease 2019 (COVID-19), for example, has been a global public health emergency unlike any other, caused by SARS-CoV-2.

Conflicts of interest

The authors declare no conflict of interests.

References

[1] Phung N L, Walter J G, Jonczyk R, Seiler L K, Scheper T and Blume C 2020 Development of an aptamer-based lateral flow assay for the detection of C-reactive protein using microarray technology as a prescreening platform *ACS Comb. Sci.* **22** 617–29

[2] Schüling T, Eilers A, Scheper T and Walter J 2018 Aptamer-based lateral flow assays *AIMS Bioeng.* **5** 78–102

[3] Modh H, Scheper T and Walter J G 2018 Aptamer-modified magnetic beads in biosensing *Sensors (Basel)* 18

[4] Ni S, Zhuo Z, Pan Y, Yu Y, Li F and Liu J *et al* 2020 Recent progress in aptamer discoveries and modifications for therapeutic applications *ACS Appl. Mater. Interfaces* **13** 9500–19

[5] Ali M H, Elsherbiny M E and Emara M 2019 Updates on aptamer research *Int. J. Mol. Sci* **10** 2511

[6] Niederlender S, Fontaine J J and Karadjian G 2021 Potential applications of aptamers in veterinary science *Vet. Res.* **52** 1–20

[7] Elskens J P, Elskens J M and Madder A 2020 Chemical modification of aptamers for increased binding affinity in diagnostic applications: current status and future prospects *Int. J. Mol. Sci.* **21** 1–31

[8] Olsen T, Zhu J, Kim J, Pei R, Stojanovic M N and Lin Q 2017 An integrated microfluidic selex approach using combined electrokinetic and hydrodynamic manipulation *SLAS Technol.* **22** 63

[9] Faulhammer D, Eschgfäller B, Stark S, Burgstaller P, Englberger W and Erfurth J *et al* 2004 Biostable aptamers with antagonistic properties to the neuropeptide nociceptin/orphanin FQ *RNA* **10** 516

[10] Lakhin A V, Tarantul V Z and Gening L V 2013 Aptamers: problems, solutions and prospects *Acta Nat.* **5** 34

[11] Ruscito A and DeRosa M C 2016 Small-molecule binding aptamers: selection strategies, characterization, and applications *Front. Chem.* **4** 14

[12] Lönne M, Zhu G, Stahl F and Walter J G 2014 Aptamer-modified nanoparticles as biosensors *Adv. Biochem. Eng. Biotechnol.* **140** 121–54

[13] Kalra P, Dhiman A, Cho W C, Bruno J G and Sharma T K 2018 Simple methods and rational design for enhancing aptamer sensitivity and specificity *Front. Mol. Biosci.* **5** 41

[14] Reinemann C and Strehlitz B 2014 Aptamer-modified nanoparticles and their use in cancer diagnostics and treatment *Swiss. Med. Wkly.* 144

[15] Khoee S and Khezrian S 2017 Applications of aptamers for the diagnosis and therapy of different diseases *Nanostructures for Novel Therapy: Synthesis, Characterization and Applications* (Amsterdam: Elsevier) 591–619

[16] Ciancio D R, Vargas M R, Thiel W H, Bruno M A, Giangrande P H and Mestre M B 2018 Aptamers as diagnostic tools in cancer *Pharmaceuticals* **11** 86

[17] Blind M and Blank M 2015 Aptamer selection technology and recent advances *Mol. Ther. Nucleic Acids* **4** e223

[18] Zhuo Z, Yu Y, Wang M, Li J, Zhang Z and Liu J *et al* 2017 Recent advances in SELEX technology and aptamer applications in biomedicine *Int. J. Mol. Sci.* **18** 2142

[19] Daniels D A, Chen H, Hicke B J, Swiderek K M and Gold L 2003 A tenascin-C aptamer identified by tumor cell SELEX: systematic evolution of ligands by exponential enrichment *Proc. Natl Acad. Sci.* **100** 15416–21

[20] Jauset-Rubio M, Botero M L, Skouridou V, Aktas G B, Svobodova M and Bashammakh A S *et al* 2019 One-pot SELEX: identification of specific aptamers against diverse steroid targets in one selection *ACS Omega* **4** 20188–96
[21] Hybarger G, Bynum J, Williams R F, Valdes J J and Chambers J P 2006 A microfluidic SELEX prototype *Anal. Bioanal. Chem.* **384** 191–8
[22] Yang J and Bowser M T 2013 Capillary electrophoresis-SELEX selection of catalytic DNA aptamers for a small-molecule porphyrin target *Anal. Chem.* **85** 1525–30
[23] Yang X, Li N and Gorenstein D G 2011 Strategies for the discovery of therapeutic aptamers *Expert Opin. Drug Discov.* **6** 75
[24] Kong H Y and Byun J 2013 Nucleic acid aptamers: new methods for selection, stabilization, and application in biomedical science *Biomol. Ther. (Seoul)* **21** 423
[25] White R, Rusconi C, Scardino E, Wolberg A, Lawson J and Hoffman M *et al* 2001 Generation of species cross-reactive aptamers using 'Toggle' SELEX *Mol. Ther.* **4** 567–73
[26] Buglak A A, Samokhvalov A V, Zherdev A V and Dzantiev B B 2020 Methods and applications of in silico aptamer design and modeling *Int. J. Mol. Sci.* **21** 1–25
[27] Chen M, Yu Y, Jiang F, Zhou J, Li Y, Liang C, Dang L, Lu A and Zhang G 2016 Development of cell-SELEX technology and its application in cancer diagnosis and therapy *Int. J. Mol. Sci.* **17** 2079
[28] Liu Y, Wang N, Chan C W, Lu A, Yu Y and Zhang G *et al* 2021 The application of microfluidic technologies in aptamer selection *Front. Cell. Dev. Biol.* **9** 2548
[29] Dickinson H, Lukasser M, Mayer G and Hüttenhofer A 2015 Cell-SELEX: *in vitro* selection of synthetic small specific ligands *Methods Mol. Biol.* **1296** 213–24
[30] Dembowski S K and Bowser M T 2017 Microfluidic methods for aptamer selection and characterization *Analyst* **143** 21–32
[31] Kim J, Olsen T R, Zhu J, Hilton J P, Yang K A and Pei R *et al* 2016 Integrated microfluidic isolation of aptamers using electrophoretic oligonucleotide manipulation *Sci. Rep.* **6** 1–10
[32] Mosing R K, Mendonsa S D and Bowser M T 2005 Capillary electrophoresis-SELEX selection of aptamers with affinity for HIV-1 reverse transcriptase *Anal. Chem.* **77** 6107–12
[33] Mosing R K and Bowser M T 2009 Isolating aptamers using capillary electrophoresis-SELEX (CE-SELEX) *Methods Mol. Biol.* **535** 33–43
[34] Wang R, Wu H, Niu Y and Cai J 2011 Improving the stability of aptamers by chemical modification *Curr. Med. Chem.* **18** 4126–38
[35] Odeh F, Nsairat H, Alshaer W, Ismail M A, Esawi E and Qaqish B *et al* 2020 Aptamers chemistry: chemical modifications and conjugation strategies *Molecules* **25** 3
[36] Nerantzaki M, Loth C and Lutz J F 2021 Chemical conjugation of nucleic acid aptamers and synthetic polymers *Polym. Chem.* **12** 3498–509
[37] Chandrasekaran R, Lee A S W, Yap L W, Jans D A, Wagstaff K M and Cheng W 2015 Tumor cell-specific photothermal killing by SELEX-derived DNA aptamer-targeted gold nanorods *Nanoscale* **8** 187–96
[38] Yu Z, Chen F, Qi X, Dong Y, Zhang Y and Ge Z *et al* 2018 Epidermal growth factor receptor aptamer-conjugated polymer-lipid hybrid nanoparticles enhance salinomycin delivery to osteosarcoma and cancer stem cells *Exp. Ther. Med.* **15** 1247–56

[39] Moosavian S A, Abnous K, Badiee A and Jaafari M R 2016 Improvement in the drug delivery and anti-tumor efficacy of PEGylated liposomal doxorubicin by targeting RNA aptamers in mice bearing breast tumor model *Colloids Surf.* B **139** 228–36

[40] Charbgoo F, Alibolandi M, Taghdisi S M, Abnous K, Soltani F and Ramezani M 2018 MUC1 aptamer-targeted DNA micelles for dual tumor therapy using doxorubicin and KLA peptide *Nanomed. Nanotechnol., Biol. Med.* **14** 685–97

[41] Ayatollahi S, Salmasi Z, Hashemi M, Askarian S, Oskuee R K and Abnous K *et al* 2017 Aptamer-targeted delivery of Bcl-xL shRNA using alkyl modified PAMAM dendrimers into lung cancer cells *Int. J. Biochem. Cell Biol.* **92** 210–7

[42] Gao S, Zheng X, Jiao B and Wang L 2016 Post-SELEX optimization of aptamers *Anal. Bioanal. Chem.* **408** 4567–73

[43] Saccà B, Lacroix L and Mergny J L 2005 The effect of chemical modifications on the thermal stability of different G-quadruplex-forming oligonucleotides *Nucleic Acids Res.* **33** 1182

[44] Chen A and Yang S 2015 Replacing antibodies with aptamers in lateral flow immunoassay *Biosens. Bioelectron.* **71** 230–42

[45] Kaiser L, Weisser J, Kohl M and Deigner H-P 2018 Small molecule detection with aptamer based lateral flow assays: applying aptamer-C-reactive protein cross-recognition for ampicillin detection OPEN *Sci. Rep.* **8** 5628

[46] Huang L, Tian S, Zhao W, Liu K, Ma X and Guo J 2021 Aptamer-based lateral flow assay on-site biosensors**186** 113279

[47] Liu J, Qin Q, Zhang X, Li C, Yu Y and Huang X *et al* 2020 Development of a novel lateral flow biosensor combined with aptamer-based isolation: application for rapid detection of grouper nervous necrosis virus *Front. Microbiol.* **11** 886

[48] Hamula C L A, Peng H, Wang Z, Tyrrell G J, Li X-F and Le X C 2016 An improved SELEX technique for selection of DNA aptamers binding to M-type 11 of *Streptococcus pyogenes* keywords: bacteria DNA binding to cells DNA library diversity PCR amplification Selection of DNA aptamers affinity binding and recognition cell SELEX for bioanalytical assays M proteins of *Streptococcus pyogenes* detection and serotyping of microbial pathogens *Methods* **97** 51–7

[49] Gao P, Wang L, He Y, Wang Y, Yang X and Fu S *et al* 2021 An enhanced lateral flow assay based on aptamer–magnetic separation and multifold AuNPs for ultrasensitive detection of *Salmonella typhimurium* in milk *Foods* **10** 1605

[50] Setlem K, Mondal B, Ramlal S and Kingston J 2016 Immuno affinity SELEX for simple, rapid, and cost-effective aptamer enrichment and identification against aflatoxin B1 *Front. Microbiol.* **7** 1909

[51] Guo X, Wen F, Zheng N, Luo Q, Wang H and Wang H *et al* 2014 Development of an ultrasensitive aptasensor for the detection of aflatoxin B1 *Biosens. Bioelectron.* **56** 340–4

[52] Ahn D G, Jeon I J, Kim J D, Song M S, Han S R and Lee S W *et al* 2009 RNA aptamer-based sensitive detection of SARS coronavirus nucleocapsid protein *Analyst* **134** 1896–901

[53] Yang G, Li Z, Mohammed I, Zhao L, Wei W and Xiao H *et al* 2021 Identification of SARS-CoV-2-against aptamer with high neutralization activity by blocking the RBD domain of spike protein 1 *Signal Transduct. Target. Ther.* **6** 1–4

[54] Shin H S, Gedi V, Kim J K and Lee D K 2019 Detection of Gram-negative bacterial outer membrane vesicles using DNA aptamers *Sci. Rep.* **9** 13167

[55] Huang Y, Chen X, Xia Y, Wu S, Duan N and Ma X *et al* 2014 Selection, identification and application of a DNA aptamer against *Staphylococcus aureus* enterotoxin A *Anal. Methods* **6** 690–7

[56] Huang Y, Chen X, Duan N, Wu S, Wang Z and Wei X *et al* 2015 Selection and characterization of DNA aptamers against *Staphylococcus aureus* enterotoxin C1 *Food Chem.* **166** 623–9

[57] Huang Y, Zhang H, Chen X, Wang X, Duan N and Wu S *et al* 2015 A multicolor time-resolved fluorescence aptasensor for the simultaneous detection of multiplex *Staphylococcus aureus* enterotoxins in the milk *Biosens. Bioelectron.* **74** 170–6

[58] Dwivedi H P, Smiley R D and Jaykus L A 2010 Selection and characterization of DNA aptamers with binding selectivity to *Campylobacter jejuni* using whole-cell SELEX *Appl. Microbiol. Biotechnol.* **87** 2323–34

[59] Sypabekova M, Dukenbayev K, Tsepke A, Akisheva A, Oralbayev N and Kanayeva D 2019 An aptasensor for the detection of *Mycobacterium tuberculosis* secreted immunogenic protein MPT64 in clinical samples towards tuberculosis detection *Sci. Rep.* **9** 1–11

[60] Liu K, Yan X, Mao B, Wang S and Deng L 2015 Aptamer-based detection of *Salmonella enteritidis* using double signal amplification by Klenow fragment and dual fluorescence *Microchim. Acta* **183** 643–9

[61] Ohk S H, Koo O K, Sen T, Yamamoto C M and Bhunia A K 2010 Antibody-aptamer functionalized fibre-optic biosensor for specific detection of *Listeria monocytogenes* from food *J. Appl. Microbiol.* **109** 808–17

[62] Hamula C L A, Zhang H, Guan L L, Li X F and Le X C 2008 Selection of aptamers against live bacterial cells *Anal. Chem.* **80** 7812–9

[63] Shim W B, Kim M J, Mun H and Kim M G 2014 An aptamer-based dipstick assay for the rapid and simple detection of aflatoxin B1 *Biosens. Bioelectron.* **62** 288–94

[64] Kulabhusan P K, Hussain B and Yüce M n.d. Pharmaceutics current perspectives on aptamers as diagnostic tools and therapeutic agents

[65] Bruno J G 2014 Application of DNA aptamers and quantum dots to lateral flow test strips for detection of foodborne pathogens with improved sensitivity versus colloidal gold *Pathogens* **3** 341–55

[66] Wang L, Ma W, Chen W, Liu L, Ma W and Zhu Y *et al* 2011 An aptamer-based chromatographic strip assay for sensitive toxin semi-quantitative detection *Biosens. Bioelectron.* **26** 3059–62

[67] Shen G, Zhang S and Hu X 2013 Signal enhancement in a lateral flow immunoassay based on dual gold nanoparticle conjugates *Clin. Biochem.* **46** 1734–8

[68] Wang C, Zhang L and Shen X 2013 Development of a nucleic acid lateral flow strip for detection of hepatitis c virus (Hcv) core antigen *Nucleos. Nucleot. Nucl.* **32** 59–68

[69] Lu C, Gao X, Chen Y, Ren J and Liu C 2019 Aptamer-based lateral flow test strip for the simultaneous detection of *Salmonella typhimurium Escherichia coli* O157:H7 and *Staphylococcus aureus Anal. Lett.* **53** 646–59

[70] Zhu Q, Liu G and Kai M 2015 DNA aptamers in the diagnosis and treatment of human diseases *Molecules* **20** 20979–97

[71] Fu Z and Xiang J 2020 Aptamer-functionalized nanoparticles in targeted delivery and cancer therapy *Int. J. Mol. Sci.* **21** 9123

[72] Huang Y F, Shangguan D, Liu H, Phillips J A, Zhang X and Chen Y *et al* 2009 Molecular assembly of an aptamer-drug conjugate for targeted drug delivery to tumor cells *Chem. Bio. Chem.* **10** 862

[73] Wang R, Zhu G, Mei L, Xie Y, Ma H and Ye M *et al* 2014 Automated modular synthesis of aptamer-drug conjugates for targeted drug delivery *J. Am. Chem. Soc.* **136** 2731–4

[74] Zhang Y, Lai B S and Juhas M 2019 Recent advances in aptamer discovery and applications *Molecules* **24** 941

[75] Chen M L, Chen J H, Ding L, Xu Z, Wen L and Wang L B *et al* 2017 Study of the detection of bisphenol A based on a nano-sized metal–organic framework crystal and an aptamer *Anal. Methods* **9** 906–9

[76] Wiedman G R, Zhao Y, Mustaev A, Ping J, Vishnubhotla R and Johnson A T C *et al* 2017 An aptamer-based biosensor for the azole class of antifungal drugs *mSphere* **2** 00274-17

[77] Hong L, Zhou F, Shi D, Zhang X and Wang G 2017 Portable aptamer biosensor of platelet-derived growth factor-BB using a personal glucose meter with triply amplified *Biosens. Bioelectron.* **95** 152–9

[78] Devi S, Sharma N, Ahmed T, Huma Z I, Kour S and Sahoo B *et al* 2021 Aptamer-based diagnostic and therapeutic approaches in animals: current potential and challenges *Saudi J. Biol. Sci.* **28** 5081–93

Chapter 7

Paper-based diagnostics for SARS-CoV-2

Nidhi Puranik and Preeti Puranik

Coronavirus disease 2019 (COVID-19), a global epidemic that swiftly spread across all countries, causing millions of people to suffer social and economic pain is caused by severe acute respiratory syndrome coronavirus 2 (SARS-CoV-2). Most nations have put in place early warning systems to detect, isolate, and treat SARS-CoV-2 patients. The most difficult aspect of the pandemic is that it is infectious and often fatal, necessitating prompt identification and treatment in order to preserve humanity. Medical specialists were able to control the harmful effects in infected persons by administering timely medicine thanks to paper-based diagnostics such as the immune-chromatography test (ICT) assay also known as lateral flow assay (LFA). However, this early test only provides an indication of the presence or absence of a target molecule based on the signal, making it a qualitative rather than quantitative test. Various LFA-based COVID-19 early diagnosis kits are now commercially available, and many more are on the way. This chapter discusses the concept of LFA, its various components, and its application in the early detection and diagnosis of SARS-CoV-2 and COVID-19, respectively.

7.1 Introduction

COVID-19, a deadly disease triggered by the SARS-CoV-2 is a dangerous disease to public health worldwide [1]. Due to initially common flu-like symptoms, the mortality rate is very high around the globe. Consequently, to control the spread of COVID-19 through communities, early detection and identification of this infectious agent is essential. For early detection and diagnosis of SARS-CoV-2 infected individuals a large number of different kinds of detection and diagnostics systems have been developed to date and are still being developed around the world. The LFA test played a crucial role in the point-of care testing of COVID-19 infected people. Nowadays, not only pharma companies but also medical institutes and research centres are rushing to develop ensitive and specific LFA assay and so LFA has become a medical priority.

doi:10.1088/978-0-7503-5820-0ch7 © IOP Publishing Ltd 2023

The immuno-chromatography assay was, for the first time, commercially used in 1984 for the confirmation of pregnancy at home as a simple urine-based test. Simple visual detection of results within 5–10 min after adding a urine sample proved this assay as an analytical platform in medical sciences, the food industry, the field of agriculture and in environmental pollution detection [2, 3]. Traditionally, a LFA result is observed by development of colour on the test lines that can be seen by the naked eye which accomplishes significant commercial success and has a noteworthy impact on various fields [4]. LFA-based point-of-care (POC) kits are very rapidly growing strategies from qualitative to quantitative analysis of various biological entities. This is a membrane-based assay performed over a strip and the different parts of this membrane assay include a nitrocellulose (NC) membrane, a sample pad, an adsorption pad and a conjugate release pad which are assembled on a plastic backing. The NC membrane is a capture membrane on which test and control lines are drawn [5]. The other main components of LFA are a reviling molecule (antigen/antibody/oligonucleotides), detection probe (nanoparticles), sample or target molecule and buffers. Each component, including capturing membrane, conjugate pad, sample pad, absorption pad, conjugation buffer, blocking buffer, wash buffer, and type of nanoparticle used in the assay are crucial in the development of the LFA kit. There are several buffers that are used in the development of LFA for antibody–nanoparticle conjugation, blocking buffer for unconjugated molecules, washing buffer for unwanted molecules and uniform flow of sample on nitrocellulose membrane. Various conditions such as the pH of the buffer, humidity, and temperature of the surroundings, nature, and stability of sample and size and stability of conjugated-nanoparticle alter the sensitivity as well as specificity of the developed LFA assay. Hence, the optimization of ideal conditions for the development and commercialization of LFA is challenging.

7.2 SARS-CoV-2

The coronavirus disease is a global public health problem that is still affecting people all over the world. In December 2019, COVID-19 was for the first time reported from a local outbreak of pneumonia caused by a previously undiscovered virus in Wuhan (Hubei, China). The whole genome sequence of COVID-19 was easily found and it showed a genetic resemblance to SARS-CoV-like coronaviruses in bats. The SARS-CoV-2 is an enveloped virus with a viral genome encased in a helicoidal capsid, like other coronaviruses. The main viral envelope proteins are spike (S), membrane (M), and envelope (E), whereas nucleocapsid (N), together with an RNA molecule, makes up the viral nucleocapsid [6]. General schematic representation of SARS-CoV-2 structure is shown in figure 7.1. COVID-19 is commonly characterized by flu-like symptoms and causes acute lung injury, known as pneumonia. The lung infection is from mild to severe stages (shown in figure 7.2) [7] by uncontrolled oxidative stress as well as the inflammatory response developed by SARS-CoV-2 in lungs [8]. Rapid screening and tight quarantine procedures have emerged as critical approaches to stop the further spread of COVID-19 all over the world [9].

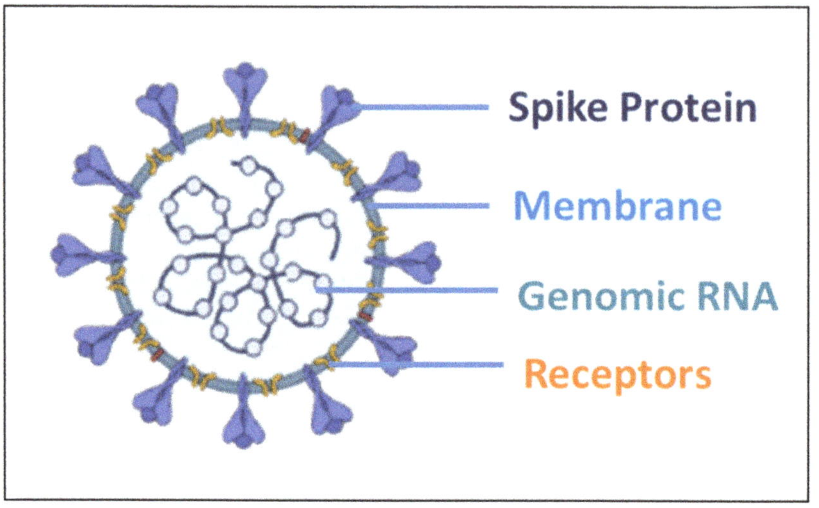

Figure 7.1. Structure of SARS-CoV-2.

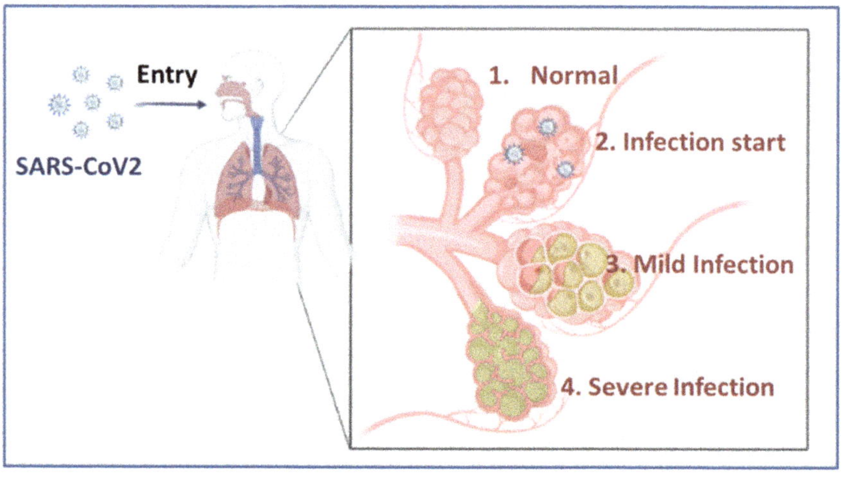

Figure 7.2. SARS-CoV-2 entry and lung infection.

SARS-CoV-2 has a number of distinct and interconnected characteristics such as high growth rate, long incubation period, large number of asymptomatic or mild symptom, and the ability of the virus to survive in various different environments. COVID-19 can spread in many ways, e.g., coughing, sneezing, and other biofluids, the first line of defence against this virus is to stop it from spreading through contaminated air, skin, or surfaces [10]. Diagnosis of COVID-19 is commonly exhibited by targeting four different SARS-CoV-2 structural proteins: membrane (M), spike (S), nucleocapsid (N), and envelope (E). However, recent studies have shown that among the four structural proteins, proteins M and E are crucial for the

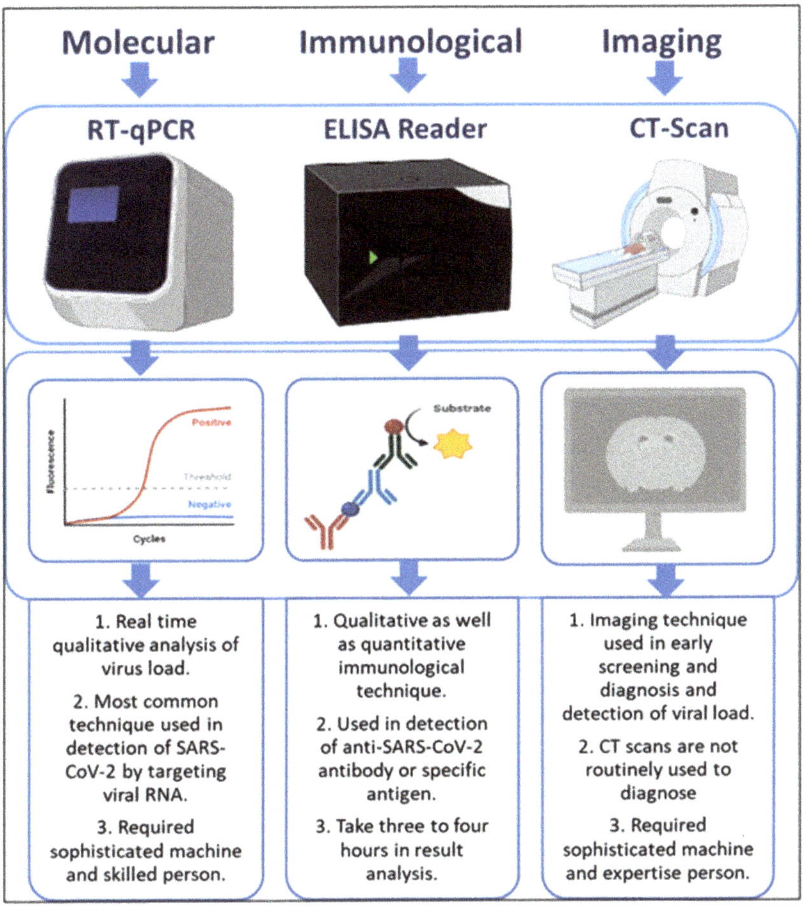

Figure 7.3. A comparative chart of the most common molecular, immunological and imaging techniques used in SARS-CoV-2 diagnosis.

assembly of the virus while the S and N proteins can be operate as essential biomarkers that might be utilized to detect SARS-CoV-2. The S-protein plays a crucial role in association with receptor-binding and host cell domains that interact with ACE2 receptors. To detect anti-SARS-CoV-2 antibodies, a patient's serum sample is used as a serological sample. Anti-SARS-CoV-2 IgM and IgG antibodies specifically generated against the S proteins by the infected patients in response to adaptive immune system activation is the most common diagnosis biomarker [11].

Commonly three types of technique are using for diagnosis and detection of viral load/COVID-19 infection including imaging techniques (x-ray, CT-scan and MRI), the molecular technique (RT-qPCR) and the immunological technique (ELISA). A basic comparison of these three techniques is shown in figure 7.3. Genes encoding protein E, S, N and RNA-dependent RNA polymerase (RdRp), and open reading frame (ORF1ab) are the current targets for nucleic acid-based diagnostic assays. Serology-based immunoassays have also been developed to detect antibodies IgM,

IgG, and IgA developed against SARS-CoV-2 specifically against S and N antigens of the COVID virus in patients [12].

LFIA has been actively explored and employed for COVID-19 diagnosis among available POC testing procedures due to its low cost, speed, and accessibility.

7.3 Lateral flow assay

LFA is usually a qualitative (gives an indication only about the presence or absence of biological entities or targets) chromatographic assay that is small, easy to carry, gives result within a minute and can be used anywhere as POC testing. Biological fluid samples, simply known as clinical samples, are applied to a sample pad that allows the sample to flow on the NC membrane and bands are observed on test and control lines after specific binding. The test is inexpensive and does not require any trained personnel, but it only yields qualitative results.

The lateral flow assay is based on the ELISA principle which means antigen (Ag) and antibody (Ab) interaction which are protein/glycoprotein in nature and therefore known as immuno-chromatography assay or lateral flow immuno-chromatography assay. However, in recent times nucleic acid (DNA/oligonucleotide) are being used instead of protein for early diagnosis which is known as nucleic acid-based lateral flow assay (NALFA) (figure 7.4). DNA also has unique properties such as it is stable, easy to isolate from the cell and can be synthesized *in vitro* easily. Therefore DNA is used to conjugate with nanoparticles and used as a recognition molecule in the assay. There are various diagnostic kits available based on DNA/ oligonucleotide as a hybridization probe for conjugation with NPs and which detect the specific nucleic acid sequences [13].

Nanoparticles (NPs) play a crucial role in enhancing the sensitivity and specificity of the developed LFA assay. For the development of sensitive and specific detection

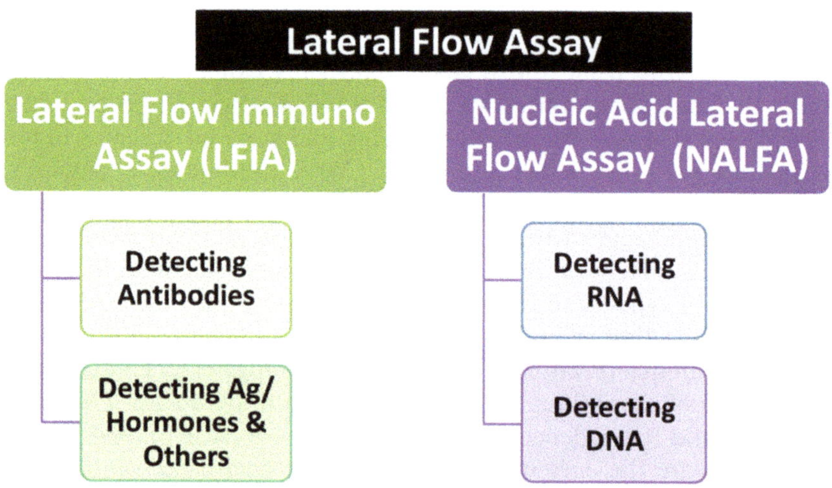

Figure 7.4. Type of lateral flow assay.

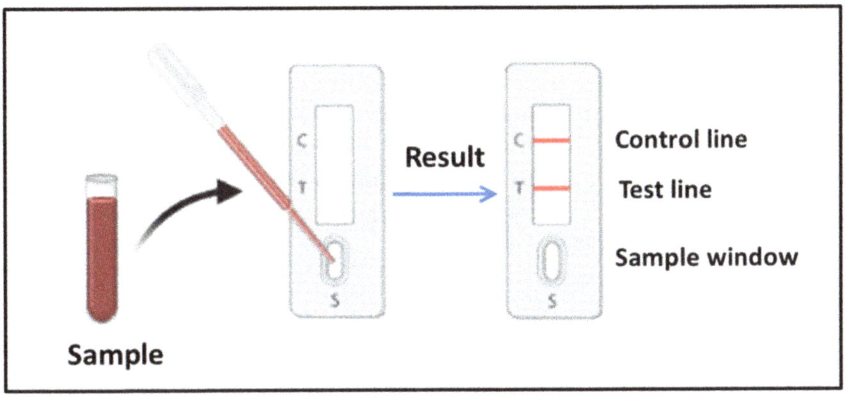

Figure 7.5. Performance of lateral flow assay and result analysis.

kits, different types of nanoparticles are using gold nanoparticles, silver nanoparticles, nanobeads, and fluorescent nanoparticles. The nanoparticles are the first choice in the development of detection assays because NPs retain many unique properties such as absorption, fluorescence, magnetic properties, as well as having a large surface-to-volume ratio, high surface-reaction activity and easy handling which allow these particles as a conjugate label in LFA [14]. The NPs could be easily conjugated with biomolecules by covalent or non-covalent bonds. For the development of rapid visual detection assay, AuNPs is the first choice due to its stability under exposure to heat and light, optical properties, ease of preparation and binding capacity, compatibility with biomolecules, low cost and visual elucidation by the naked eye [15]. The result analysis by bands observed on test and control lines as shown in figure 7.5.

7.3.1 Biological reagents in LFAs

7.3.1.1 The target molecules

The target molecule of LFA has a wide variety including proteins, glycoprotein, carbohydrate, nucleic acids, glycolipids, whole bacteria and may be a complex. These target molecules should be a specific biomarker. This target molecule could be purified native protein, recombinant protein, or artificially-produced molecules. The target molecule preferably produced in the laboratory. Bacterial or mammalian cell culture, molecular biology, protein expression, and purification and other biophysical techniques are used to prepare the target molecule. The target molecule used in LFA should be specific for clinical diagnosis purposes.

7.3.1.2 Recognition molecules

Commonly antibodies are used as recognition elements in the immuno-chromatography assay. The antibody used in the assay may be monoclonal, polyclonal or engineered by different methods (phage display). Polyclonal antibodies are generated in an animal model by immunizing with a specific Ag. However, the immunized animal sera consist of various antibodies that have different specificity and binding affinity. Therefore, the use of a polyclonal antibody in LFA has less sensitivity and specificity. Nowadays, monoclonal antibodies are used in detection assays over the polyclonal antibodies. A monoclonal antibody is derived by specific B-cell hybridoma because antibodies produced from this have a single affinity for the target Ag. The advantage of polyclonal antibodies is easy to produce and also obtained a large yield amount of antisera while the screening and isolation of a monoclonal antibody-secreting cell line are labour-intensive and a smaller amount is gained [16].

7.3.1.3 Clinical samples

The clinical sample is directly applied to a sample pad for detection/diagnosis of infection. The clinical sample has a wide variety including whole, blood, plasma, serum, nasal swab, body fluid and urine depending upon the infection. These clinical samples have variability in salt, pH and protein content [17].

7.3.2 Labels for ICT assay

The sensitivity of the developed assay is the main concern. However, the low limit of detection and specificity are often required at clinical diagnosis and another field of analysis [18]. Along with recognizing and target molecules, the conjugate label is a component of the developing detection assay. For onsite immune-detection assays, visual detection by the naked eye or using an optical reader is most common; however, there are various types of label available such as fluorescent, chemiluminescent, and magnetic measurement systems. Reporter particles, such as colorimetric ones (such as gold nanoparticles and colloidal carbon), luminescent ones (such as fluorescent probes, quantum dots, upconversion nanoparticles, and bioluminescent markers), electroactive compounds, and paramagnetic ones are used in LFA to transform the detection signal [19]. A general summary of the advantages and disadvantages of various labels used in the detection assay is listed in table 7.1.

Gold nanoparticles are still the most popular labels among all labels that are used in the development of LFA due to low cost, easy preparation and ease of use [24]. The gold nanoparticle is briefly described here.

7.3.2.1 Gold nanoparticles

AuNPs are most frequently used as a conjugate label in LFA assay due to their unique properties. The AuNPs can be easily synthesized in a laboratory and can be manipulated accordingly. They are stable with time, having large variety in size from 5 to 100 nm, biocompatible, intense surface plasmon resonance and have a concentrated red colour which is easy to detect even by the naked eye [25]. Of these properties, AuNPs are the most reported nanomaterial used as optical labels in the development of LFA [26]. AuNPs are not only used as detection probes in LFA assays, they have multiple attributes that make them powerful in imaging applications, as a biosensor and drug delivery and also have therapeutics use [27]. AuNPs have a strong binding affinity to amines, thiols, and disulfides which facilitate their conjugation with biomolecules (e.g., protein, hormone, antibodies, and DNA) [28].

Table 7.1. Advantages and disadvantages of various labels used in detection assays.

Label	Advantages	Disadvantages	References
Colloid gold	Well-characterized conjugation methods, comparatively high sensitivity	Difficult to suspend once dried; changing in pH and salt concentration leads to instability	[20, 21]
Cellulose nanobeads	High intensity colour; various colours, blue, green, black and red are available commercially could be used in multiplexing visual assays	Passive conjugation	[22]
Fluorescent particles	Highly uniform and reproducible, more highly sensitive in most cases than visual labels	Result can be analysed by reader only	[21, 23]
Coloured latex particles	Various known conjugation techniques are available, characterization is easy	Conjugate stability is the chief disadvantage, requires more concentration of antibody than Au	[21]

AuNPs have a wide range of sizes. The AuNPs with <5 nm exhibit high catalytic activities [29] while larger-sized AuNPs possess stronger optical absorbance because of the higher molar extinction coefficient of the larger size. The extinction coefficient of 80 nm size AuNPs is approximately 200 times higher than that of 15 nm size AuNPs. Therefore, the use of a large-sized AuNPs as a probe is advantageous to improving the sensitivity of the LFA assay. In detection assays, 20–40 nm AuNPs are commonly used. They have a maximum signal and also give a red colour that can be easily visualized [30]. The size, concentration, and quality of synthesized AuNPs are characterized by two different methods viz. absorption and fluorescence [25] by using different techniques: absorption spectroscopy; UV–visible spectroscopy [31], transmission electron microscopy [32], and dynamic light scattering [33].

Conjugation of recognition molecules to AuNPs is the most critical step in the development of LFA assay. The specificity and sensitivity of the assay are remarkably dependent on the level of conjugation. Various methods are established for conjugation based on the physical and chemical properties of AuNPs. There could be covalent or non-covalent bonds formed between protein/antibody and AuNP listed in table 7.2.

The biological activities of the conjugated gold colloid are evaluated by electrochemical measurements and immunoassay format [35].

Table 7.2. A table showing physical and chemical interaction between ligand and AuNPs surface [34].

Physical interaction	Chemical interaction
Hydrophobic interactions	By chemisorption via thiol derivatives
Ionic interactions	Through biolinkers or mediator linkers, e.g., polyethylene glycol (PEG)
Native binding	By using adaptor molecules: like Streptavidin

7.4 Principle of LFA

The principle of LFA is based on ELISA where antigen–antibody interaction occurs and antibody conjugated colloid gold allows the band on test and control line to be seen by the naked eye. As in ELISA the antibody is coated in a multiwall ELISA plate overnight, as in LFA the test and control antibody is coated on the NC membrane and is dryed overnight at room temperature or at 37 °C for 2–4 h. On the test line, a conjugate release pad is placed over the conjugated pad, the sample pad is placed over that and the adsorbent pad is placed at the end the LFA strip. The sample is applied on a sample pad which is presoaked with a buffer with a suitable composition of salts and surfactants that makes the sample suitable for interaction with the conjugate and capture molecule present on the conjugation pad and NC membrane, respectively. The sample with wash buffer or running buffer migrates through the conjugate release pad, which contains antibodies conjugated colloid gold or fluorescent particles (antibody is specific to the target analyte). The sample is bound to the antibody and forms the sample–antibody conjugated label complex and together with the conjugated antibody bound to the target analyte, migrates along the strip. The strip is porous and by capillary action the sample containing complex run towards the test and control line. The sample reacts with the test line which contains a recognition molecule (specific Ab generated against sample Ag) and reacts with the analyte bound to the conjugated antibody. Recognition of the sample analyte results in an appropriate interaction and colours the test line, while a response on the control line indicates the proper liquid flow through the strip. The result is represented by lines appearing on the test and control lines. The liquid flows across the strip and moves to an absorbent pad attached at the end of the strip and can be judged by eye or using a dedicated reader. The absorbent pad plays two important role: the first is to wick the excess reagents and the second is to prevent backflow of the liquid. The presence of the control line gives the idea of functionality of assay. If a band is observed on both test and control positions, the result is evaluated as positive while if a band is only observed on the control band it is considered negative. However, when no band is observed on the control line that indicates the assay is not working and cannot be used for sample analysis. The intensity of the test line is directly proportional to the concentration of the analyte. But visual detection is only a qualitative assay, not quantitative. For the multiplex assay, multiple test lines are drawn on the NC membrane [20].

There are two basic formats of LFA: sandwich and competitive [36]. In a sandwich format, a conjugate label (nanoparticles or magneto particle or fluorescence dyes) coated antibody or oligonucleotide is immobilized on the pretreated conjugate pad. A primary antibody or oligonucleotide specific for target analyte is immobilized over the test line. A secondary antibody or probe against labelled conjugate antibody/oligonucleotide is immobilized at the control zone. A sample containing the target molecule is applied to the sample pad and subsequently buffer is added (if required). However, the competitive format (also known as inhibition immunoassay) is commonly used for small molecular weight analyte with single antigenic determinants [37].

7.5 LFA-based diagnosis of SARS - Cov-2

To stop the disease from spreading further within the population, it is crucial to identify pathogens at an early stage. The most extensively used approach for COVID-19 diagnosis is real-time-qPCR that involves the reverse transcription of RNA and amplification of particular complementary DNA (cDNA) fragments. However, it can offer quantitative information of viral loads in a highly sensitive and selective manner, therefore, this approach has become the gold standard of clinical diagnosis of COVID-19 [38, 39]. However, this assay is time consuming and requires sophisticated equipment and trained users so this test cannot be performed in field conditions. For a rapidly spreading and contageous disease early detection needs to be easy, at point-of-care and performed at home or in the field. Paper-based ICT is one of the best point-of-care testing assays. From 2020 to date various paper-based ICT/LFIA have been developed worldwide in research laboratories as well as by many pharmaceutical companies. This LFA could target anti-SARS-CoV-2 IgM and IgG antibodies in clinical serum which is the primary choice of sample while a few assays target the antigen such as nucelocapsid protein. Many research and review papers are available which have validated or evaluated this commercially available LFIA for their sensitivity and specificity for anti-SARS-CoV-2 antibody or antigen [40–45]. In a study, clinical validation of an open-access LFA (OA-LFA) design was reported using the commercially available materials and reagents [42] while review papers are available that have compared the various detection assays including molecular and immunological system for detection of SARS-CoV-2 [46, 47]. A list of various different types of LFAs developed for diagnosis of COVID-19 is listed in table 7.3.

7.6 Discussion

The deadly repercussions of the current COVID-19 outbreak are still being felt around the world. The extremely communicable nature of this respiratory disease puts current viral detection technology to the test in terms of speed, scalability, affordability, and accuracy. Immunoassays have been utilized in the surveillance of individuals by detecting anti-SARS-CoV-2 Abs, whereas molecular assays have been the gold standard for direct detection of viral RNA in suspected individuals [12]. SARS and MERS, two viruses from the same taxonomic group, were

Table 7.3. List of developed LFA-based kit for diagnosis of SARS - Cov-2.

Lateral flow	Label used	Target	Sample	Detection sensitivity	References
Half-strip LFA	Latex bead	SARS-CoV-2	N protein samples	0.65 ng ml^{-1} (Genemedi N protein) 3.03 ng ml^{-1} (Genscript N protein)	[48]
Microfluidic-integrated LF RPA assay	Biotin- and FAM-labelled	RNA	Throat/nasopharyngeal swabs	30 copies per sample	[49]
Competitive LFA	Gold nanoparticles	Anti-N IgM and IgG antibodies	Serum	94% and 96% for IgM and IgG antibodies, respectively	[50]
Sandwich LFA	Europium-chelate-based fluorescent nanoparticles	ORF1ab, E and N regions of RNA	Throat swab or sputum sample	Sensitivities of 100% and specificities of 99% for both samples	[51]
Paper-based electrochemical LFA	Label-free	SARS-CoV-2 antibodies	Clinical sera	1 ng ml^{-1}	[52]
NG Biotech LFIA kit	Gold nanoparticle	Anti-SARS-CoV-2 IgG and IgM antibodies	Serum/plasma	IgM LFIA (95.8%)	[53]
NG Biotech LFIA kit	Gold nanoparticle	Anti-SARS-CoV-2 IgG and IgM	Serum/plasma	Sensitivity 85% and the specificity 98.3% for both IgG and IgM	[54]
Competitive LFA	Gold nanoparticle	Anti-SARS-CoV-2 IgG	Serum/plasma	Assure Tech Rapid Test showed a sensitivity 93.8%, the IFA and PRNT of 100%	[55]
Clungene	Gold nanoparticle	Anti-SARS-CoV-2 IgG and IgM	Plasma	Sensitivity	[56]

(*Continued*)

Table 7.3. (*Continued*)

Lateral flow	Label used	Target	Sample	Detection sensitivity	References
SARS-CoV-2-IgG/IgM Rapid Test				IgG- 87.3%, IgM- 50.8% and specificity 100.0% and 80.0% for IgG and IgM, respectively	
Competitive LFA	Gold nanoparticle	Anti-SARS-CoV-2 IgG and IgM	Blood	Sensitivity was 88.66% and specificity was 90.63%.	[57]
Sandwich and Competitive LFA	Dye-loaded polymersome	SARS-CoV-2 Antigen and antibody	Nasal swab and serum	93 and 92.2% sensitivity for antigen and antibody	[58]

responsible for past regional outbreaks. SARS-CoV-2 is a zoonotic virus, identical to the viruses that exaggerated the earlier viral outbreaks [59].

A huge number of detection and diagnostic systems and assays have been developed to date worldwide for early diagnosis of COVID-19 including SERS-based aptasensor [60], RT-LAMP [61, 62], reverse transcription recombinase polymerase amplification [63], paper-based electrochemical biosensor [52], electrochemical biosensor [64], CRISPR-Cas13a [65]. Test papers, such as pH test strips and urine test strips, are the most typical examples of paper used as a diagnostic tool. The purpose of the urine test strips is to identify certain metabolic products in the urine that are frequently used pathological markers [66]. LFAs are an appealing choice for monitoring disease prevalence and assessing vaccine responsiveness due to their cost-effectiveness, scalable manufacturing process, and appropriateness for self-testing. LFA is widely used in medical science, food analysis, environmental issues (for pollutants) and detection of biomarkers. Various LFAs have been developed for detection of bacterial pathogens—*Clostridium botulinum* [67], *Yersinia pestis* [68], *Bacillus anthracis* [69], *Brucella melitensis* [70] and for viruses including the influenza virus [71, 72], African swine fever virus [73], foot-and-mouth disease virus [74], ebola virus [75] and many more. To track SARS-CoV-2 transmission, LFA can detect anti-SARS-CoV-2 antibodies [76] and S and N antigen of SARS-CoV-2. Due to its quick reading, low cost, and convenience of use, LFA remains one of the most used POC tests worldwide, with noteworthy limitations including limited sensitivity, low specificity, and lack of quantitation [77].

7.7 Conclusion

The COVID-19 pandemic was caused by SARS-CoV-2 a deadly virus affected the life of people around the world. There are currently several different detection methods in use, and numerous new ones are also being created for the quick and in-the-moment diagnosis of COVID-19 infection in the wake of this pandemic. The improvement of reporter systems that would deliver test findings in real-time is a recent focus in immunological approaches for quick testing. For rapid detection and diagnosis, LFAs have been developed. LFA assay is simple, sensitive, specific, easy to handle and could be used for onsite detection. Colloid gold or gold nanoparticles are the most commonly used reporting system to date but to enhance the sensitivity of assays, new reporter systems need to be discovered. Early diagnosis is necessary for effective prevention and patient management. Thus, LFA assay could be an accurate, sensitive, and convenient method for the detection and diagnosis to achieve an effective result on the spot within few minutes.

References

[1] Yu S, Nimse S B, Kim J, Song K S and Kim T 2020 Development of a lateral flow strip membrane assay for rapid and sensitive detection of the SARS-CoV-2 *Anal. Chem.* **92** 14139–44

[2] Jiang X and Lillehoj P B 2021 Lateral flow immunochromatographic assay on a single piece of paper *Analyst* **146** 1084–90

[3] Mak W C, Beni V and Turner A P F 2016 Lateral-flow technology: from visual to instrumental *TrAC Trends Anal. Chem.* **79** 297–305

[4] Deng Y, Jiang H, Li X and Lv X 2021 Recent advances in sensitivity enhancement for lateral flow assay *Microchim. Acta* **188** 1–15

[5] Sajid M, Kawde A N and Daud M 2015 Designs, formats and applications of lateral flow assay: a literature review *J. Saudi Chem. Soc* **19** 689–705

[6] Pinheiro T, Cardoso A R, Sousa C E A, Marques A C, Tavares A P M and Matos A M *et al* 2021 Paper-based biosensors for COVID-19: a review of innovative tools for controlling the pandemic *ACS Omega* **6** 29268–90

[7] Bösmüller H, Matter M, Fend F and Tzankov A 2021 The pulmonary pathology of COVID-19 *Virchows Arch.* **478** 137

[8] Martín Giménez V M, Inserra F, Tajer C D, Mariani J, Ferder L and Reiter R J *et al* 2020 Lungs as target of COVID-19 infection: protective common molecular mechanisms of vitamin D and melatonin as a new potential synergistic treatment *Life Sci.* **254** 117808

[9] Chen P Y, Ko C H, Wang C J, Chen C W, Chiu W H and Hong C *et al* 2021 The early detection of immunoglobulins via optical-based lateral flow immunoassay platform in COVID-19 pandemic *PLoS One* **16** e0254486

[10] Chaudhary V, Royal A, Chavali M and Yadav S K 2021 Advancements in research and development to combat COVID-19 using nanotechnology *Nanotechnol. Environ. Eng.* **6** 1–15

[11] Singh K R B, Rathee S, Nagpure G, Singh J and Singh R P 2022 Smart and emerging nanomaterials-based biosensor for SARS-CoV-2 detection *Mater. Lett.* **307** 131092

[12] Habli Z, Saleh S, Zaraket H and Khraiche M L 2021 COVID-19 in-vitro diagnostics: state-of-the-art and challenges for rapid, scalable, and high-accuracy screening *Front. Bioeng. Biotechnol.* **8** 1562

[13] Corstjens P, Zuiderwijk M, Brink A, Li S, Feindt H and Niedbala R S *et al* 2001 Use of up-converting phosphor reporters in lateral-flow assays to detect specific nucleic acid sequences: a rapid, sensitive DNA test to identify human papillomavirus type 16 infection *Clin. Chem.* **47** 1885–93

[14] Huang X, Aguilar Z P, Xu H, Lai W and Xiong Y 2015 Membrane-based lateral flow immunochromatographic strip with nanoparticles as reporters for detection: a review *Biosens. Bioelectron.* **75** 166–80

[15] Lee L G, Nordman E S, Johnson M D and Oldham M F 2013 A low-cost, high-performance system for fluorescence lateral flow assays *Biosensors* **3** 360–73

[16] Christopher P, Robinson N and Shaw M K 2005 Antibody-label conjugates in lateral-flow assays *Drugs Abuse* (Totowa, NJ: Humana Press), pp 87–98

[17] Hsieh H V, Dantzler J L and Weigl B H 2017 Analytical tools to improve optimization procedures for lateral flow assays *Diagnostics (Basel, Switzerland)* **2** 29

[18] Oliveira-Rodríguez M, López-Cobo S, Reyburn H T, Costa-García A, López-Martín S and Yáñez-Mó M *et al* 2016 Development of a rapid lateral flow immunoassay test for detection of exosomes previously enriched from cell culture medium and body fluids *J. Extracell. Vesicles* **1** 31803

[19] Hu J, Choi J R, Wang S, Gong Y, Feng S and Pingguan-Murphy B *et al* 2017 Multiple test zones for improved detection performance in lateral flow assays *Sensors Actuators* B **243** 484–8

[20] Koczula K M and Gallotta A 2016 Lateral flow assays *Essays Biochem.* **60** 111–20

[21] Chun P 2009 Colloidal gold and other labels for lateral flow immunoassays *Lateral Flow Immunoassay* 1–19

[22] Choi E S, Lee S G, Lee S J and Kim E 2015 Rapid detection of 6 ×-histidine-labeled recombinant proteins by immunochromatography using dye-labeled cellulose nanobeads *Biotechnol. Lett.* **37** 627–32

[23] Xie Q Y, Wu Y H, Xiong Q R, Xu H Y, Xiong Y H and Liu K *et al* 2014 Advantages of fluorescent microspheres compared with colloidal gold as a label in immunochromatographic lateral flow assays *Biosens. Bioelectron.* **54** 262–5

[24] O'Farrell B 2015 Lateral flow technology for field-based applications-basics and advanced developments *Top. Companion Anim. Med.* **30** 139–47

[25] Zuber A, Purdey M, Schartner E, Forbes C, Van Der Hoek B and Giles D *et al* 2016 Detection of gold nanoparticles with different sizes using absorption and fluorescence based method *Sensors Actuators* B **227** 117–27

[26] Quesada-González D and Merkoçi A 2015 Nanoparticle-based lateral flow biosensors *Biosens. Bioelectron.* **73** 47–63

[27] Yeh Y C, Creran B and Rotello V M 2012 Gold nanoparticles: preparation, properties, and applications in bionanotechnology *Nanoscale* **4** 1871–80

[28] Das M, Shim K H, An S S A and Yi D K 2011 Review on gold nanoparticles and their applications *Toxicol. Environ. Heal. Sci.* **3** 193–205

[29] Balasubramanian S K, Yang L, Yung L Y L, Ong C N, Ong W Y and Yu L E 2010 Characterization, purification, and stability of gold nanoparticles *Biomaterials* **31** 9023–30

[30] Li J, Duan H, Xu P, Huang X and Xiong Y 2016 Effect of different-sized spherical gold nanoparticles grown layer by layer on the sensitivity of an immunochromatographic assay *RSC Adv.* **6** 26178–85

[31] Amendola V and Meneghetti M 2009 Size evaluation of gold nanoparticles by UV–vis spectroscopy *J. Phys. Chem.* C **113** 4277–85

[32] Busch R T, Karim F, Weis J, Sun Y, Zhao C and Vasquez E S 2019 Optimization and structural stability of gold nanoparticle-antibody bioconjugates *ACS Omega* **4** 15269–79

[33] Fagúndez P, Botasini S, Tosar J P and Endez E M 2017 Systematic process evaluation of the conjugation of proteins to gold nanoparticles *Heliyon* **6** e07392

[34] Jazayeri M H, Amani H, Pourfatollah A A, Pazoki-Toroudi H and Sedighimoghaddam B 2016 Various methods of gold nanoparticles (GNPs) conjugation to antibodies *Sens. Bio-Sensing Res.* **9** 17–22

[35] Thobhani S, Attree S, Boyd R, Kumarswami N, Noble J and Szymanski M *et al* 2010 Bioconjugation and characterisation of gold colloid-labelled proteins *J. Immunol. Methods* **356** 60–9

[36] Hsiao W W W, Le T N, Pham D M, Ko H H, Chang H C and Lee C C *et al* 2021 Recent advances in novel lateral flow technologies for detection of COVID-19 *Biosensors* **9** 295

[37] Raeisossadati M J, Danesh N M, Borna F, Gholamzad M, Ramezani M and Abnous K *et al* 2016 Lateral flow based immunobiosensors for detection of food contaminants *Biosens. Bioelectron.* **86** 235–46

[38] Zhou Y, Wu Y, Ding L, Huang X and Xiong Y 2021 Point-of-care COVID-19 diagnostics powered by lateral flow assay *TrAC Trends Anal. Chem.* 145

[39] Xi H, Juhas M and Zhang Y 2020 G-quadruplex based biosensor: a potential tool for SARS-CoV-2 detection *Biosens. Bioelectron.* **167** 112494

[40] Owen S I, Williams C T, Garrod G, Fraser A J, Menzies S and Baldwin L *et al* 2022 Twelve lateral flow immunoassays (LFAs) to detect SARS-CoV-2 antibodies *J. Infect.* **84** 355–60
[41] Mahmoudinobar F, Britton D and Montclare J K 2021 Protein-based lateral flow assays for COVID-19 detection *Protein Eng. Des. Sel.* **34** 1–10
[42] Bachman C M, Grant B D, Anderson C E, Alonzo L F, Garing S and Byrnes S A *et al* 2021 Clinical validation of an open-access SARS-COV-2 antigen detection lateral flow assay, compared to commercially available assays *PLoS One* **16** e0256352
[43] Flower B, Brown J C, Simmons B, Moshe M, Frise R and Penn R *et al* 2020 Clinical and laboratory evaluation of SARS-CoV-2 lateral flow assays for use in a national COVID-19 seroprevalence survey *Thorax* **75** 1082–8
[44] Fischer P U, Fischer K, Curtis K C, Huang Y, Fetcho N and Goss C W *et al* 2021 Evaluation of commercial rapid lateral flow tests, alone or in combination, for SARS-CoV-2 antibody testing *Am. J. Trop. Med. Hyg.* **105** 378–86
[45] Peto T, Affron D, Afrough B, Agasu A, Ainsworth M and Allanson A *et al* 2021 COVID-19: rapid antigen detection for SARS-CoV-2 by lateral flow assay: a national systematic evaluation of sensitivity and specificity for mass-testing *EClinicalMedicine* **36** 100924
[46] Mohit E, Rostami Z and Vahidi H 2021 A comparative review of immunoassays for COVID-19 detection *Expert Rev. Clin. Immunol.* **17** 573–99
[47] Eftekhari A, Alipour M, Chodari L, Dizaj S M, Ardalan M R and Samiei M *et al* 2021 A comprehensive review of detection methods for SARS-CoV-2 *Microorganism* **9** 232
[48] Grant B D, Anderson C E, Williford J R, Alonzo L F, Glukhova V A and Boyle D S *et al* 2020 SARS-CoV-2 coronavirus nucleocapsid antigen-detecting half-strip lateral flow assay toward the development of point of care tests using commercially available reagents *Anal. Chem.* **92** 11305–9
[49] Liu D, Shen H, Zhang Y, Shen D, Zhu M and Song Y *et al* 2021 A microfluidic-integrated lateral flow recombinase polymerase amplification (MI-IF-RPA) assay for rapid COVID-19 detection *Lab Chip* **21** 2019–26
[50] Alhabbab R Y, Alfaleh M A, Alsulaiman R M, Alamri S S, Eyouni M S and ElAssouli M-Z *et al* 2022 Amplifying lateral flow assay signals for rapid detection of COVID-19 specific antibodies *Glob. Challenges* **7** 2200008
[51] Wang D, He S, Wang X, Yan Y, Liu J and Wu S *et al* 2020 Rapid lateral flow immunoassay for the fluorescence detection of SARS-CoV-2 RNA *Nat. Biomed. Eng.* **4** 1150–8
[52] Yakoh A, Pimpitak U, Rengpipat S, Hirankarn N, Chailapakul O and Chaiyo S 2021 Paper-based electrochemical biosensor for diagnosing COVID-19: detection of SARS-CoV-2 antibodies and antigen *Biosens. Bioelectron.* **176** 112912
[53] Nicol T, Lefeuvre C, Serri O, Pivert A, Joubaud F and Dubée V *et al* 2020 Assessment of SARS-CoV-2 serological tests for the diagnosis of COVID-19 through the evaluation of three immunoassays: two automated immunoassays (Euroimmun and Abbott) and one rapid lateral flow immunoassay (NG Biotech) *J. Clin. Virol.* **129** 104511
[54] Garlantézec R, Heslan C, Tadie E, Tattevin P, Thibault V and Paris C 2020 A lateral flow immunoassay test performance in SARS-CoV-2 seroprevalence surveys: a validation study among healthcare workers *Emerg. Microbes Infect.* **9** 2547–9
[55] Kohmer N, Westhaus S, Rühl C, Ciesek S and Rabenau H F 2020 Clinical performance of different SARS-CoV-2 IgG antibody tests *J. Med. Virol.* **92** 2243–7

[56] Ragnesola B, Jin D, Lamb C C, Shaz B H, Hillyer C D and Luchsinger L L 2020 COVID19 antibody detection using lateral flow assay tests in a cohort of convalescent plasma donors *BMC Res. Notes* **1** 1–7
[57] Li Z, Yi Y, Luo X, Xiong N, Liu Y and Li S *et al* 2020 Development and clinical application of a rapid IgM–IgG combined antibody test for SARS-CoV-2 infection diagnosis *J. Med. Virol.* **92** 1518–24
[58] Ghorbanizamani F, Tok K, Moulahoum H, Harmanci D, Hanoglu S B and Durmus C *et al* 2021 Dye-loaded polymersome-based lateral flow assay: rational design of a COVID-19 testing platform by repurposing SARS-CoV-2 antibody cocktail and antigens obtained from positive human samples *ACS Sens.* **6** 2988–97
[59] Singh D and Yi S V 2021 On the origin and evolution of SARS-CoV-2 *Exp. Mol. Med.* **53** 537–47
[60] Chen H, Park S G, Choi N, Kwon H J, Kang T and Lee M K *et al* 2021 Sensitive detection of SARS-CoV-2 using a SERS-based aptasensor *ACS Sens.* **6** 2378–85
[61] Sherrill-Mix S, Hwang Y, Roche A M, Glascock A, Weiss S R and Li Y *et al* 2021 Detection of SARS-CoV-2 RNA using RT-LAMP and molecular beacons *Genome Biol.* **22** 1–17
[62] Agarwal S, Warmt C, Henkel J, Schrick L, Nitsche A and Bier F F 2022 Lateral flow–based nucleic acid detection of SARS-CoV-2 using enzymatic incorporation of biotin-labeled dUTP for POCT use *Anal. Bioanal. Chem.* **414** 3177–86
[63] Yu Y, Su G, Zhang W S, Pan J, Li F and Zhu M *et al* 2021 Reverse transcription recombinase polymerase amplification coupled with CRISPR-Cas12a for facile and highly sensitive colorimetric SARS-CoV-2 detection *Anal. Chem.* **93** 4126–33
[64] Chaibun T, Puenpa J, Ngamdee T, Boonapatcharoen N, Athamanolap P and O'Mullane A P *et al* 2021 Rapid electrochemical detection of coronavirus SARS-CoV-2 *Nat. Commun.* **12** 1–10
[65] Fozouni P, Son S, Díaz de León Derby M, Knott G J, Gray C N and D'Ambrosio M V *et al* 2021 Amplification-free detection of SARS-CoV-2 with CRISPR-Cas13a and mobile phone microscopy *Cell* **184** 323–33 .e9
[66] Hui Q, Pan Y and Yang Z 2020 Paper-based devices for rapid diagnostics and testing sewage for early warning of COVID-19 outbreak *Case Stud. Chem. Environ. Eng.* **2** 100064
[67] Gessler F, Pagel-Wieder S, Avondet M A and Böhnel H 2007 Evaluation of lateral flow assays for the detection of botulinum neurotoxin type A and their application in laboratory diagnosis of botulism *Diagn. Microbiol. Infect. Dis.* **57** 243–9
[68] Hsu H L, Chuang C C, Liang C C, Chiao D J, Wu H L and Wu Y P *et al* 2018 Rapid and sensitive detection of *Yersinia pestis* by lateral-flow assay in simulated clinical samples *BMC Infect. Dis.* **18** 1–12
[69] Puranik N, Pal V, Tripathi N K N K and Goel A K A K 2020 Development of a rapid immunochromatographic assay for detection of surface array protein (Sap), a potent biomarker of *Bacillus anthracis Biologia (Bratisl)* **75** 613–7
[70] Ge L, Wang D, Lian F, Zhao J, Wang Y and Zhao Y *et al* 2021 Lateral flow immunoassay for visible detection of human brucellosis based on blue silica nanoparticles *Front. Vet. Sci.* **8** 1396
[71] Han M Y, Xie T A, Li J X, Chen H J, Yang X H and Guo X G 2020 Evaluation of lateral-flow assay for rapid detection of influenza virus *BioMed Res. Int.* 2020
[72] Kim S K, Sung H, Hwang S H and Kim M N 2022 A new quantum dot-based lateral flow immunoassay for the rapid detection of influenza viruses *Biochip J.* **16** 175–82

[73] Zhu W, Meng K, Zhang Y, Bu Z, Zhao D and Meng G 2022 Lateral flow assay for the detection of african swine fever virus antibodies using gold nanoparticle-labeled acid-treated p72 *Front. Chem.* **9** 1164

[74] Jae K O, Ferris N P, Lee K N, Joo Y S, Hyun B H and Park J H 2009 Simple and rapid lateral-flow assay for the detection of foot-and-mouth disease virus *Clin. Vaccine Immunol.* **16** 1660–4

[75] Phan J C, Pettitt J, George J S, Fakoli L S, Taweh F M and Bateman S L *et al* 2016 Lateral flow immunoassays for ebola virus disease detection in liberia *J. Infect. Dis.* **214** S222–8

[76] Trombetta B A, Kandigian S E, Kitchen R R, Grauwet K, Webb P K and Miller G A *et al* 2021 Evaluation of serological lateral flow assays for severe acute respiratory syndrome coronavirus-2 *BMC Infect. Dis.* **21** 1–14

[77] Liu Y, Zhan L, Qin Z, Sackrison J and Bischof J C 2021 Ultrasensitive and highly specific lateral flow assays for point-of-care diagnosis *ACS Nano* **15** 3593–611

Chapter 8

Development of paper-based assay for detection of miRNA in various diseases

Rohit Kumar Singh, Bijayananda Panigarhi and Uday Suryakant

8.1 Introduction

Nanobiotechnology is an innovative and exciting area of science, which includes numerous fields such as chemistry, biology, biotechnology, agriculture, biomedical sciences, etc. Biosensor-based technology has advanced greatly in recent years, particularly for biomedical diagnostics and environmental pollution detection [1]. In comparison to laboratory-based big equipment, biosensing devices are often fast, sensitive, selective, and user-friendly, and do not require lengthy pre-treatment of materials or skilled staff [2]. Thus, the rapid development of nanotechnology-based research lead to the development of new nanomaterials that have been widely applied in biosensor application especially in the detection of antibiotics, heavy metals, pesticide, fungicide, rare earth metals, and pathogenic biomarkers [3–7] because of the exclusive biochemical, biophysical properties of the nanomaterials. In addition, the size of the nanomaterials has played a crucial role in the different biosensing applications. Nanomaterials, such as carbon nanoparticles [8], metal nanoparticles [9], silica nanoparticles [10], quantum dots (QDs) [11], proteins, peptides [12], and other functionalized nanoparticles, have been investigated for biomedical applications such as drug delivery, tissue engineering, antimicrobial agents [13], biosensors [14] and immunosensors [15]. For an economical diagnostic kit, the combination of nanomaterials with biosensors offers significant promise for monitoring biomolecules and sensitive detection of target analytes. When utilized as functional materials on electrode surfaces, nanomaterials have been reported to act as carriers to load signal markers or directly as signal reporters for selective detection of biomarkers, and they can speed up electron transmission. Various disease biomarkers such as protein, enzyme, nucleic acid, or any small molecule have been used in day-to-day life for diagnosis. However, detecting disease through traditional methods leads to lower efficiency, lower sensitivity, etc. Therefore,

doi:10.1088/978-0-7503-5820-0ch8

© IOP Publishing Ltd 2023

molecular-based diagnosis infrastructure was developed for the diagnosis of sex--linked disease, cancer, and viral disease. Nowadays everybody needs a first diagnostic report and rapid testing is a major concern in today's rapidly growing world. This was realized during the COVID-19 pandemic, where rapid diagnosis with high accuracy was a major need. Molecular diagnosis of viral nucleic acid detection with RT-PCR was a time-consuming, costly procedure, needing trained people and high-quality BSL 3 level lab facilities. Therefore, developing these types of diagnostic tools at low cost, which are easy to operate to detect pathogenic biomarkers like microRNAs (miRNAs) have been recent hot topics. A miRNA is a group of small non-coding RNAs which perform a vital role in gene regulation during post transcription which leads to mRNA degradation [16]. Therefore, these types of macromolecule are used as potential biomarker contestants for the diagnosis of different diseases [17]. Especially, quantitative real-time PCR (qPCR) is a commonly used technique for miRNA for quantification and validation. However, developing highly sensitive and selective miRNA detection methods remains difficult. Due to their distinct properties, such as low abundance, tiny size, and high sequence homology among family members, they are rare [18]. Besides, the cost of setting up a lab with qPCR and ready availability everywhere is a major challenge. These methods are time-consuming because of the complex process needed to isolate miRNA and the time-consuming PCR cycle processes. Therefore, to solve this problem, this chapter gathers nanomaterial-based biosensors. In order to gain significant benefits in miRNA detection, it is critical to create low cost, transferrable, and less costly technologies for POC and in-field assays. As a result, paper-based biosensors for detecting mRNA-based disease biomarkers, such as lateral flow test-strips (LFTSs) and developing paper microfluidics, provide important diagnostic platforms to address this need. These nanomaterial-based LFTSs and paper microfluidic devices show significant promise for improving detection sensitivity and selectivity by combining with various types of NPs.

8.2 MicroRNA and its role

MicroRNAs (miRNAs) are naturally transcribed single-strand nucleic acid molecules of 18–27 nucleotide base and are considered non-expressive or non-coding RNAs, which is not responsible for protein synthesis for gene expression [19]. According to some research, the bulk of human genomes is translated into non-coding RNAs. While the bulk of ncRNAs has uncertain functions. The majority of miRNAs are found in split gene regions, with about 30% of miRNA genes found in intergenic areas or the antisense orientation of genes, each with its promoter and regulatory units [20]. In the nucleus, an 80 nt primary or pri-miRNA is translated from the genome and broken by the nuclear RNase III enzyme Drosha [21]. As a result, a 60–70 nucleotide stem-loop intermediate called pre-miRNA is produced, and Ran-GTP and Exportin-5 aggressively traffic it to the cytoplasm. Further, pre-miRNA is processed by a nuclease such as RNase III endonuclease forming Dicer complex in the cytoplasmic region, and form 20–22 nt double-stranded fragment which is fused into RNA-induced silencing complex (RISC) [19]. miRNAs' 5′ region binds to the 3′ untranslated region (3′ UTR) on target messenger RNA (mRNA) transcripts, causing translational suppression or mRNA destruction in many cases [22] miRNA expression patterns range from universal to cell/tissue-specific, and its role is determined by the substances of the cell and the obtainability of targets inside the cell [23].

8.3 The involvement of microRNAs in disease

Lin-4 miRNA was the first microRNA identified in 1993. It has been about 30 years since the first microRNA (miRNA) was discovered, and microRNAs are now involved in a wide range of physiological and pathological processes. It has been postulated that mutations impacting miRNA activity may have a role in the development of human illnesses since the discovery of miRNAs' significant effect on biological processes. MicroRNAs have been discovered to have a crucial impact in a variety of human disorders in recent years. Furthermore, several researchers have attempted to use miRNAs in human illnesses for diagnostic and therapeutic purposes. We review the significance of miRNAs in pathological processes and discuss how miRNAs may be employed as disease biomarkers in this chapter.

8.4 Different miRNA detection methods

8.4.1 Electrochemical detection of miRNA

Electrochemical biosensors are a good choice for diagnostics purposes and are fast, simple, and economical for the study of nucleic acid. A characteristic electrochemical biosensor consists of a solid electrode with an immobilized short single-stranded nucleotide probe on it and electroactive hybridization indicators. The efficiency of electrochemical biosensors depends on the annealing of the probe and the complementary sequence [24].

Electrochemical detection of miRNA is found in the literature depending on the hybridization method. After the hybridization process takes place, there are different techniques to convert the annealing result into a calculable signal. Sensitivity is one of the challenging factors for developing an electrochemical sensor. When the targeted gene exists in the form of a distinct copy in the genome of the organism, the quantity of DNA/RNA is detected at the attomolar to femtomolar level [25, 26].

There are various methods such as miRNA microarrays, mass spectrometry, optical, northern blotting, sequencing, (PCR)-based techniques, and electrochemical methods that are being studied for sensitive and selective detection of miRNA [27]. Comparing all the methods, electrochemical detection methods are cost-effective and, also offer higher selectivity and sensitivity detection [28]. Electrochemical techniques can be used for developing paper-based sensors integrated with it [29]. These collective systems consist of permutations of different electrodes, like ion-selective or microelectrodes [30]. They deliver signal amplification while working in flow injection systems. As well, paper-based analytical devices can also be combined with several electrochemical methods, such as amperometry, coulometer, cyclic voltammetry, impedimetric detection, and potentiometric techniques [31].

Eskin *et al* reported a gold nanoparticle (AuNPs) converted paper-based electrode platform used to sense target microRNA-155 by the electrochemical impedance spectroscopy method. The impedimetric sensing of miRNA-155 was achieved by determining the fractional change at the charge transfer resistance (Rct), the limit of detection in PBS was found to be 33.8 nm in foetal bovine serum, the medium was 93.4 nm. The selectivity of the developed paper-based biosensor was compared to non-complementary and mismatch miRNA sequences in the presence of a mixture sample containing miRNA:NC (1:1) and miRNA:MM (1:1) in PBS (pH 7.40) or FBS (Paper-based electrode assemble for impedimetric detection of miRNA) [32].

Wang *et al* developed a novel paper-based biosensor for the simultaneous detection of different miRNA(miRNA-155 and miRNA-126). The developed paper-based sensing microfluidic platform was made by the combination of a screen-printing method, wax printing technology, and *in situ* AuNPs development to form hydrophobic boundaries, hydrophilic areas, driving electrode regions, waterproof electronic bridge, and parallel bipolar electrode regions. They used CdTe quantum dots (QDs)-H2 and Au@g-C_3N_4nanosheets (NSs)-DNA1 as dual electrochemiluminescence signal probes and carboxylated Fe_3O_4 magnetic nanoparticles existed as carriers. CdTe QDs-H_2/$S_2O_8^{2-}$ and Au@g-C_3N_4 NSs-DNA1/ $S_2O_8^{2-}$ provided different tough and constant emissions when voltages of 9 and 12 v were delivered respectively, this helped in forming operative potential-resolved signal tags. Additionally, the developed 3D DNA nanomachine model and the target miRNA cycle strategy helped in achieving dual amplification of electrochemiluminescence intensity. The unique design of the electrode system and multi-target electrochemiluminescence method helped in reducing the spatial interference between substances. The limit of detection was 5.7 and 4.2 fM for miRNA-155 and miRNA-126 respectively for the proposed ECL biosensor. With the unique design of the system, great selectivity, and sensitivity, the developed paper-based biosensor is an efficient system for clinical application, especially in the detection of different targets [33] (figure 8.1).

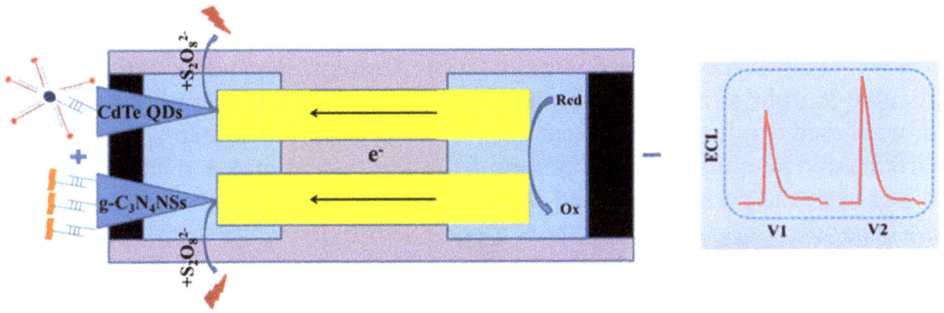

Figure 8.1. Schematic illustration of detection of multiple miRNAs (miRNA-155 and miRNA-126) by CdTe quantum dots (QDs)-H2 and Au@g-C3N4 nanosheets (NSs)-DNA1.

Torul *et al* developed a paper-based electrochemical biosensor for detecting microRNAs (miRNA-155 and miRNA-21) associated with the initial diagnosis of lung cancer. Wax printing was used for developing hydrophobic barriers for creating electrode space, the electrode system was made by a simple model approach. The system consisted of a carbon-based functioning electrode that was reformed using either reduced graphene oxide or molybdenum disulfide nanosheets reformed with gold nanoparticles (AuNPs/RGO, AuNPs/MoS_2) hybrid structures. The final developed paper-based biosensors showed excellent efficiency in sensing miRNA-155 and miRNA-21 by differential pulse voltammetry (DPV) of only 5.0 µl samples. The total duration of detection of miRNA along with electrode modification was completed within in 35 min The LOD for miRNA-21 and miRNA-155 was found to be 12.0 and 25.7 nM for AuNPs/RGO and 51.6 and 59.6 nM for AuNPs/MoS_2 sensors. The paper-based electrochemical biosensors developed were sensitive and specific enough to differentiate the specifically targeted miRNA in presence of single-base mismatch miRNA or non-complementary miRNA sequences [34].

8.4.2 Optical detection of miRNA

Some of the nanoparticles, such as AuNPs and quantum dots (QDs) due to their optical properties are used as optical signal reporters in the paper-based trip biosensor, AuNPs particularly have many distinct advantages, good compatibility, chemically stability, easy surface modification, and also have great naked-eye visibility and are extremely good at specificity and sensitivity of the analytes. This makes them a better choice as signal indicators for colorimetric sensing of the analytes in paper-based trip biosensors. Similarly, QDs are efficient enough to be labelled due to their better fluorescent and optical properties, as well as size-tunable light emission and various excitations of multiple fluorescence colours [35]. The lateral flow strip biosensors and AuNPs, QDs are considered as favourable methods due to their rapid analysis, low costs, high sensitivity, and specificity for detection of specific miRNA [36].

Deng *et al* developed a quantum dot-labelled strip biosensor for the very first time centred on a target-recycled, non-enzymatic amplification approach for miRNA detection. The strip biosensor system was developed using commercial quantum dots from Wuhan Jiayuan Quantum Dots Co., Ltd. (Wuhan, China) as they delivered better photostable signal labels, which helps the system with better sensing efficiency. This target-recycled amplification strategy depends on the sequence particular hairpin strand displacement method without the support of enzymes, and was used to further increase the sensitivity of the system; removing the environment-susceptible enzyme protein from the system makes it easy to preserve and increases the permanency and reproducibility of this sensor. The sensors with these many exceptional features show a good sensitivity range from 2 to 200 fmol, with LOD as 200 amol. The biosensor has proved to be 10 fold more sensitive than gold nanoparticles-based paper strip biosensor for detection of miRNA. Therefore, the developed biosensor has great potential for point of care applications and early cancer diagnosis [37] (figure 8.2).

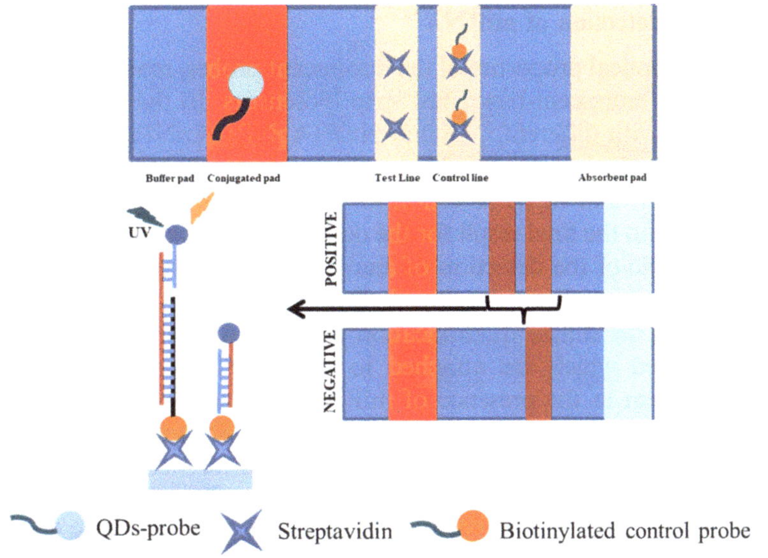

Figure 8.2. Schematic illustration of the QDs-labelled strip biosensor for the amplification products detection.

These are some of the novel approaches of gold nanoparticle, paper-based strip biosensors. Gao *et al* made DNA–GNP based biosensor for very specific, sensitive and optical sensing of miRNA-215. The specific miRNA sensing can be done simply by seeing the colour change and quantifying it using a simple paper-based strip instrument. Considering the conditions a quantitative detection limit of 60 pM within 20 min was obtained. The intervention of other constituents in the real biological samples is minor during analysis. The specific miRNA-215 could be well detected in A549 lysate without any complex purification or separation methods [36]. Hou *et al* developed a method that uses lateral flow nucleic acid strips and AuNPs can sense and quantify miRNA with a limit of detection of 1 fmol and 5 amol without and with silver enhancement respectively. The method is different from other sandwich processes; the tested microRNA and the detection probe perfectly match the capture probe in this study. The unique design of the system allows miRNA to crosslink its capture probe at room temperature. The assay takes about 70 min after the probe and sample preparations. But, the assay was reported for detecting miRNA-21 very effectively [38]. Zheng *et al* reported a low cost approach for multiplex miRNA assay on lateral flow nucleic acid biosensor. The biosensor was based on the nucleic acid hybridization reactions principle to develop gold nanoparticle GNP-attached complexes (ssDNA-microRNA–ssDNA/GNPs), which are caught and pictured on the test zone of lateral flow nucleic acid biosensor (LFNAB). The biosensor design consists of three different test zones on the strip, for instantaneous sensing of microRNA-21, microRNA-155 and microRNA-210 were attained with the addition of measuring model employing GNP as the visual tag. The test strip is a valued technique for clinical application and biomedical diagnosis [39].

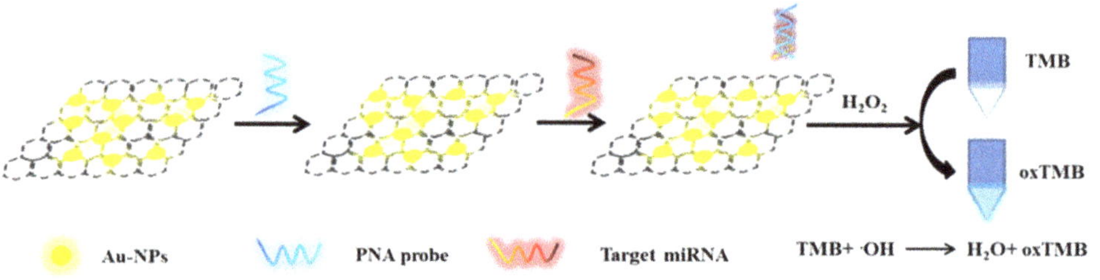

Figure 8.4. Schematic of the label-free visible sensor for miRNA detection based on the peroxidase-like catalytic ability of graphene/AuNP hybrids.

range from 1 to 700 pM, with LOD of 0.6 pM, another assay was carried on a Y-shaped paper-based microfluidic device to use the characteristic features of micro-channels such as short response time, low production cost, with very low reagent volume, etc. This paper-based assay produced a good linear range of 10–1000 pM with a detection limit of 4.1 pM. This biosensor is very efficient in the detection of miRNA-21 in the real sample (human urine sample) and proves the colorimetric method is an acceptable method [46].

S. No.	Material	Type	Analyte	Diagnosis disease	LOD	Reference
1.	AuNPs@BHQ2	Fluorescence-based	miRNA (miR-5010, miR-331	Parkinson disease	3.42×10^{-15} mol l^{-1}	[41]
2.	Quantum dots (λ_{ex} = 605 nm) coated with streptavidin	Optical-based biosensor	miRNA-21	Various cancer diseases	200 amol	[37]
3.	AuNPs	Electrochemical detection	miRNA (miRNA-155)	Lung diseases (asthma, cystic fibrosis)	33.8 nM in PBS 93.4 nM in foetal bovine serum	[32]
4.	Luminescent reporter (PT) impregnated PVDF paper	Optical detection/ colorimetric detection	miRNA-21	Lung cancer		[45]
5.	CdTe (QDs)	Electrochemiluminescence based	miRNA (miRNA-155 and miRNA-126)	Lung diseases, digestive system cancer	miRNA-155–5.7 fM miRNA-126–4.2 fM	[33]

(*Continued*)

(Continued)

S. No.	Material	Type	Analyte	Diagnosis disease	LOD	Reference
6.	AuNPs/RGO AuNPs/MoS_2	Electrochemical-based biosensor	miRNA (miRNA-155 and miRNA-21) miRNA (miRNA-155 and miRNA-21)	Lung cancer	miRNA-155–25.7 nM miRNA-21–12.0 nM miRNA-155–59.6 nM miRNA-21–51.6 nM	[34]
7.	Ag@Au core–shell/GQD conductive nano ink	Electrochemical-based	miRNA-21 in human plasma samples	Cancer	5 pM	[47]
8.	Cu-MOFS modified with AuNPs	Electrochemical-based biosensor	miRNA-155 in serum samples	Lung cancer	0.35 fM	[48]
9.	DNA–AgNCs	Fluorescence-based	miRNA-155	Cancer	0.1 nM	[49]
10.	Graphene/ AuNP hybrid	Colorimetric-based sensor	miRNA-21 detection in human serum	Lung disease in premature infants	3.2 nM	[44]
11.	DNA–Ag/Pt NCs	Colorimetric-based sensor	miRNA-21 detection in human sample	Cancer	0.6 pM	[46]
12.	DNA–GNP	Optical-based detection	miRNA-215 in aqueous solutions and biological samples	Breast cancer	60 pM	[36]
13.	S1-Cyt c-p-TiO2@PtNPs	Electrochemical-based biosensor	miRNA-155	Lung cancer	0.35 fM	[50]
14.	OsO2 nanoparticles (osmium oxide)	Electrochemical-based biosensor	miRNA		80 fmol l^{-1} in 2.5-μl Droplets,	[51]
15.	DNA–gold nanoparticle	Fluorescence-based	miR-203	Breast cancer	0.2 fmol	[40]
16.	Gold nanoparticle (GNP)-attached complexes (ssDNA-microRNA-ssDNA/GNPs)	Optical-based detection	microRNA-21, microRNA-155, miRNA-210	Lung and breast cancer	miRNA-21–0.073 nM, miRNA-155–0.061 nM, miRNA-210–0.085 nM	[39]

17.	AuNPs-thiol DNA	Optical-based detection	miRNA-21	Lung disease	1 fmol without Ag attachment 5 amo with Ag attachment	[38]
18.	P1/P2–CNNS-carbon nitride nanosheet	Fluorescence-based biosensor	miR-106a	Alzheimer's disease	0.10 pM	[42]
19.	mf-CNNS/ ssDNA, folate assembled	Fluorescence-based biosensor	miRNAs in a living cell		(In Live cells)	[43]

8.5 Future prospective paper-based assay for detection of miRNA

MicroRNAs (miRNAs) are a promising class of molecules that affect gene expression, and their level and type are linked to early detection, focused therapy, and disease prognosis [52]. Improving the accuracy of miRNA detection would result in extraordinary breakthroughs in early treatment [53]. Many approaches have been proposed to enhance sensitivity, and have recently proven invaluable in the detection of miRNAs [54]. However, there is a scarcity of research that focuses on improving detection specificity. This chapter provides a retrospective summary of the most common detection methods, including northern blot, quantitative polymerase chain reaction reverse transcription, next-generation sequencing, and microarrays which are among the most popular detection methods covered in this category [55]. Because of their maturity and stability, common approaches play a significant role in a variety of ways. The difficulty of specificity, however, persists. As a result, this chapter brings together the findings of classic procedures that are closely related to progressive strategies for increasing specificity. Therefore, this chapter summarizes the results of traditional techniques which are closely related to progressive methods to improve specificity [56]. Furthermore, much research is targeted on improving accuracy and is looking for a realistic recipe of common methods and strategies to help enhance precision [57]. This objective of this chapter is to demonstrate the significance of detection accuracy and explore how to improve the specificity in the detection of miRNAs, especially homologous families [58].

8.6 Conclusion

Understanding the importance of miRNA in the human body and complex gene regulatory networks is very important because these effector molecules could be applicable in diagnosis via nano-based sensing methods. The combination of biomaterials and antisense miRNA technology will be the new future dimensions of the therapeutic tool. Biosensing in new nanotechnology-based platforms will become the new diagnostic tools for different diseases. Thus, nano-based biomaterials synthesis and its potential biomedical application have been gaining momentum to establish a solid understanding of the development of new miRNA sensing in cancer and viral disease. The above mentioned miRNA detection methods such as electrochemical, optical, colorimetric, fluorescent, and other detection techniques play an incredible role in the development of nano biomaterials to translate a paper-based diagnosis of infectious and non-infectious diseases. This will be cost-effective, rapid, easy to use, and extremely sensitive in biomedical research.

References

[1] Nikolelis D P and Nikoleli G P 2018 eds *Nanotechnology and Biosensors* (Amsterdam: Elsevier)

[2] Teles F S R R 2011 Biosensors and rapid diagnostic tests on the frontier between analytical and clinical chemistry for biomolecular diagnosis of dengue disease: a review *Anal. Chim. Acta* **687** 28–42

[3] Anand K P and Panigrahi B 2021 Green synthesized nanoparticles: a way to produce novel nano-biosensor for agricultural application *Nanotechnology in Sustainable Agriculture.* (Boca Raton, FL: CRC Press)

[4] Singh R K, Mishra S, Jena S, Panigrahi B, Das B and Jayabalan R *et al* 2018 Rapid colorimetric sensing of gadolinium by EGCG-derived AgNPs: the development of a nanohybrid bioimaging probe *Chem. Commun.* **54** 3981–4

[5] Singh R K, Panigrahi B, Mishra S, Das B, Jayabalan R and Parhi P K *et al* 2018 pH triggered green synthesized silver nanoparticles toward selective colorimetric detection of kanamycin and hazardous sulfide ions *J. Mol. Liq.* **269** 269–77

[6] Kerry R G, Ukhurebor K E, Kumari S, Maurya G K, Patra S and Panigrahi B *et al* 2021 A comprehensive review on the applications of nano-biosensor-based approaches for non-communicable and communicable disease detection *Biomater. Sci.* **9** 3576–602

[7] Mandal D, Singh R K, Maharana U S, Panigrahi B and Mishra S 2021 Microbial gold nanoparticles and their biomedical applications *Microbial Interactions at Nanobiotechnology Interfaces* (New York: Wiley), pp 303–36 (https://onlinelibrary.wiley.com/doi/abs/10.1002/9781119617181.ch9)

[8] Chakrabarti M, Kiseleva R, Vertegel A and Ray S K 2015 Carbon nanomaterials for drug delivery and cancer therapy *J. Nanosci. Nanotechnol.* **15** 5501–11

[9] Panigrahi B, Mishra S, Singh R K, Siddiqui N, Bal R and Mandal D 2019 Peptide generated anisotropic gold nanoparticles as efficient siRNA vectors *Int. J. Pharm.* **563** 198–207

[10] Trewyn B G, Giri S, Slowing I I and Lin V S-Y 2007 Mesoporous silica nanoparticle based controlled release, drug delivery, and biosensor systems *Chem. Commun.* **31** 3236–45

[11] Singh R K, Bhol P, Mandal D and Mohanty P S 2019 Stimuli-responsive photoluminescence soft hybrid microgel particles: synthesis and characterizations *J. Phys. Condens. Matter* **32** 044001

[12] Panigrahi B, Singh R K, Mishra S and Mandal D 2018 Cyclic peptide-based nanostructures as efficient siRNA carriers *Artif. Cells Nanomed. Biotechnol.* **46** S763–73

[13] Singh R K, Behera S S, Singh K R, Mishra S, Panigrahi B and Sahoo T R *et al* 2020 Biosynthesized gold nanoparticles as photocatalysts for selective degradation of cationic dye and their antimicrobial activity *J. Photochem. Photobiol.,* A **400** 112704

[14] Patra S, Kerry R G, Maurya G K, Panigrahi B, Kumari S and Rout J R 2020 Emerging molecular prospective of SARS-CoV-2: feasible nanotechnology based detection and inhibition *Front. Microbiol.* **11** 2098

[15] Mani V, Chikkaveeraiah B V, Patel V, Gutkind J S and Rusling J F 2009 Ultrasensitive immunosensor for cancer biomarker proteins using gold nanoparticle film electrodes and multienzyme-particle amplification *ACS Nano.* **3** 585–94

[16] Stefani G and Slack F J 2008 Small non-coding RNAs in animal development *Nat. Rev. Mol. Cell Biol.* **9** 219–30

[17] Shin V Y and Chu K-M 2014 MiRNA as potential biomarkers and therapeutic targets for gastric cancer *World J. Gastroenterol.* **20** 10432–9

[18] Shabaninejad Z, Yousefi F, Movahedpour A, Ghasemi Y, Dokanehiifard S and Rezaei S *et al* 2019 Electrochemical-based biosensors for microRNA detection: nanotechnology comes into view *Anal. Biochem.* **581** 113349

[19] Ying S-Y, Chang D C and Lin S-L 2008 The MicroRNA (miRNA): overview of the RNA genes that modulate gene function *Mol. Biotechnol.* **38** 257–68

[20] Leigh-Ann M and Paul R M 2010 MicroRNA: biogenesis, function and role in cancer *Curr. Genomics.* **11** 537–61

[21] Hata A and Davis B N 2010 Regulation of pri-miRNA processing through Smads *Adv. Exp. Med. Biol.* **700** 15–27

[22] Palanisamy V, Jakymiw A, Van Tubergen E A, D'Silva N J and Kirkwood K L 2012 Control of cytokine mRNA expression by RNA-binding proteins and microRNAs *J. Dent. Res.* **91** 651–8

[23] Spaethling J M, Na Y-J, Lee J, Ulyanova A V, Baltuch G H and Bell T J *et al* 2017 Primary cell culture of live neurosurgically resected aged adult human brain cells and single cell transcriptomics *Cell Rep.* **18** 791–803

[24] Hamidi-Asl E, Palchetti I, Hasheminejad E and Mascini M 2013 A review on the electrochemical biosensors for determination of microRNAs *Talanta.* **115** 74–83

[25] Tosar J P, Brañas G and Laíz J 2010 Electrochemical DNA hybridization sensors applied to real and complex biological samples *Biosens. Bioelectron.* **26** 1205–17

[26] Lucarelli F, Tombelli S, Minunni M, Marrazza G and Mascini M 2008 Electrochemical and piezoelectric DNA biosensors for hybridisation detection *Anal. Chim. Acta* **609** 139–59

[27] Kilic T, Erdem A, Ozsoz M and Carrara S 2018 microRNA biosensors: opportunities and challenges among conventional and commercially available techniques *Biosens. Bioelectron.* **99** 525–46

[28] Sage A T, Besant J D, Lam B, Sargent E H and Kelley S O 2014 Ultrasensitive electrochemical biomolecular detection using nanostructured microelectrodes *ACC Chem. Res.* **47** 2417–25

[29] Lee S H, Lee J H, Tran V-K, Ko E, Park C H and Chung W S *et al* 2016 Determination of acetaminophen using functional paper-based electrochemical devices *Sensors Actuators* B **232** 514–22

[30] Ding R, Fiedoruk-Pogrebniak M, Pokrzywnicka M, Koncki R, Bobacka J and Lisak G 2020 Solid reference electrode integrated with paper-based microfluidics for potentiometric ion sensing *Sensors Actuators* B **323** 128680

[31] Fu L-M and Wang Y-N 2018 Detection methods and applications of microfluidic paper-based analytical devices *TrAC, Trends Anal. Chem.* **107** 196–211

[32] Eksin E, Torul H, Yarali E, Tamer U, Papakonstantinou P and Erdem A 2021 Paper-based electrode assemble for impedimetric detection of miRNA *Talanta.* **225** 122043

[33] Wang F, Liu Y, Fu C, Li N, Du M and Zhang L *et al* 2021 Paper-based bipolar electrode electrochemiluminescence platform for detection of multiple miRNAs *Anal. Chem.* **93** 1702–8

[34] Torul H, Yarali E, Eksin E, Ganguly A, Benson J and Tamer U *et al* 2021 Paper-based electrochemical biosensors for voltammetric detection of miRNA biomarkers using reduced

graphene oxide or MoS_2 nanosheets decorated with gold nanoparticle electrodes *Biosensors* **11** 236
[35] Ge X, Asiri A M, Du D, Wen W, Wang S and Lin Y 2014 Nanomaterial-enhanced paper-based biosensors *TrAC, Trends Anal. Chem.* **58** 31–9
[36] Gao X, Xu H, Baloda M, Gurung A S, Xu L-P and Wang T *et al* 2014 Visual detection of microRNA with lateral flow nucleic acid biosensor *Biosens. Bioelectron.* **54** 578–84
[37] Deng H, Liu Q, Wang X, Huang R, Liu H and Lin Q *et al* 2017 Quantum dots-labeled strip biosensor for rapid and sensitive detection of microRNA based on target-recycled non-enzymatic amplification strategy *Biosens. Bioelectron.* **87** 931–40
[38] Hou S-Y, Hsiao Y-L, Lin M-S, Yen C-C and Chang C-S 2012 MicroRNA detection using lateral flow nucleic acid strips with gold nanoparticles *Talanta* **99** 375–9
[39] Zheng W, Yao L, Teng J, Yan C, Qin P and Liu G *et al* 2018 Lateral flow test for visual detection of multiple MicroRNAs *Sensors Actuators* B **264** 320–6
[40] Degliangeli F, Kshirsagar P, Brunetti V, Pompa P P and Fiammengo R 2014 Absolute and direct MicroRNA quantification using DNA–gold nanoparticle probes *J. Am. Chem. Soc.* **136** 2264–7
[41] Chen M, Li H, Shi Z, Peng W, Qin Y and Luo R *et al* 2020 High fluorescence quenching probe-based reverse fluorescence enhancement LFTS coupling with IS-primer amplification reaction for the rapid and sensitive Parkinson disease-associated MicroRNA detection *Biosens. Bioelectron.* **165** 112278
[42] Liao X, Li L, Pan J, Peng T, Ge B and Tang Q 2018 In situ biosensor for detection miRNA in living cells based on carbon nitride nanosheets with catalytic hairpin assembly amplification *Luminescence* **33** 190–5
[43] Liao X, Wang Q and Ju H 2014 Simultaneous sensing of intracellular microRNAs with a multi-functionalized carbon nitride nanosheet probe *Chem. Commun.* **50** 13604–7
[44] Zhao H, Qu Y, Yuan F and Quan X 2016 A visible and label-free colorimetric sensor for miRNA-21 detection based on peroxidase-like activity of graphene/gold-nanoparticle hybrids *Anal. Methods* **8** 2005–12
[45] Yildiz U H, Alagappan P and Liedberg B 2013 Naked eye detection of lung cancer associated miRNA by paper based biosensing platform *Anal. Chem.* **85** 820–4
[46] Fakhri N, Abarghoei S, Dadmehr M, Hosseini M, Sabahi H and Ganjali M R 2020 Paper based colorimetric detection of miRNA-21 using Ag/Pt nanoclusters *Spectrochim. Acta Part* A **227** 117529
[47] Farshchi F, Saadati A, Fathi N, Hasanzadeh M and Samiei M 2021 Flexible paper-based label-free electrochemical biosensor for the monitoring of miRNA-21 using core–shell Ag@Au/GQD nano-ink: a new platform for the accurate and rapid analysis by low cost lab-on-paper technology *Anal. Methods* **13** 1286–94
[48] Wang H, Jian Y, Kong Q, Liu H, Lan F and Liang L *et al* 2018 Ultrasensitive electrochemical paper-based biosensor for microRNA via strand displacement reaction and metal-organic frameworks *Sensors Actuators* B **257** 561–9
[49] Hosseini M, Akbari A, Ganjali M R, Dadmehr M and Rezayan A H 2015 A novel label-free microRNA-155 detection on the basis of fluorescent silver nanoclusters *J. Fluoresc.* **25** 925–9
[50] Wu X, Chai Y, Zhang P and Yuan R 2015 An electrochemical biosensor for sensitive detection of microrna-155: combining target recycling with cascade catalysis for signal amplification *ACS Appl. Mater. Interfaces* **7** 713–20

[51] Gao Z and Yang Z 2006 Detection of MicroRNAs using electrocatalytic nanoparticle tags *Anal. Chem.* **78** 1470–7

[52] Fujii T, Shimada K, Nakai T and Ohbayashi C 2018 MicroRNAs in smoking-related carcinogenesis: biomarkers, functions, and therapy *J. Clin. Med.* **7** 98

[53] Hassanein M, Callison J C, Callaway-Lane C, Aldrich M C, Grogan E L and Massion P P 2012 The state of molecular biomarkers for the early detection of lung cancer *Cancer Prev. Res.* **5** 992–1006

[54] Moody L, He H, Pan Y-X and Chen H 2017 Methods and novel technology for microRNA quantification in colorectal cancer screening *Clin. Epigenet.* **9** 119

[55] Ouyang T, Liu Z, Han Z and Ge Q 2019 MicroRNA detection specificity: recent advances and future perspective *Anal. Chem.* **91** 3179–86

[56] Zheng-Xing G, Shi-Hao L, Zi-Mei Z, Dan Z, Hui Y and Hui D 2019 A brief survey for MicroRNA precursor identification using machine learning methods *Curr. Genom.* **21** 11–25

[57] Shandilya R, Ranjan S, Khare S, Bhargava A, Goryacheva I Y and Mishra P K 2021 Point-of-care diagnostics approaches for detection of lung cancer-associated circulating miRNAs *Drug Discov. Today* **26** 1501–9

[58] Kandhro A H 2016 MicroRNAs from diagnosis to therapy: future perspective *Transl. Biomed* **7** 4

Chapter 9

PCR and other nucleic acid amplification technique based lateral flow assay for detection of the infectious agents

Meenu Jain, Vaibhav Misra, Jyoti Jain, Rishika Khetan, Urmila Jarouliya, Sushil Kumar Sharma, Pramod Kumar and Savita Bharat Jain

Polymerase chain reaction (PCR) is a well-established molecular technique for the rapid diagnosis of infectious diseases. It is a widely accepted tool in the diagnostic realm of clinical healthcare facilities, for viral and bacterial infections, food pathogens, oncogenic mutations, biomedical research, genetic diseases, forensic investigations and agricultural biotechnology. It is a highly sensitive and specific method. However, the conventional PCR lacks end point analysis as instrumentation is needed and time consuming agarose gel electrophoresis is the conventional method for visualization of results. Real-time PCR addresses this issue but it further adds to the very high cost in terms of instrumentation and reagents, moreover, the real-time PCR setting requires highly skilled manpower in specialized laboratory settings. PCR accompanied with lateral flow assay (LFA) offers an easy, time saving, inexpensive and point-of-care replacement. Thus, the PCR accompanied with LFA can be seen as a benefit to the diagnostic world for fast, sensitive, specific, cost-effective, and easy-to-use nucleic acid based point-of-care (POC) diagnosis of the diseases in low-resource settings.

9.1 Introduction

Infectious diseases are a major public health concern affecting billions of people worldwide. During the last few decades, many advanced molecular diagnostic techniques have been developed for early diagnosis of infectious diseases, which successfully participated in timely patient management and reduced the spread of disease. The emerging molecular tools have concentrated on keynote measures such as rapidity, being user-friendly, specificity, sensitivity, accuracy, cost-effective, eliminating the need for well-trained persons, and can be used in limited resource

doi:10.1088/978-0-7503-5820-0ch9 © IOP Publishing Ltd 2023

settings, and tests can be done at the bedside (POCT) especially suitable in outbreaks, epidemic and pandemic conditions. In the modern era, protein- and DNA-based diagnostic methods are the crucial tools for identification of infectious diseases. Diagnostic tools including electrophoresis, chromatography, ELISA, lateral flow immunoassays, neutralization assay, SPR-based biosensor test, luminescent immunoassay, protein microarray and rapid antigen test, are employed as effective protein-based diagnostic assays [1, 2]. On the other hand, DNA-based assays and nucleic acid amplification tests (NAATs) such as isothermal amplification technologies (rolling circle amplification (RCA), cross priming amplification (CPA), loop-mediated isothermal amplification (LAMP), recombinase polymerase amplification (RPA)), clustered regularly interspaced short palindromic repeats (CRISPR), DNA hybridization, species-specific polymerase chain reaction (PCR), real-time PCR, PCR-RFLP, DNA microarray and sequencing, are being employed owing to their high sensitivity and specificity [3–8]. Among them, species-specific PCR and isothermal amplification are the promising tools for diagnosis with paramount advantages over other DNA-based techniques in term of simplicity, speed, accuracy, sensitivity, and specificity. Additionally, isothermal amplification can be employed in low-resource settings even as point-of-care testing (POCT). The nucleic acid amplified products can be detected by different mechanisms, including electrophoresis, EvaGreen and/or SYBR Green fluorescent dyes, turbidimetry, fluorimetry, and pH-sensitive dyes etc, those usually required extensive time and sophisticated equipment [9–12]. Hence, there is an urgent requirement for an alternative technique that is fast, simple, accurate, and portable. Lateral flow assay (LFA) is a well-established screening detection tool to detect the DNA amplification products [13]. It is a one-step process, analogous to ELISA, depends on antigen–antibody interaction or probe-target DNA hybridization, and the results can be visualized in few minutes with the naked eye [14]. PCR and other isothermal amplification methods combined with LFA enhances the diagnostic province to maintain the simplicity, user-friendly, rapidity, cost-effective and thus are capable of successfully detecting the infectious diseases with high sensitivity and specificity [7, 15–18]. In this chapter, we discussed the PCR, isothermal amplification methods, other NAATs techniques, LFA, PCR/NAATs combined with LFA, their applications and advantages.

9.2 Polymerase chain reactions

PCR, invented by Kary Mullis in 1983, is a rapid nucleic acid amplification technique that generates unlimited copies of DNA templates. This technique is being employed for the specific and sensitive detection of mutations, and various types of pathogens from clinical as well as from environmental specimens. It is known to be valuable to diagnose those particular pathogens that are tough to culture in *in vitro* conditions or need a long period of time to culture. The specificity and sensitivity of the technique may vary depending on DNA extraction methodology, primers, probes, thermal profile, and amplicon detection techniques. PCR assay follows the main steps of DNA extraction, PCR amplification and detection of amplified products. PCR perform three processing steps for DNA amplification, (a) denaturation (double stranded target DNA breaks into single stranded DNA), (b) annealing (primers bind to complementary sequence in the single stranded DNA), (c) extension (polymerization of target DNA by enzymes). The targeted DNA sequence is amplified in multiple copies by repeated cycles (35–40 cycles) of PCR within 2–3 h without culture enrichment [19]. A PCR reaction contains buffered solution, oligonucleotide primers, DNA template, four nucleotides (dATPs, dGTPs, dCTPs, dTTPs), $MgCl_2$, DNA polymerase (Taq polymerase, pfu polymerase etc) [20]. There are two primers used, one forward primer binds to the sense strand of DNA template, and other reverse primer attaches to the anti-sense strand. The DNA polymerases used in the PCR, have revolutionized the technology by their thermostable property. Taq polymerase is the most common thermostable enzyme used in PCR, and is isolated from hot spring bacteria, *Thermus aquaticus* [21]. PCR reaction is carried out in a machine called a thermocycler that conducts multiple temperature cycles of heating and cooling. Its first step denaturation double stranded (ds) DNA is separated into single strand (ss) DNA by heating to temperature 92 °C–95 °C. In the next step (annealing), the primers anneal to the complementary DNA strand at low temperature 55 °C–70 °C. Primer concentration and annealing temperature should be optimized for more primers binding to the DNA template. During the third step (extension) the temperature again rises to 72 °C–75 °C for activity of DNA polymerase enzyme that recognizes the template and adds nucleotides (complementary to DNA template) at 3′ end of primers, and finally extend the new DNA strand. After finishing the final step, two copies of the DNA template will be prepared. These three steps repeat in multiple cycles (35–40 cycles) to produce multiple copies of the desired DNA template. The target DNA is amplified exponentially by multiple cooling and heating cycles of the denaturation, annealing and extension steps. PCR is more sensitive, highly specific, fast, user-friendly, cost-effective and can use in POC settings for detection of infectious agents, including *Plasmodium falciparum* [17], *Mycobacterium tuberculosis* [18], bird flu virus [16], *Yersinia pestis* [7] and *Escherichia coli* [15]. It is a well-recognized technique, and has a wide range of applications in different clinical and medical fields, including early diagnosis of biothreat pathogens, evolving mutations, antimicrobial resistance profiling, phylogenetic analysis, surveillance studies [22, 23]. Multiple genes can be simultaneously detected by multiplex PCR through multiple sets of primers in a reaction [22, 23].

9.2.1 Detection methods for PCR products

The amplified PCR products can be detected by employing various detection methodologies, i.e., electrophoresis, southern hybridization with specific radioisotope or non-radioisotope labelled probe, PCR-immunoassays, digoxigenin (DIG)-PCR-enzyme-linked immunosorbent assay (ELISA), sequencing, LFA, lateral flow biosensor (LFB) and LFA-NanoSuit method (LNSM). All the detection methodologies have their inherent merits and demerits. Electrophoresis is a traditional method for the detection of amplified PCR products. The amplified DNA fragments are separated on agarose gel and comprise a matrix of pores that assist in segregating the fragments based on their size. The gel placed in a tank fills with electrolyte aqueous solution, with the opposite ends having a positive and a negative electrode. DNA molecules run from the negative to positive electrode due to their negative charge. Longer DNA fragments move slower than shorter fragments. Once the electrophoresis is completed, the DNA molecules are stained with coloured or ethidium bromide dyes will be visualized as a specific colour in visible light or will show fluorescence under ultraviolet light [24]. Ethidium bromide (EtBr) is an intercalating dye. Its mutagenic property causes severe health risks by intercalating between the strands of DNA and deforms it [25, 26]. Other harmless alternative nucleic acid stains to the EtBr dye are Midori Green DNA Stain, Safelook Load-Green, and SYBR green, which can work in the same manner and sensitive as agarose gel electrophoresis [27–30]. The southern hybridization method shows the high sensitivity than EtBr detection method, but it requires additional steps of blotting and hybridization [31]. The target DNA, which has to be detected, is transferred on the membrane, and further the complementary probe (labelled with either radioactive or fluorescent or colorimetric dye) bound to the target DNA. The immuno-PCR (I-PCR) assays improves the detection sensitivity from 10 to 10^9-fold times compared to the conventional approaches of immunoassays (e.g., ELISA) by associating the nucleic acid amplification with antibody-based methods [32]. I-PCR follows the same pattern as ELISA, however it detects the DNA-antibody conjugate instead of enzyme-conjugated antibody [33]. In this method, the antibody is conjugated with the amplified PCR product (DNA). The I-PCR improves the sensitivity, assay set-ups and readout methods. The PCR-DIG-ELISA diagnostic method is accomplished via PCR and ELISA [34]. It illustrates 10–100 fold higher sensitivity as compared to the conventional electrophoresis method. PCR reaction comprises digoxigenin (DIG)-11-dUTP and biotinylated primers, thus the primers and dUTPs are incorporated into the PCR amplified product. The biotinylated PCR product is bound to the streptavidin that is coated on microtiter plate. An enzyme-conjugated anti-DIG antibody further binds to the hybrid (biotin–streptavidin conjugate). These hybrids provide the colour by the colorimetric substrates.

Sequencing is the standard method for detection of the PCR product by sequencing and comparing with the known reference sequence and heightening the specificity [35]. However, sequencing is not the routine diagnostic procedure due to its limitations of high cost, requirement for equipment and well-trained personnel. Conversely, the LFA is a simple, rapid and most appropriate point-of-care diagnostic test for the detection of infectious diseases. It does not require specific instruments/infrastructure or trained personnel, however it shows low specificity and sensitivity. Hence, the latest lateral flow biosensors (LFBs) enhance the specificity by detecting micro- and nanoparticles [36]. The signal is monitored for quantitative evaluation by luminescence, magnetic characteristics, colorimetric, electrochemical signals, and surface-enhanced Raman spectroscopy (SERS) [36–38]. A newer diagnostic technique, the LFA-NanoSuit method (LNSM), exhibits higher sensitivity and specificity than visual detection of individual LFA by grabbing the high resolution images of the immunocomplexes, e.g., gold/platinum-labelled antibody against the pathogenic antigens [39]. In this method, LFA is combined with a desktop scanning electron microscope (SEM) for direct detection of the metal particles avoiding cellulose deformities and conductive treatments in traditional SEM.

9.3 Other PCR techniques

Some additional PCR techniques, including nested PCR and real-time PCR, enhance the sensitivity and specificity of the microbial diagnosis. In nested PCR, primarily original primers amplify the PCR product, which is used as template for the second PCR reaction [40]. A second pair of primers amplify the internal region of this amplified product and increase the diagnostic sensitivity. Nested PCR is a valuable tool in suboptimal or very low quantity nucleic acid samples and also decreases the amplification of non-specific products. Real-time PCR is a more sensitive, effective and quantitative method for detecting DNA on the basis of SYBR green dye or fluorescent probes [41, 42]. Its readout method is easy, real-time, quantitative and based on the Ct (cycle threshold) value. However, it is costly, time consuming, requires expensive equipment and professional personnel. These drawbacks reduce its POCT utility as well as routine usefulness. Therefore, there is a increasing need for a simple and cost-effective diagnostic method that can be used in low-resource settings such as LMICs.

9.4 Other nucleic acid amplification techniques

In recent times, a variety of nucleic acid (NA)-based diagnostic platforms have been developed for the detection of biological contaminants, because the requirement for highly specific, more sensitive and faster techniques than the culture-based method [43]. There are two different approaches: hybridization and amplification, performed for NA-based detection. In nucleic acid hybridization, the fluorescent or radioactive labelled ss oligonucleotide probe binds to the complementary sequence of the target gene [44, 45]. The drawback of the test is the need for a high concentration of the target gene for a measurable signal. This problem can be solved by using NAATs, including PCR and isothermal amplifications, which amplify the number of specific target genes [9, 46].

9.4.1 Loop-mediated isothermal amplification

Loop-mediated isothermal amplification (LAMP) is a fast, simple, specific, and money saving isothermal nucleic acid amplification technique. The technique depends on the auto-cycling strand displacement DNA synthesis with the help of Bst DNA polymerase (synthesized by *Bacillus stearothermophilus*) at 60 °C–65 °C for 45–60 min. There are the four sets of primers (two inner and two outer) used that bind to six different target sequences and amplify the DNA in three major steps: production of starting material, cycling amplification, and elongation, further recycling [47]. LAMP enables the amplification from minimal number of DNA with high precision without using expensive instruments. It also amplifies the RNA by association with reverse transcription (RT) with high efficiency. Its product can be detected by measuring direct turbidity or by detecting fluorescence or gel electrophoresis [48, 49]. Visual signals of the amplified products can be increased by using fluorescent dyes, SYBR green and pico [50]. LAMP has been applied as POCT and used in the fields of research, medical diagnosis, environmental pollutants and hygiene, infectious disease diagnosis [51].

9.4.2 Nucleic acid sequence based amplification

Nucleic acid sequence based amplification (NASBA) is a transcription-mediated amplification method [52], also called self-sustained sequence replication (3SR) [53]. The technique was fabricated for RNA amplification, however DNA can also be detected. Initially, it was used for the diagnosis of HIV but now it is being used for other RNA viruses. The overall reaction is maintained at a constant temperature of 41 °C. The reaction contains two primers (P1 and P2) and three thermolabile enzymes, RNase H, T7 DNA dependent RNA polymerase (DdRp), and avian myeloblastosis virus (AMV) reverse transcriptase [54], amplify the ssRNA. The RNA product is sequenced with the help of reverse transcription and a oligonucleotide primer. The amplified target sequence length is approximately 100–250 nucleotides. NASBA amplified products are detected through electrophoresis, electro-chemiluminescence (ECL), enzyme-linked gel assay (ELGA), enzymatic bead based assay, molecular beacon technique and fluorescent correlation spectroscopy [55]. The technique represents high analytical sensitivity and can differentiate the viable cells with specific and sensitive amplification of mRNA [56].

9.4.3 Recombinase polymerase amplification

Recombinase plymerase amplification (RPA) is a probe-based isothermal DNA amplification method. It contains the two enzymes, recombinase and DNA polymerase with DNA-binding proteins for recombination, synthesis and repair of the DNA. There is no need for thermal or pre-treatment for denaturation of the DNA because recombinase enzyme performs the task [57]. Recombinase enzyme accomplishes the primer binding through recombinase-attached primers scanning the complementary sequence of target DNA. Recombinase separates the strands of DNA, and single strand binding (SSB) proteins inhibit the reannealing of the strands. Once the primer properly hybridizes to the DNA strand, the recombinase detaches from the complex and remove from the 3′ end. Extension takes place by the DNA polymerase and two dsDNA are prepared. Repeated cycles will produce many copies of the DNA. The amplified product is detected by the real-time fluorescence or gel electrophoresis [57]. The method is successfully applied in the detection of several infectious diseases. Apart from this, RPA lateral flow dipstick (RPA-LFD) has been efficaciously used in the diagnosis of diseases in fish such as cyprinid herpesvirus 2 (CyHV-2), that shows 100 times higher sensitivity and 50 min faster as compared to PCR [45].

9.4.4 Rolling circle amplification

Rolling circle amplification (RCA) is an isothermal technique based on rolling circle replication. It is also known as cascade RCA and ramification amplification (RAM) [58, 59]. It amplifies the short RNA or DNA oligonucleotides (primers or probe) from circularized DNA template through RNA or DNA polymerase to achieve more than 10^9 copies at a specific temperature. There are various polymerase enzymes used in the technique, like Φ29, Bst and Vent exo-DNA polymerases, however, Φ29 is most commonly used [60]. In the reaction, primers bind to circularized DNA, then Φ29 DNA polymerase further extends the primer sequence continuously around the template DNA and produces a long ssDNA which has tandem repeat sequences [61, 62]. When compared to the PCR and other isothermal amplification techniques, it shows resistant to contamination, does not require temperature changes, can perform in liquid or solid or in *in vivo* or *in vitro*, needs less assay optimization, and is capable of better multiplexing. RCA is simple, easy-to-use, efficacious, can be prepare for portability and automation of high-throughput analysis [63].

9.4.5 Strand displacement amplification

Strand displacement amplification (SDA) is an isothermal amplification method, which contains DNA polymerase I (exo-klenow) that is a deficient exonuclease activity with four distinct primers. Of them, two primers (S1 and S2) have a restriction site that recognizes the HincII exonuclease, binds to 5′ end of the complementary sequence of the target. The other two primers (B1 and B2) are called the bumper primers. SDA follows the different steps: (1) primers bind to displaced target sequence, (2) primer/target complex is extended by DNA polymerase, and simultaneously extend the S1 and S2 strands occurred displacement have HincII restriction sites, (3) dsDNA form that have HincII restriction sites, (4) unmodified original extended strand is nicked by the enzyme, (5) HincII dissociate from the nicked site, (6) 3′ end of the newly synthesized strand further extend by polymerase and results in the displacement of downstream strand, (7) exponential amplification of the target [64]. SDA is operated at high temperature and can produce 10^9 copies of the target sequence in a reaction within an hour. The robustness of the technique makes it efficacious for POC criteria as well as for clinical purposes.

9.4.6 Multiple displacement amplification

Multiple displacement amplification (MDA) is an isothermal amplification and highly processive method based on the strand-displacing method. The reaction consists of modified random primers with a polymerase with strand displacement capability isolated bacteriophage Φ29. It is highly sensitive and yields more DNA. The method is suitable in cases where there is a very small amount of the initial target material [65]. The 20–30 μg of DNA can be generated from 1 to 10 copies of

DNA [66]. The method is favourable for qualitative multiplex detection and its several attributes make it useful in forensics and single cell clinical diagnostics [67].

9.4.7 Clustered regularly interspaced short palindromic repeats

Clustered regularly interspaced short palindromic repeats (CRISPR) is an RNA-guided endonuclease (RGEN)-based nucleic acid editing tool. CRISPR RNA is associated with Cas protein that employs endonuclease activity. Nucleases are named 'Cas' for 'CRISPR-associated'. CRISPR (repetitive DNA sequences) array (often palindromic) separated by unique spacer sequences are found on the bacterial genome. The CRISPR RNA (crRNA) also known as guide RNA, is designed against specific target DNA or RNA through binding to the complementary sequence [68]. Upon binding of guide crRNA to a cognate target (RNA for Cas13a, dsDNA for Cas12a, ssDNA for Cas14a), nuclease of Cas proteins is activated, leading to target cleavage and catalytic cleavage of nearby nucleic acids (ssRNA for Cas13a, ssDNA for Cas12a and Cas14a). This 'collateral' nuclease activity is turned into an amplified signal by providing reporter probes with a fluorophore (usually FAM) linked to a quencher (or biotin for later flow assay) by a short oligonucleotide. During CRISPR/Cas cleavage, the reporter molecule is cleaved by the activated nuclease activity. The cleaved reporter molecules can be detected by fluorescence measurements and colored band appearance on lateral flow assay strips by employing FAM and biotin detection, respectively.

There are various types of CRISPR–Cas systems in different bacteria and show several applications, including editing in epigenomes, genomes and transcriptomes, detailing the cellular events, bioimaging of nucleic acids, and detection of DNA/RNA [69–73]. The CRISPR–Cas technique has shown potential to increase the specificity, sensitivity, and rapidity and when accompanied with LFA is a promising nucleic acid based diagnostic tool that has been used for several viruses and bacteria [74–76].

9.5 Lateral flow assay

Lateral flow assay is a quick and efficacious analytical method originating from the latex agglutination test established by Singer and Plotz in 1956 [77]. It is also known as immunochromatographic tests (ICT). The principle is based on paper chromatography, which was developed by Rosalyn S Yalow and Solomon A Berson in 1959 [78]. The lateral flow tests (strip assay) were commercially released by Unipath in 1984 [79]. The first successful LFA was the pregnancy test that diagnoses the human chorionic gonadotropin (HCG) hormone present in urine [80]. Presently, they are an appropriate alternative to existing analytical equipment based diagnostic techniques. The method is a simplified version of the modern biosensors and its popularity is continuously increasing in the clinical and healthcare industries, especially where resources are inadequate and a rapid, low-priced and door to door POC test is required. The speed and cost-effectiveness of the technique make it suitable for conducting diagnostic surveillance programs. Its simplicity and easy visual readout within a few minutes make it attractive as a portable diagnostic tool. According to

WHO, LFA accomplishes the context of ASSURED (affordable, sensitive, specific, user-friendly, robust, equipment-free and deliverable) [81].

9.5.1 Principle and structure of LFA

LFA devices comprise of four pads (sample pad, conjugate pad, nitrocellulose membrane and absorbent pad), which are arranged in a particular sequence, and are bordered by a plastic backing card as well as other components, including adhesive strip and cover tape, which are associated for better endurance and firmness. The principle of the LFA is based on the movement of the analytes present in the liquid samples through capillary action via different pads of the strip, on which antibodies and detector molecules interact with the analyte and diagnose it [82]. The pads are organized in different ways according to detection of the target analyte type [83]. The sample pad is soaked with surfactants and buffer salts which would be appropriate for sample detection and confirm that the sample analytes will interact with the captured reagents. The absorbed sample moves towards the conjugate pad, that has antibodies against the target analyte. These antibodies conjugated with fluorescent or coloured dyes. Further, the complex of target analyte and conjugated antibody move forward to the nitrocellulose membrane (also called the detection zone). This is the porous region containing specific immobilized antigens and antibodies attached at the test line and control line. These immobilized antigens and antibodies interact with the target analytes bound to the conjugated antibody. Results will be observed as a response seen at the test line. The control line denotes the appropriate flow of the reagents on the strip and test quality. In a strip, multiple analytes can be detected simultaneously by adding multiple test lines coated with either specific antibodies for different analytes or the same antibody for quantitative analysis of an analyte [84–87]. Finally on the strip, an absorbent pad is situated, which avoids backflow of the liquid and wicks the excessive reagents. It increases the test's capacity to take large volume of samples that helps to increase the sensitivity of test.

There are two types of LFAs routinely used, (1) direct assay, and (2) competitive assay. A direct test is useful for larger analytes (e.g., p24 antigen for HIV test) or those having multiple epitopes or several antigenic determinants (e.g., hCG for pregnancy tests) [88, 89]. The hCG test is based on a sandwich assay, in which target analyte is sandwiched between two different antibodies, which are associated with distinct epitopes of the analyte. Usually, monoclonal antibodies (anti-analyte Ab) against the target analyte act as a capture molecule, and are labelled on the test line present on nitrocellulose membrane. Other polyclonal antibodies (Ab-conjugated) are situated on the conjugate pad and act as detector molecules. Additional species-specific anti-IgG antibodies are placed on the control line. First the extracted sample is applied on the sample pad, the liquid moves forward towards the conjugate pad by capillary action, where the analytes bind to the detection antibody and prepared the Ab-conjugated. On the test line, bound and unbound analytes interact with the capture antibody, where the bound analytes (Ab-conjugated) give the positive results. The test line intensity is directly proportional to the sample analyte concentration [90, 91]. On the other hand, competitive assay is advantageous for the cases when target analytes are small molecules and show single antigenic determinant, those cannot be bound with two antibodies simultaneously [92]. In the assay, the analytes bind to the conjugated Ab that present on the conjugate pad, and prevent the interaction of coloured conjugate to antibodies on the test line. In the positive results, a coloured line is not formed on the test line, in contrast a visible line appears at the control line. However, in negative results, two lines, one at the test line and another at the control line will appear.

9.6 PCR and other nucleic acid amplification technique based LFA

During last few decades, new innovations have been implemented in the LFA diagnostic tests for improving sensitivity and specificity to develop nucleic acid amplification (NAA) based LFA [93–95]. There are various ways for detection of PCR and other NAA based LFA, including antibody-dependent or antibody-independent methods. Antibody-dependent is known as 'nucleic acid lateral flow immunoassay (NALFIA)', where the antibodies are used as detecting components. It contains the lines labelled with antibodies, and amplicons and probes labelled with tag-specific antibodies. Another, antibody-independent method is called the nucleic acid lateral flow test strip (NALFT), which uses two high affinity partners, i.e., biotin (tags the target amplicon or probe) and streptavidin participate. In these detection systems, primers and oligonucleotides tagged with the different molecules such as biotin, digoxigenin, FAM/fluorescence isothiocyanate (FITC) etc are applied to diagnose the amplified nucleic acid.

In figure 9.1(A), two differently tagged primers (biotin and FITC/FAM) amplify the target specific dsDNA, which recognize the tag-specific antibody (anti-FITC/anti-FAM antibody) at one side and its biotinylated end bind to avidin tagged with gold nanoparticles at another end and visualize the colour [96]. In another approach

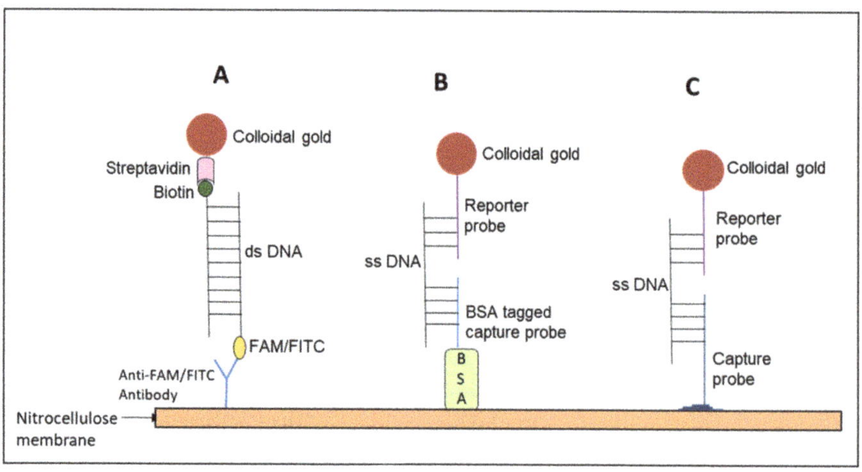

Figure 9.1. Schematic representation of different approaches of the detection methods on lateral flow strips, (A) anti-FAM/FITC antibody immobilized on the nitrocellulose membrane and detect dsDNA, (B) BSA bind to the membrane tagged with capture probe that can detect the ssDNA, (C) capture probe directly attach to the membrane and detect ssDNA.

(figure 9.1(B)), BSA tagged with oligonucleotide probe, passively absorb on the surface of nitrocellulose membrane. The target single strand (ss) nucleic acid binds to the oligonucleotide probe at one end and reporter probe at the other end through the complementary sequences. The reporter molecule gives a response via gold nanoparticles. In figure 9.1(C), a oligonucleotide capture probe directly immobilizes on the membrane via passive adsorption that detects the complementary sequence of the target ss nucleic acid in the same way as in figure 9.1(B). The colour of the reporter molecule is directly proportional to the analyte concentration [97].

There are several ways for detection of the product of CRISPR/Cas reaction (figure 9.2). The control line is coated with streptavidin and the test line is layered with rabbit polyclonal anti-IgG antibody. The ss oligonucleotide probe (target analyte) either cleaved or intact molecules bind to the anti-FAM-Ab tagged with gold nanoparticles. The uncleaved (intact) reporter molecules bind to streptavidin through biotin and give the colour. On the other hand, cleaved reporter molecules interact with anti-IgG antibody and visualize the signal [74, 98].

PCR amplified the amplicon can be detected by the lateral flow strips, is more appropriate alternative for diagnosis of the target analyte of infectious diseases [7, 91]. Target specific primers that amplify the PCR product, are tagged with biotin and FAM dyes at 5′ end. Therefore, the amplified products are labelled with biotin and FAM at both 5′ end [7]. The PCR product is detected in the same manner as figure 9.1(A). PCR-LFA method enhances the sensitivity, specificity, and reduces the need of cost, time and electrophoresis.

There are a few new approaches like silver enhancement technology, or an enzyme associated with gold nanoparticles (GNPs) that intensify the signal generated by GNPs [99–101]. Some reagents such as magnetic particles of immuno-nanoparticles or nano-gold particles increase the detection sensitivity and reduce the limit of detection (LOD) [102]. Furthermore, a few devices, including laser or light-emitting diode (LED), and thermal contrast etc, amplify the signals up

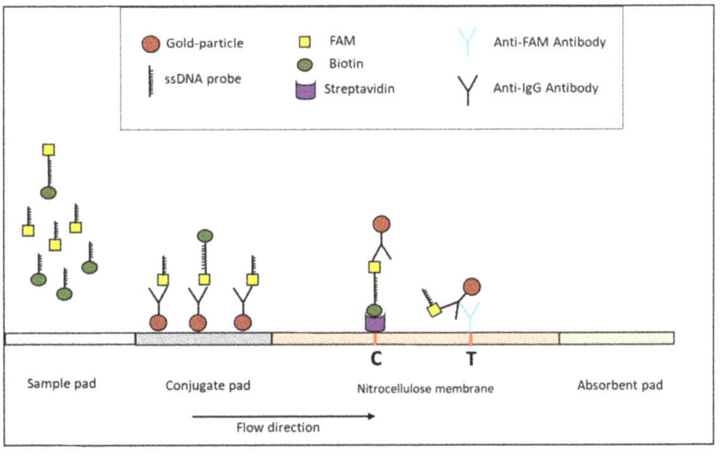

Figure 9.2. Schematic diagram of the detection of the product of CRISPR/Cas reaction on lateral flow strip.

to 1000 fold [103]. Additionally, LFA associated with computational methods like electronic logic gates, deliver a new logic-sensing platform [104].

9.7 Pros and cons of PCR and other NAATs based LFA

The LFA test has many advantages, including that it is fast, easy-to-use, cost-effective, results can be visualized easily and read by any untrained person, no requirement for additional equipment and the test can be performed at the bedside (POCT). However, it has a few disadvantages like sensitivity, specificity, LOD and quantification etc. These drawbacks could be overcome by the addition of the PCR and nucleic acid amplification tests (NAATs). Because of the sensitivity and specificity, these NAATs and PCR techniques are used as the gold standard test for most of the diagnostics tests in clinical and healthcare facilities. Although detection of the amplified nucleic acid is a major problem with the NAATs LFA has solved the problem and simplified the PCR technology by eliminating the need for other detection techniques (electrophoresis, southern hybridization, DIG-PCR-ELISA) which are costly, time consuming, equipment and trained manpower demanding. These advantages make the test well suited for LMICs. The advantages and disadvantages of LFA are summarizedin figure 9.3 [82, 105].

9.8 Applications of PCR-based LFA

The test can be used in various fields of clinical and healthcare diagnosis, food safety investigation, quality control and environmental monitoring. LFA-based tests are mainly applied for quantitative and qualitative diagnostic analysis of antibodies, antigens, and amplified nucleic acid product, that can screen for infectious diseases, cardio vascular diseases, cancer biomarkers, chemicals, environmental pollutants, toxins, metabolites and small molecule drugs etc [106–114]. PCR-based LFA has been efficaciously used with high sensitivity and specificity for diagnosis of pork components [115], bird flu virus [16], *E. coli* [15], *P. falciparum* [17], *M. tuberculosis* [18] and *Y. pestis* [7].

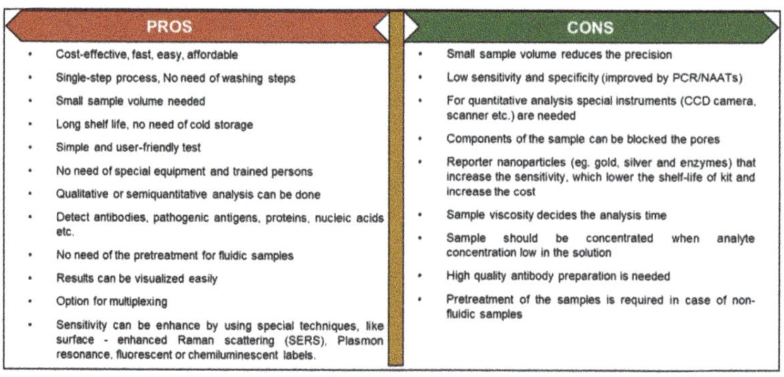

Figure 9.3. Pros and cons of PCR and other NAATs based LFA.

9.9 Future aspects

PCR and other NAATs based lateral flow assays are capable of developing more sensitive, specific and portable devices for diagnosis of aetiological agents. The test could be employed in various fields, including clinical, medical, food safety, agriculture and environmental monitoring. Scientific efforts towards development of NAATs accompanied LFA would encourage fast, accurate, and cost-effective testing that could be conducted at POC/bedside and thus deliver considerable advantages for timely disease management especially in LMICs.

References

[1] Carter L J *et al* 2020 Assay techniques and test development for COVID-19 diagnosis *ACS Cent. Sci.* **6** 591–605

[2] Shaffaf T and Ghafar-Zadeh E 2021 COVID-19 diagnostic strategies part II: protein-based technologies *Bioengineering (Basel)* **8** 54

[3] Amaral J S, Santos C G, Melo V S, Costa J, Oliveira M B P and Mafra I 2015 Identification of duck, partridge, pheasant, quail, chicken and turkey meats by species-specific PCR assays to assess the authenticity of traditional game meat *Alheira* sausages *Food Control* **47** 190–5

[4] Cottenet G, Sonnard V, Blancpain C, Ho H Z, Leong H L and Chuah P F A 2016 DNA macro-array to simultaneously identify 32 meat species in food samples *Food Control* **67** 135–43

[5] Bertolini F, Ghionda M C, D'Alessandro E, Geraci C, Chiofalo V and Fontanesi L 2015 A next generation semiconductor-based sequencing approach for the identification of meat species in DNA mixtures *PLoS One* **10** e0121701

[6] Jolany Vangah S, Katalani C, Booneh H A, Hajizade A, Sijercic A and Ahmadian G 2020 CRISPR-based diagnosis of infectious and noninfectious diseases *Biol. Proced. Online* **22** 22

[7] Singh R, Pal V, Kumar M, Tripathi N K and Goel A K 2021 Development of a PCR-lateral flow assay for rapid detection of *Yersinia pestis*, the causative agent of plague *Acta Trop.* **220** 105958

[8] Tombuloglu H, Sabit H, Al-Suhaimi E, Al Jindan R and Alkharsah K R 2021 Development of multiplex real-time RT-PCR assay for the detection of SARS-CoV-2 *PLoS One* **16** e0250942

[9] Yadava J P, Jain M and Goel A K 2013 Detection and confirmation of toxigenic *Vibrio cholerae* O1 in environmental and clinical samples by a direct cell multiplex PCR *Water SA* **39** 611–4

[10] Houzet L, Deleage C, Satie A P, Merlande L, Mahe D and Dejucq-Rainsford N 2015 A new method for rapid screening of end-point PCR products: application to single genome amplified HIV and SIV envelope amplicons *PLoS One* **10** e0128188

[11] Mori Y, Kitao M, Tomita N and Notomi T 2004 Real-time turbidimetry of LAMP reaction for quantifying template DNA *J. Biochem. Biophys. Methods* **59** 145–57

[12] Tanner N A, Zhang Y and Evans T C Jr. 2015 Visual detection of isothermal nucleic acid amplification using pH-sensitive dyes *Biotechniques* **58** 59–68

[13] Lo Y T and Shaw P C 2018 DNA-based techniques for authentication of processed food and food supplements *Food Chem.* **240** 767–74

[14] Bahadır E B and Sezgintürk M K 2016 Lateral flow assays: principles, designs and labels *TrAC Trends Analyt. Chem.* **82** 286–306

[15] Noguera P, Posthuma-Trumpie G A, van Tuil M, van der Wal F J, de Boer A, Moers A P and van Amerongen A 2011 Carbon nanoparticles in lateral flow methods to detect genes encoding virulence factors of Shiga toxin-producing *Escherichia coli Anal. Bioanal. Chem.* **399** 831–8

[16] Nagatani N, Yamanaka K, Ushijima H, Koketsu R, Sasaki T, Ikuta K, Saito M, Miyahara T and Tamiya E 2012 Detection of influenza virus using a lateral flow immunoassay for amplified DNA by a microfluidic RT-PCR chip *Analyst* **137** 3422–6

[17] Ongagna-Yhombi S Y, Corstjens P, Geva E, Abrams W R, Barber C A, Malamud D and Mharakurwa S 2013 Improved assay to detect *Plasmodium falciparum* using an uninterrupted, semi-nested PCR and quantitative lateral flow analysis *Malar. J.* **12** 74

[18] Sun Y, Chen J, Li J, Xu Y, Jin H, Xu N, Yin R and Hu G 2017 Novel approach based on one-tube nested PCR and a lateral flow strip for highly sensitive diagnosis of tuberculous meningitis *PLoS One* **12** e0186985

[19] Saiki R K, Gelfand D H, Stoffel S, Scharf S J, Higuchi R, Horn G T, Mullis K B and Erlich H A 1988 Primer-directed enzymatic amplification of DNA with a thermostable DNA polymerase *Science* **239** 487–91

[20] Erlich H A 1989 Basic methodology ed H A Erlich *PCR Technology.* 1st edn (New York: Stockton Press), pp 1–5

[21] Erlich H A, Gelfand D and Sninsky J J 1991 Recent advances in the polymerase chain reaction *Science* **252** 1643–51

[22] Kumar P, Jain M, Goel A K, Bhadauria S, Sharma S K, Kamboj D V, Singh L, Ramamurthy T and Nair G B 2009 A large cholera outbreak due to a new cholera toxin variant of the *Vibrio cholerae* O1 El Tor biotype in Orissa, Eastern India *J. Med. Microbiol.* **58** 234–8

[23] Jain M, Kushwah K S, Kumar P and Goel A K 2013 Molecular characterization of *Vibrio cholerae* O1 reveals continuous evolution of its new variants in India *Indian J. Microbiol* **53** 137–41

[24] Huang Q and Fu W L 2005 Comparative analysis of the DNA staining efficiencies of different fluorescent dyes in preparative agarose gel electrophoresis *Clin. Chem. Lab. Med.* **43** 841–2

[25] Waring M J 1965 Complex formation between ethidium bromide and nucleic acids *J. Mol. Biol.* **13** 269–82

[26] Lowe D 2016 The myth of ethidium bromide *In the Pipeline* 18 April 2016

[27] Abid H A, Ong J W, Lin E S, Song Z, Liew O W and Ng T W 2022 Low-cost imaging of fluorescent DNA in agarose gel electrophoresis using Raspberry Pi cameras *J Fluoresc* **32** 443–8

[28] Motohashi K 2019 Development of highly sensitive and low-cost DNA agarose gel electrophoresis detection systems, and evaluation of non-mutagenic and loading dye-type DNA-staining reagents *PLoS One* **14** e0222209

[29] Kirsanov K I, Lesovaya E A, Yakubovskaya M G and Belitsky G A 2010 SYBR Gold and SYBR Green II are not mutagenic in the Ames test *Mutat. Res.* **699** 1–4

[30] Haines A M, Tobe S S, Kobus H J and Linacre A 2015 Properties of nucleic acid staining dyes used in gel electrophoresis *Electrophoresis* **36** 941–4

[31] Yamamoto Y 2002 PCR in diagnosis of infection: detection of bacteria in cerebrospinal fluids *Clin. Diagn. Lab Immunol.* **9** 508–14

[32] Chang L, Li J and Wang L 2016 Immuno-PCR: an ultrasensitive immunoassay for biomolecular detection *Anal. Chim. Acta* **910** 12–24

[33] Mehta P K, Raj A, Singh N P and Khuller G K 2014 Detection of potential microbial antigens by immuno-PCR (PCR-amplified immunoassay) *J. Med. Microbiol.* **63** 627–41

[34] Luk J M, Kongmuang U, Tsang R S and Lindberg A A 1997 An enzyme-linked immunosorbent assay to detect PCR products of the rfbS gene from serogroup D salmonellae: a rapid screening prototype *J. Clin. Microbiol.* **35** 714–8

[35] Sharma S *et al* 2021 Emergence and expansion of highly infectious spike protein D614G mutant SARS-CoV-2 in central India *Sci. Rep.* **11** 18126

[36] Huang Y, Xu T, Wang W, Wen Y, Li K, Qian L, Zhang X and Liu G 2019 Lateral flow biosensors based on the use of micro- and nanomaterials: a review on recent developments *Mikrochim. Acta* **187** 70

[37] Urusov A E, Zherdev A V and Dzantiev B B 2019 Towards lateral flow quantitative assays: detection approaches *Biosensors (Basel)* **9** 89

[38] Ye H, Liu Y, Zhan L, Liu Y and Qin Z 2020 Signal amplification and quantification on lateral flow assays by laser excitation of plasmonic nanomaterials *Theranostics* **10** 4359–73

[39] Kawasaki H, Suzuki H, Maekawa M and Hariyama T 2021 Combination of the NanoSuit method and gold/platinum particle-based lateral flow assay for quantitative and highly sensitive diagnosis using a desktop scanning electron microscope *J. Pharm. Biomed. Anal.* **196** 113924

[40] Green M R and Sambrook J 2019 Screening colonies by polymerase chain reaction (PCR) *Cold Spring Harb. Protoc* **2019** 6

[41] Ponchel F *et al* 2003 Real-time PCR based on SYBR-Green I fluorescence: an alternative to the TaqMan assay for a relative quantification of gene rearrangements, gene amplifications and micro gene deletions *BMC Biotechnol* **3** 18

[42] Tajadini M, Panjehpour M and Javanmard S H 2014 Comparison of SYBR Green and TaqMan methods in quantitative real-time polymerase chain reaction analysis of four adenosine receptor subtypes *Adv. Biomed. Res.* **3** 85

[43] Jofre J and Blanch A R 2010 Feasibility of methods based on nucleic acid amplification techniques to fulfil the requirements for microbiological analysis of water quality *J. Appl. Microbiol.* **109** 1853–67

[44] Saccà M L *et al* 2019 Chemical mixtures and fluorescence *in situ* hybridization analysis of natural microbial community in the Tiber River *Sci. Total Environ.* **673** 7–19

[45] Wang H, Sun M, Xu D, Podok P, Xie J, Jiang Y and Lu L 2018 Rapid visual detection of cyprinid herpesvirus 2 by recombinase polymerase amplification combined with a lateral flow dipstick *J. Fish Dis.* **41** 1201–6

[46] Mendes Silva D and Domingues L 2015 On the track for an efficient detection of *Escherichia coli* in water: a review on PCR-based methods *Ecotoxicol. Environ. Saf.* **113** 400–11

[47] Notomi T, Okayama H, Masubuchi H, Yonekawa T, Watanabe K, Amino N and Hase T 2000 Loop-mediated isothermal amplification of DNA *Nucleic Acids Res.* **28** E63

[48] Mori Y, Kitao M, Tomita N and Notomi T 2004 Real-time turbidimetry of LAMP reaction for quantifying template DNA *J. Biochem. Biophys. Methods* **59** 145–57

[49] Obande G A and Banga Singh K K 2020 Current and future perspectives on isothermal nucleic acid amplification technologies for diagnosing infections *Infect. Drug Resist.* **13** 455–83

[50] Tomita N, Mori Y, Kanda H and Notomi T 2008 April Loop-mediated isothermal amplification (LAMP) of gene sequences and simple visual detection of products *Nat. Protoc.* **3** 877–82

[51] Fakruddin M 2011 Loop mediated isothermal amplification-an alternative to polymerase chain reaction (PCR) *Bang. Res. Pub. J.* **5** 425–39

[52] Gill P and Ghaemi A 2008 Nucleic acid isothermal amplification technologies: a review *Nucleosides Nucleotides Nucleic Acids* **27** 224–43

[53] Guatelli J C, Whitfield K M, Kwoh D Y, Barringer K J, Richman D D and Gingeras T R 1990 Isothermal, *in vitro* amplification of nucleic acids by a multienzyme reaction modelled after retroviral replication *Proc. Natl Acad. Sci. USA* **87** 1874–8

[54] Deiman B, van Aarle P and Sillekens P 2002 Characteristics and applications of nucleic acid sequence-based amplification (NASBA) *Mol. Biotechnol.* **20** 163–79

[55] Sergentet-Thevenot D, Montet M P and Vernozy-Rozand C 2008 Challenges to developing nucleic acid sequence based amplification technology for the detection of microbial pathogens in food *Rev. Med. Vet.* **159** 514–27

[56] Fakruddin M, Mazumdar R M, Chowdhury A and Mannan K S B 2012 Nucleic acid sequence-based amplification (NASBA)-prospects and applications *Int. J. Life Sci. Pharma Res* **2** 106–21

[57] Piepenburg O, Williams C H, Stemple D L and Armes N A 2006 DNA detection using recombination proteins *PLoS Biol.* **4** e204

[58] Thomas D C, Nardone G A and Randall S K 1999 Amplification of padlock probes for DNA diagnostics by cascade rolling circle amplification or the polymerase chain reaction *Arch. Pathol. Lab Med* **123** 1170–6

[59] Zhang D Y, Brandwein M, Hsuih T and Li H B 2001 Ramification amplification: a novel isothermal DNA amplification method *Mol. Diagn* **6** 141–50

[60] Ali M M, Li F, Zhang Z, Zhang K, Kang D K, Ankrum J A, Le X C and Zhao W 2014 Rolling circle amplification: a versatile tool for chemical biology, materials science and medicine *Chem. Soc. Rev.* **43** 3324–41

[61] Demidov V V 2002 Rolling-circle amplification in DNA diagnostics: the power of simplicity *Expert Rev. Mol. Diagn.* **2** 542–8

[62] Cho E J, Yang L, Levy M and Ellington A D 2005 Using a deoxyribozyme ligase and rolling circle amplification to detect a non-nucleic acid analyte, ATP *J. Am. Chem. Soc.* **127** 2022–3

[63] Gusev Y *et al* 2001 Rolling circle amplification: a new approach to increase sensitivity for immunohistochemistry and flow cytometry *Am. J. Pathol.* **159** 63–9

[64] Walker G T, Fraiser M S, Schram J L, Little M C, Nadeau J G and Malinowski D P 1992 Strand displacement amplification—an isothermal, *in vitro* DNA amplification technique *Nucleic Acids Res.* **20** 1691–6

[65] Dean F B, Nelson J R, Giesler T L and Lasken R S 2001 Rapid amplification of plasmid and phage DNA using Phi 29 DNA polymerase and multiply-primed rolling circle amplification *Genome Res* **11** 1095–9

[66] Dean F B *et al* 2002 Comprehensive human genome amplification using multiple displacement amplification *Proc. Natl Acad. Sci. USA* **99** 5261–6

[67] Morisset D, Stebih D, Cankar K, Zel J and Gruden K 2008 Alternative DNA amplification methods to PCR and their application in GMO detection: review *Eur. Food Res. Technol.* **227** 1287–97

[68] Makarova K S *et al* 2011 Evolution and classification of the CRISPR-Cas systems *Nat. Rev. Microbiol.* **9** 467–77

[69] Hilton I B, D'Ippolito A M, Vockley C M, Thakore P I, Crawford G E, Reddy T E and Gersbach C A 2015 Epigenome editing by a CRISPR-Cas9-based acetyltransferase activates genes from promoters and enhancers *Nat. Biotechnol.* **33** 510–7

[70] Cong L *et al* 2013 Multiplex genome engineering using CRISPR/Cas systems *Science* **339** 819–23

[71] Cox D B T, Gootenberg J S, Abudayyeh O O, Franklin B, Kellner M J, Joung J and Zhang F 2017 RNA editing with CRISPR-Cas13 *Science* **358** 1019–27

[72] Sheth R U, Yim S S, Wu F L and Wang H H 2017 Multiplex recording of cellular events over time on CRISPR biological tape *Science* **358** 1457–61

[73] Chen B *et al* 2013 Dynamic imaging of genomic loci in living human cells by an optimized CRISPR/Cas system *Cell* **155** 1479–91

[74] Bai J *et al* 2019 Cas12a-based on-site and rapid nucleic acid detection of African swine fever *Front. Microbiol.* **10** 2830

[75] Yuan T *et al* 2020 A rapid and sensitive CRISPR/Cas12a based lateral flow biosensor for the detection of Epstein-Barr virus *Analyst* **145** 6388–94

[76] Mukama O *et al* 2020 An ultrasensitive and specific point-of-care CRISPR/Cas12 based lateral flow biosensor for the rapid detection of nucleic acids *Biosens. Bioelectron.* **159** 112143

[77] Plotz C M and Singer J M 1956 The latex fixation test. I. Application to the serologic diagnosis of rheumatoid arthritis *Am. J. Med.* **21** 888–92

[78] Yalow R S and Berson S A 1960 Immunoassay of endogenous plasma insulin in man *J. Clin. Invest.* **39** 1157–75

[79] O'Farrell B 2013 Lateral flow immunoassay systems: evolution from the current state of the art to the next generation of highly sensitive, quantitative rapid assays The Immunoassay Handbook: Theory and Applications of Ligand Binding, ELISA and related Techniques. (Amsterdam: Elsevier) pp 89–107

[80] Leuvering J H, Thal P J, van der Waart M and Schuurs A H 1980 Sol particle immunoassay (SPIA) *J. Immunoassay* **1** 77–91

[81] Kosack C S, Page A L and Klatser P R 2017 A guide to aid the selection of diagnostic tests *Bull. World Health Organ* **95** 639–45

[82] Koczula K M and Gallotta A 2016 Lateral flow assays *Essays Biochem.* **60** 111–20

[83] Posthuma-Trumpie G A, Korf J and van Amerongen A 2009 Lateral flow (immuno)assay: its strengths, weaknesses, opportunities and threats. A literature survey *Anal. Bioanal. Chem.* **393** 569–82

[84] Xu Y, Liu Y, Wu Y, Xia X, Liao Y and Li Q 2014 Fluorescent probe-based lateral flow assay for multiplex nucleic acid detection *Anal. Chem.* **86** 5611–4

[85] Yen C W, de Puig H, Tam J O, Gómez-Márquez J, Bosch I, Hamad-Schifferli K and Gehrke L 2015 Multicolored silver nanoparticles for multiplexed disease diagnostics: distinguishing dengue, yellow fever, and Ebola viruses *Lab Chip* **15** 1638–41

[86] Fang C, Chen Z, Li L and Xia J 2011 Barcode lateral flow immunochromatographic strip for prostate acid phosphatase determination *J. Pharm. Biomed. Anal.* **56** 1035–40

[87] Leung W, Chan C P, Rainer T H, Ip M, Cautherley G W and Renneberg R 2008 InfectCheck CRP barcode-style lateral flow assay for semi-quantitative detection of C-reactive protein in distinguishing between bacterial and viral infections *J. Immunol. Methods* **336** 30–6

[88] Workman S, Wells S K, Pau C P, Owen S M, Dong X F, LaBorde R and Granade T C 2009 Rapid detection of HIV-1 p24 antigen using magnetic immuno-chromatography (MICT) *J. Virol. Methods* **160** 14–21

[89] Butler S A, Khanlian S A and Cole L A 2001 Detection of early pregnancy forms of human chorionic gonadotropin by home pregnancy test devices *Clin. Chem.* **47** 2131–6

[90] Peng D, Hu S, Hua Y, Xiao Y, Li Z, Wang X and Bi D 2007 Comparison of a new gold-immunochromatographic assay for the detection of antibodies against avian influenza virus with hemagglutination inhibition and agar gel immunodiffusion assays *Vet. Immunol. Immunopathol.* **117** 17–25

[91] Peng F, Wang Z, Zhang S, Wu R, Hu S, Li Z, Wang X and Bi D 2008 Development of an immunochromatographic strip for rapid detection of H9 subtype avian influenza viruses *Clin. Vaccine Immunol.* **15** 569–74

[92] Qian S and Bau H H 2004 Analysis of lateral flow biodetectors: competitive format *Anal. Biochem.* **326** 211–24

[93] Barnard R, George C, Jacobs K, Wu A C K, Nagasaki T K, Shan J, Greenwood K and Kachab E 2005 *Point-of Care* **4** 108–18

[94] Carter D J and Cary R B 2007 Lateral flow microarrays: a novel platform for rapid nucleic acid detection based on miniaturized lateral flow chromatography *Nucleic Acids Res.* **35** e74

[95] Edwards K A and Baeumner A J 2009 Liposome-enhanced lateral-flow assays for the sandwich-hybridization detection of RNA *Methods Mol. Biol.* **504** 185–215

[96] Amerongen V A and Koets M 2005 Simple and rapid bacterial protein and DNA diagnostic methods based on signal generation with colloidal carbon particles ed A van Amerongen, D Barug and M Lauwaars *Rapid Methods for Biological and Chemical Contaminants in Food and Feed* (Wageningen: Wageningen Academic Publishers), pp 105–26

[97] Corstjens P L, Zuiderwijk M, Nilsson M, Feindt H, Sam Niedbala R and Tanke H J 2003 Lateral-flow and up-converting phosphor reporters to detect single-stranded nucleic acids in a sandwich-hybridization assay *Anal. Biochem.* **312** 191–200

[98] Lee R A, Puig H, Nguyen P Q, Angenent-Mari N M, Donghia N M, McGee J P, Dvorin J D, Klapperich C M, Pollock N R and Collins J J 2020 Ultrasensitive CRISPR-based diagnostic for field-applicable detection of *Plasmodium* species in symptomatic and asymptomatic malaria *Proc. Natl Acad. Sci. USA* **117** 25722–31

[99] Anfossi L, Di Nardo F, Giovannoli C, Passini C and Baggiani C 2013 Increased sensitivity of lateral flow immunoassay for ochratoxin A through silver enhancement *Anal. Bioanal. Chem.* **405** 9859–67

[100] Lai W, Tang D, Que X, Zhuang J, Fu L and Chen G 2012 Enzyme-catalyzed silver deposition on irregular-shaped gold nanoparticles for electrochemical immunoassay of alpha-fetoprotein *Anal. Chim. Acta* **755** 62–8

[101] Parolo C, de la Escosura-Muñiz A and Merkoçi A 2013 Fe Enhanced lateral flow immunoassay using gold nanoparticles loaded with enzymes *Biosens. Bioelectron.* **40** 412–6

[102] Tang D, Sauceda J C, Lin Z, Ott S, Basova E, Goryacheva I, Biselli S, Lin J, Niessner R and Knopp D 2009 Magnetic nanogold microspheres-based lateral-flow immunodipstick for rapid detection of aflatoxin B2 in food *Biosens. Bioelectron.* **25** 514–8

[103] Qin Z, Chan W C, Boulware D R, Akkin T, Butler E K and Bischof J C 2012 Significantly improved analytical sensitivity of lateral flow immunoassays by using thermal contrast *Angew. Chem. Int. Ed. Engl.* **51** 4358–61

[104] Chen J, Fang Z, Lie P and Zeng L 2012 Computational lateral flow biosensor for proteins and small molecules: a new class of strip logic gates *Anal. Chem.* **84** 6321–5

[105] Andryukov B G 2020 Six decades of lateral flow immunoassay: from determining metabolic markers to diagnosing COVID-19 *AIMS Microbiol* **6** 280–304

[106] McPartlin D A and O'Kennedy R J 2014 Point-of-care diagnostics, a major opportunity for change in traditional diagnostic approaches: potential and limitations *Expert Rev. Mol. Diagn.* **14** 979–98

[107] Fu X, Wen J, Li J, Lin H, Liu Y, Zhuang X, Tian C and Chen L 2019 Highly sensitive detection of prostate cancer specific PCA3 mimic DNA using SERS-based competitive lateral flow assay *Nanoscale* **11** 15530–6

[108] Zhao Y, Wang H, Zhang P, Sun C, Wang X, Wang X, Yang R, Wang C and Zhou L 2016 Rapid multiplex detection of 10 foodborne pathogens with an up-converting phosphor technology-based 10-channel lateral flow assay *Sci. Rep.* **6** 21342

[109] Sastre P, Gallardo C, Monedero A, Ruiz T, Arias M, Sanz A and Rueda P 2016 Development of a novel lateral flow assay for detection of African swine fever in blood *BMC Vet. Res.* **12** 206

[110] Boisen M L, Oottamasathien D, Jones A B, Millett M M, Nelson D S and Bornholdt Z A *et al* 2015 Development of prototype filovirus recombinant antigen immunoassays *J. Infect. Dis.* **212** *S* 359–67

[111] Nielsen K, Yu W L, Kelly L, Bermudez R, Renteria T, Dajer A, Gutierrez E, Williams J, Algire J and de Eschaide S T 2008 Development of a lateral flow assay for rapid detection of bovine antibody to *Anaplasma marginale J. Immunoassay Immunochem.* **29** 10–8

[112] Rohrman B A, Leautaud V, Molyneux E and Richards-Kortum R R 2012 A lateral flow assay for quantitative detection of amplified HIV-1 RNA *PLoS One* **7** e45611

[113] Ngom B, Guo Y, Wang X and Bi D 2010 Development and application of lateral flow test strip technology for detection of infectious agents and chemical contaminants: a review *Anal. Bioanal. Chem.* **397** 1113–35

[114] Kuang H, Xing C, Hao C, Liu L, Wang L and Xu C 2013 Rapid and highly sensitive detection of lead ions in drinking water based on a strip immunosensor *Sensors (Basel)* **13** 4214–24

[115] Yin R, Sun Y, Wang K, Feng N, Zhang H and Xiao M 2020 Development of a PCR-based lateral flow strip assay for the simple, rapid, and accurate detection of pork in meat and meat products *Food Chem.* **318** 126541

IOP Publishing

Paper-Based Diagnostic Devices for Infectious Diseases

Nidhi Puranik, Arpana Parihar and Raju Khan

Chapter 10

Plasmonic thermal based lateral flow assay for detection and quantification of antibody/antigen

Agrata Singh, Bandi Lokesh Reddy and Ankit Sharma

In resource limited areas, the use of large instruments and the time devoted to collecting and analyzing the data, should be minimized. The use of LFA has increased drastically in the past few years. There are several experiments that have been conducted in order to maximize the accuracy and the specificity of the instruments. This will further lead to early detection of the diseases and allow proper treatment to reduce morbidity. The main principle behind this instrument is the collection of emitted light and its use in quantitative detection. By transmitting, reflecting, or scattering light out of an external source, optical information is gained, that is captured in the optical reader which will carry out the quantification. The main advantage of this instrument is the simple yes/no result based on the colour change. The light source that is used can also improve the sensitivity of the instrument; it was observed that when green light was used, it increased the sensitivity 32-fold. Gold nanoparticles were also introduced in the instruments to increase efficiency. These gold particles act as analysts which can be used to increase the heat generated which can be detected by the transducer. The use of this device has increased as a result of the various developments made to boost its sensitivity.

10.1 Introduction

Recent COVID-19 infection outbreaks around the world have shown the most recent advancements in lateral flow assay (LFA) technology, which is based on surface-enhanced Raman scattering (SERS) and used for infectious disease diagnostics. Quick detection of the virus is crucial in order to stop the spread of disease and ensure that pandemic preparation is undertaken. A state-of-the-art point-of-care diagnostic strategy is essential in this situation. Recently, the medical world has covered a lot of SERS-based assay system news. On the other hand, its multimodal detection ability and high-sensitivity LFAs offer a user-friendly and approachable

doi:10.1088/978-0-7503-5820-0ch10 © IOP Publishing Ltd 2023

sensing platform. The earlier a disease is detected, the easier it is to treat. Because traditional medical tests take longer, large instruments are required, as well as additional time to collect and analyze the sample/data. As a result, point-of-care testing (POCT) is now required. In resource-constrained communities, standard medical tests might be a barrier. The POCT takes less time and includes all of the basic instruments needed to produce a useful result. This will allow clinicians and patients to make decisions more quickly, resulting in better medical conditions in all areas. Consequently, combining LFAs with such a SERS detecting system results in a new diagnostic approach for a precise and quick diagnosis of infectious diseases. In this context, we will examine the recent use of LFA platforms for SARS-CoV-2 POC diagnosis (figure 10.1). The development of SERS-based LFA systems for the rapid diagnosis of infectious diseases will next be discussed, along with how useful they are for the rapid detection of SARS-CoV-2. Finally, important issues that need to be resolved are explored in order to hasten the practical implementation of SERS-based LFA systems first from lab to the bedside.

The lateral flow assay is one of the greatest examples of PCOT, and it has undergone extensive development to improve its ability to identify disease. LFA is a paper-based device with a biosensor that detects the target analyte [1, 2]. An adsorption pad, nitrocellulose pad, conjugate pad, and sample pad make up the paper-based strip used in LFA. The detection is straightforward, yielding a yes or no

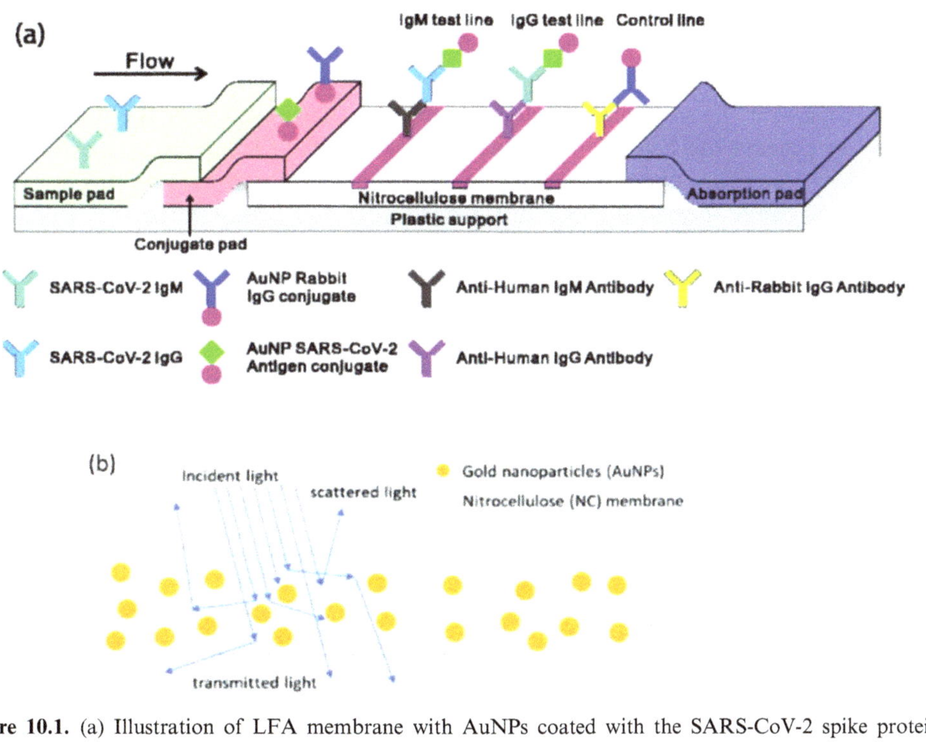

Figure 10.1. (a) Illustration of LFA membrane with AuNPs coated with the SARS-CoV-2 spike protein. (b) Process of absorption and scattering of light inside the strip with AuNPs. Reprinted from [3], with the permission of AIP Publishing.

answer based on a colour shift on the test line that can be seen with the naked eye. The images are acquired in the strip reader using sensors such as complementary metal-oxide semiconductors and charged coupled devices. Image processing software is required to obtain accurate quantitative findings [2].

To analyze the LFA strip, the reader collects the colour intensity, such as the grey value, and compares it to the control. Fluorescence readers are also incorporated in the system; these can be employed with organic fluorophores that emit fluorophore when exposed to a certain excitable wavelength [4, 5]. The light that is emitted can then be captured and used to make quantitative measurements. However, because the fluorophores utilized in this detection can be photobleached and chemically degraded with time, they must be kept in proper storage and handled with care.

The primary premise of an LFA is signal creation and detection, as we already know. As a result, stronger signals are currently utilized to improve LFA diagnostics, such as quantum dots, upconverting nanoparticles, caron NPPs, non-metal NPs, latex beads, magnetic NPs, and so on, and the range of LFA applications has been expanded. Attempts to incorporate additional reagents, such as enzyme-based catalytic processes, have been unsuccessful since they enhance the LFA's complexity. When plasmonic gold particles (GNPs) were first used, it provided a great boost to the application of LFA. They generate far stronger signals than colour-coded ones, making them more useful and detectable.

10.2 Plasmonic thermal sensing LFA

There has been a recent transition in LFA to thermal sensors. A heat transducer is used in this, and the heat created is enhanced by the presence of the analyte. The transducer detects the heat that is generated. Polo and Qin investigated this area, with the former using plasmonic heating with the use of a cancer biomarker called carcinoembryonic antigen (CEA) and a near-infra-red light source to induce heat generation by using the plasmonic property of the gold nanoparticle [6]. Qin, on the other hand, used thermal contrast to quantify LFA. His light source was green light, which increased LFA's analytical sensitivity by 32 times. It was also discovered that the light source utilized can be set to a precise wavelength to assure the detection's specificity [7–9]. This will eliminate the impediment imposed by other molecules that do not absorb light at the specified wavelength. The light sources in the NIR areas allow light from a wide spectrum of molecules, especially blood, to pass through, making the plasmonic thermal LFA very effective [10].

However, until recently, there was no such portable thermal LFA produced with NIR as a light source. This increases the assay's analytical sensitivity without causing significant differences in the strips. In this case, NIR laser irradiation was employed to amplify the signal, resulting in better and more precise results. The heat created was then measured either by radiation or conduction by the thermal sensor. The amount of heat produced is related to the irradiation power or the number of nanoparticles in the test line [11]. Conduction, convection, and radiation are the three types of heat transport. Nanoparticles were immediately placed onto the strips for device verification, and the strips were subsequently measured using a traditional visual detector. Because the system was temperature-dependent in this experiment, careful attention was paid to the outside temperature. An incubator was used to keep the temperature between 27.5 °C and 40 °C. During the experiment, it was also discovered that the temperature's negative influence affected the radiation mode more than the conduction (contact) mode. Human chorionic gonadotrophins were utilized as a biomarker to test the detection capabilities of thermal sensing (HCG). With the use of this biomarker, it was also determined that the radiation mode had a higher sensitivity than the conduction mode. The limit-of-detection (LOD) in thermal sensing was lowered 2-fold when using the radiation mode, whereas it was the same as visual detection when using the conduction method. With the help of all of these findings, it can be stated that thermal sensing is more practical for early detection than other methods.

10.3 Advancement of LFA

Apart from the thermal sensor, there have been many other advancements in this field, which have led to the improvement of the usage of LFA. Some of them are discussed in more detail below the table (table 10.1).

10.3.1 SERS enhanced signal

The basic idea behind this method is to amplify and generate inelastic light that is scattered and absorbed by metals. The efficiency of a nanoparticle can be improved by modulating the frequency of the excitation light along with the nanoparticle's LSPR. The known tags of Raman fingerprints are used as detection agents in this technique. This, in combination with nanoparticles, will aid in the detection of analytes. The Raman molecules can be conjugated together [12, 13] to apply this approach with several targets, although this can result in overlapping peaks, which can reduce the sensitivity of the technique [14]. Parallel test bands can be designed to prevent this, allowing correct peaks to be observed [15]. If the sample's response time needs to be shortened, microarrays of LFA strips can be created. It is critical to choose the right Raman fingerprints or reporter so that the right analyses and findings may be produced in less time.

10.3.2 Sensitivity enhancement based on sample pretreatment

Saliva and serum are the sample matrices most often used for diagnosing illnesses. The matrix of serum and saliva, which contains proteins, nucleic acids, and other substances, may cause AuNPs to clump, lowering the specificity and sensitivity of detection. LFA introduces numerous sample pretreatment techniques, such as isothermal replication for nucleic acid detection or sample enrichment for protein detection, to get rid of interfering elements. The example pretreatment in conjunction with LFA will be the main topic of the sections that follow.

10.3.2.1 Sensitivity enhancement based on isothermal nucleic acid amplification

Nucleic acids are increasingly being categorized as biomarkers for disease diagnosis, microbiological detection, and environmental monitoring because they are more

Table 10.1. The advancement of LFA.

	Advancement of LFA	Property
1	SERS enhanced signal	Efficiency of a nanoparticle is improved by modulating the frequency of the excitation light along with the nanoparticle's LSPR. The known tags of Raman fingerprints are used as detection agents in this technique.
2	Based on sample pretreatment	Sample pretreatment reduce the chances of AuNPs clumping.
2a	Based on isothermal nucleic acid amplification	Even while nucleic acid is less sensitive, it is more stable. To increase the sensitivity of LFA for nucleic acid detection, isothermal amplification techniques like RCA and LAMP are employed.
2b	Sensitivity enhancement based on RCA	A short DNA or RNA primer is amplified to create a lengthy single-stranded circular DNA template using the isothermal PCR technique known as RCA, which also uses particular DNA or RNA polymerases to create the DNA or RNA. 100 times more sensitive than a regular PCR.
2c	Based on RPA	RPA is a form of isothermal PCR. The detection of harmful bacteria and viruses in food safety, environmental monitoring, and other applications have been made possible by the widespread use of RPA.
2d	Based on LAMP	For six regions of the target gene segment, LAMP generates two or three pairs of primers. LAMP's use of several primers ensured precise and effective specificity. Paper was added to the LAMP microfluidic system, and the outcomes were more consistent.
3	Sensitivity enhancement based on sample enrichment	Amplification cannot increase the amount of proteins, hence sample enrichment is required.
3a	Based on electrophoresis	To increase the detection sensitivity of LFA, paper-based preconcentrates for ion concentration polarization (ICP) are used. The target analyte can be concentrated to increase LFA sensitivity.
3b	Based on extraction	In order to concentrate the target in a smaller volume, an aqueous two-phase system is developed. To examine diluted samples, 3D paper might be employed.
3c	Based on dialysis	Magnetic bead-based separation, which employs super magnetism, is a method to perform sample pretreatment and remove the impact of food matrices in LFA. A semi-permeable membrane is used.

(Continued)

Table 10.1. (*Continued*)

	Advancement of LFA	Property
4	Sensitivity enhancement based on the change of flow rate	The sensitivity is increased by using a paper-based shunt and a polydimethylsiloxane (PDMS) barrier with LFA to create the proper fluidic delays.
5	Sensitivity enhancement based on NC membrane size change	In order to alter the membrane's size, a constriction barrier is placed in the flow channel. Sensitivity is increased by size restriction.
6	Sensitivity enhancement based on dual AuNPs	Use of AuNPs as the labelling nanomaterial with higher particle size is more conducive to improving sensitivity
7	Sensitivity enhancement based on enzymatic amplification	Nanocarrier enzyme probes have been used in LFA to increase the detection performance. Enzyme accelerated signal amplification improves the sensitivity.
8	Sensitivity enhancement based on photothermal method	A thermal contrast-based approach improves the sensitivity of LFA.

stable in extreme environments than other biomarkers. LFA for nucleic acid identification has drawn more interest as the need for diagnosis in environments with limited resources has increased because of its lower cost and ease of use. However, the sensitivity of the present LFA for nucleic acid screening is low, which restricts its usefulness.

Pathogenic bacteria that cause disease can exist in concentrations as low as a few CFU ml^{-1}, in contrast to protein biomarkers which exist at nanomolar or picomolar levels. Rolling circle amplification (RCA), motion isothermal overexpression (LAMP), recombinase polymerase amplification (RPA), nucleic acid series amplification (NASBA), and helicase dependent isothermal DNA amplification are some of the isothermal amplification techniques used to increase the sensitivity of LFA for nucleic acid detection (HDA).

10.3.2.2 Sensitivity enhancement based on RCA

In RCA, a short DNA or RNA primer is amplified to create a long single-stranded circular DNA template, and particular DNA or RNA polymerases are utilized to create DNA or RNA. This is an isothermal enzymatic process. A significant number of capturing or signal-generating sites are produced by the RCA product, which is a concatemer made up of tens to hundreds of tandem repetitions that are complimentary to the circular template. Researchers simultaneously identified miRNA21 and miRNA let-7a using RCA in conjunction with AuNP-based LFA [16]. For one, the detection limit (LOD) was as low as 40 pM, and for the other, it was 20 pM. When compared to the results of Kor *et al* [17], the sensibility of miRNA21 was improved by 7.5 times. Additionally, RCA in conjunction with LFA was used to find Karenia mikimotoi (hyperbranched RCA, HRCA) and Karlodinium venefcum (exponential RCA, E-RCA). While E-RCA-LFA had a LOD of 0.01 cell per mL and a sensitivity of 100-fold that of pcr technique, HRCA-LFA had a sensitivity of 100-fold of that of PCR. Additionally, RCA-based LFA has been used to find antibodies, enzymes, metal ions, and tiny molecules.

10.3.2.3 Based on RPA

RPA falls under the category of isothermal PCR. Recombinase and single-stranded binding proteins are used to replace the PCR's planned temperature changes. The single-stranded binding protein maintains the single-chain so that the DNA polymerase may finish the primer extension process. The recombinase completes the separation of the template and the combining of primers and templates. Most importantly, it is a successful approach in terms of sensitivity, specificity, and multiplexing. Using cluster frequently interspaced short palindromic repeats (CRISPR), Zhang's team [18] created a diagnostic tool called specialized high-sensitivity enzymatic reporter unlocking that combined RPA and LFA with CRISPR-Cas enzymology for the precise detection of specified DNA or RNA sequences. The template performed RPA's isothermal amplified response to amplify the signal. In order to transform the goal from DNA to RNA for detection, a T7 promoter for RPA *in vitro* transcription was simultaneously inserted. After identifying the RNA target location, Cas13a would fragment molecular beacons on the fly to produce signals. The RNA target required reverse transcription. The detection of harmful microorganisms and viruses in food security, environmental control, and other applications has been made possible by the widespread use of RPA.

10.3.2.4 Sensitivity enhancement based on LAMP

The primary idea behind LAMP is to design two or three pairs of primers for each of the six regions of the target gene fragment in order to achieve quick and effective amplification. Similar to nested PCR, the use of several primers in LAMP ensured precise and effective specificity. Target DNA is not infected by non-target DNA or PCR inhibitors that closely resemble the target DNA. Dou and colleagues coupled a polydimethylsiloxane (PDMS)/paper hybrid microfluidic chip with LAMP for Neisseria meningitidis detection. When compared to earlier experiments, the microfluidic device for LAMP with paper in it produced more reliable findings than a paperless microfluidic system. The LOD was less than in earlier research, at roughly three copies of DNA.

A research team developed STOPCovid, an improved version of the new coronavirus detection algorithm based on SHERLOCK [18], in response to COVID-19. The RNA in the sample was enhanced by the addition of magnetic beads during sample preparation, which increased the amount of original RNA in LMAP and increasing detection sensitivity. Additionally, TOPCovid version 2.0 simplified the magnetic bead RNA enrichment operating procedures, did away with the ethanol washing and eluting step, and cut the RNA enrichment procedure's overall time to under 15 min. In addition, the use of LAMP in conjunction with LFA has allowed the detection of *Escherichia coli*, plasmodium, *Pseudomonas aeruginosa*, and SARS-CoV-20.

10.3.3 Sensitivity enhancement based on sample enrichment

Protein cannot be amplified to produce more of it, unlike nucleic acids. Protein detection can be used with enrichment techniques like iso-electric electrophoresis, dialysis, and magnetic enrichment, for instance, to increase concentration and boost detection sensitivity.

10.3.3.1 Sensitivity enhancement based on electrophoresis

The identification sensitivity of human chorionic gonadotropin is increased when LFA is used with paper-based ion concentration polarization (ICP) preconcentrates hCG. When compared to the commercial LFA for hCG, the preconcentration factor was manufactured utilizing a straightforward 9 V battery with little power consumption (about 81 W), and the detection sensitivity was raised by 2.69 times. Target analytes were concentrated by isotachophoresis (ITP) into a thin band and then given to the LFA test line, which significantly increased the rate of surface response and equilibrium binding. With respect to commercial LFAs, this approach can increase LFA sensitivity for hCG by 400 times.

10.3.3.2 Sensitivity enhancement based on extraction

Kamei's team developed an aqueous two-phase system (ATPS) to concentrate a specific biomarker into a smaller volume before loading it onto LFA [19]. Using this technique, the overall detection capability of LFA for bacteriophage M13 and transferrin (Tf) was increased 10-fold. According to the focusing phenomenon [20], this recently discovered paper membrane also accelerated the macroscopic phase separation of ATPS. The cross-sectional area of the paper device was increased vertically to take advantage of gravity's impact on macroscopic separation. In addition to accelerating phase separation, this 3D component enhanced the capability to process larger and much more diluted quantities of sample. A 3D paper that successfully combined ATPS and LFA increased transferrin detection by ten times.

10.3.3.3 Sensitivity enhancement based on dialysis

Tang *et al* used a semi-permeable membrane, glass fibre, and PEG buffer with LFA for sample enrichment. PEG-loaded glass fibre was used as the dialysate to concentrate the sample. HIV detection had a 10-fold signal improvement over the baseline LFA, while myoglobin detection had a 4-fold improvement. Super magnetism-based magnetic bead-based separation is an easy method to carry out sample pretreatment and get rid of the impact of food matrices in LFA. Aptamers or antibodies are frequently marked with magnetic beads for target capture. Brown coloured magnetic nanoparticles or magnetic beads with less background noise are excellent LFA label materials. Fe_3O_4 superparamagnetic nanosphere (SPMN) probes were used to build a multiple immunoassay test strip that was used to enrich specimens and quench the fluorescence of several fluorescent species on the test line [21]. The simultaneous detection of carbohydrate antigen (CA153) and carcinoembryonic antigen (CEA) was accomplished with LODs of 0.06 ng ml^{-1} and 0.6 U ml^{-1}.

10.3.4 Sensitivity enhancement based on the change of flow rate

Another crucial factor impacting LFA sensitivity is the duration of the immunoreaction between the analyte and the capture antibody pre-deposited on the test line, which is reliant on the sample migration time over the test line. The reported techniques of enzyme augmentation, temperature and humidity control, and fluidic control via hydrophobic barriers all produced results that were comparable to or even better than those obtained with a test that should be long enough to allow for a sufficient antibody–antigen limit of 100 copies of dengue virus RNA [14]. The wax barrier on the NC membrane of the LFA, however, might melt when heated. A paper-based shunt and a polydimethylsiloxane barrier were combined with LFA to create the proper fluidic delays, and this resulted in a 10-fold increase in signal strength for detecting hepatitis B virus (HBV) nucleic acid. Because of its high permeability, superior mechanical qualities, ease of fluid control, and variable pore size and porosity, agarose was chosen as the barrier in following testing. Surprisingly, with a detection period of only a few minutes, this method of detection boosted sensitivity by roughly ten times. Synthesis of 100 copies of dengue viral RNA yielded results that were comparable to or more sensitive than those previously reported for techniques to fluidic control using hydrophobic barriers, temperature and humidity control, and enzyme augmentation (figure 10.2).

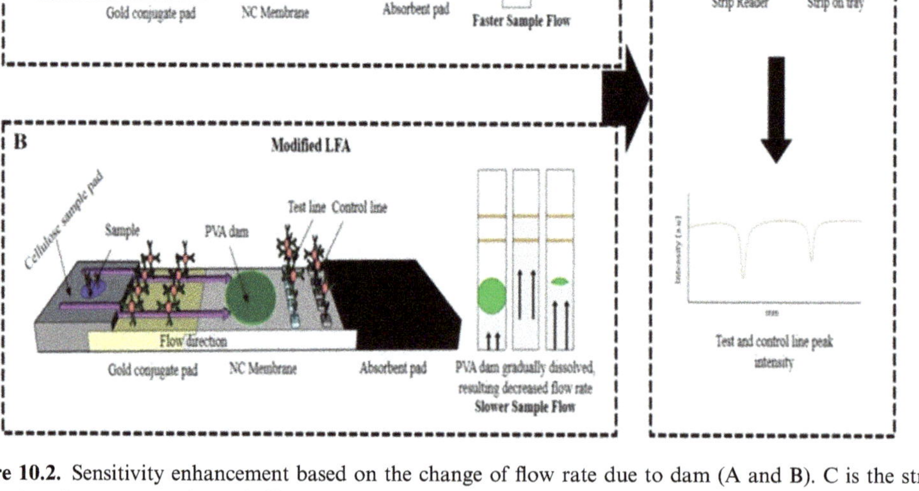

Figure 10.2. Sensitivity enhancement based on the change of flow rate due to dam (A and B). C is the strip reader for a better comparison of different strips [22] (2021) (Copyright © 2021, The Author(s), under exclusive licence to Springer Nature B.V.). With permission of Springer.

10.3.5 Sensitivity enhancement based on NC membrane size change

Katis *et al* [23] used spatial constrictions in the flow route as a strategy to increase sensitivity and lower the LOD of LFA due to the slower flow velocity and smaller test zone area. The liquid photopolymer was applied with a deposition nozzle to the paper substrate. A laser beam then followed the deposition head (figure 10.3). By shining light on the patterns that had been deposited, the polymer underwent photopolymerization. The polymerized patterns served as demarcation barriers to hold and transport liquids inside the paper device, defining the fluidic walls. Compared to the conventional LFA with a 5 mm wide constriction, the C-reactive protein (CRP) LOD was 5 ng ml^{-1} with a 1 mm wide constriction.

10.3.6 Sensitivity enhancement based on dual AuNPs

As particle size grows, the molar extinction coefficient of gold nanoparticles (AuNPs) rises noticeably. As a result, it is easier to increase sensitivity when utilizing AuNPs, a labelling nanomaterial with a larger particle size [14]. Researchers used two distinct sizes of AuNPs to successfully detect cardiac troponin I (cTnI) via LFA. The first conjugate consisted of AuNPs (10 nm) coated with anti-troponin I antibody and blocked with BSA, while the second conjugate consisted of AuNPs (40 nm) coated with anti-BSA antibody and blocked with human serum albumin. A double AuNP-based LFA may detect cTnI in as little as 0.01 ng ml^{-1} in 10 min, which is 100 times more accurate than Posthuma-findings. Then, Trumpie's [24] dual-labelling technique was made more sensitive and practical for on-site melamine detection. Later, procalcitonin, mercury, and bisphenol A (BPA) were detected using this method (PCT). Sensitivity is increased through silver staining. Silver staining, which was developed to alter the form of AuNPs, was inspired by GNSs. Silver staining, which involves a colour change at the test line as a result of chemical interactions, is another technique for signal amplification. As a result of these processes, which include the catalytic reduction of silver ions on gold nanoparticles, the LFA test lines exhibit darker colours and greater gold nanoparticle absorbance values. Yang *et al* [25] employed silver staining in LFA for the first time. The reducer pad was then placed on top of the $AgNO_3$ pad-coated NC membrane,

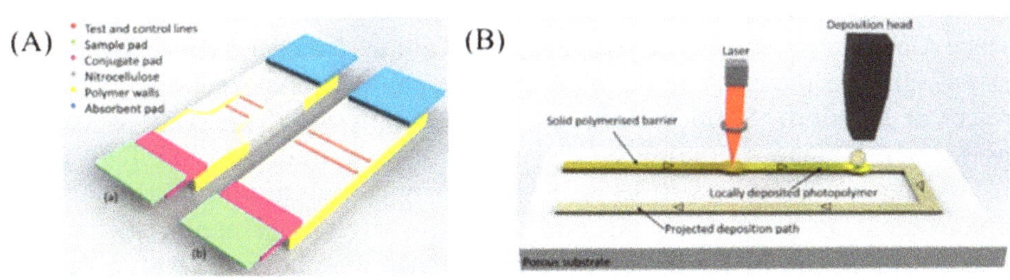

Figure 10.3. Based on the constriction on the flow path better sensitivity detected. (A) Sensitivity due to change in NC pore size. (B) Laser based direct write procedure [19] (2021) (Copyright © 2021, The Author(s), under exclusive licence to Springer-Verlag GmbH Austria, part of Springer Nature). With permission of Springer.

and a clear red hue resulted. In order to highlight the contrast, the detection line's colour was changed from red to black using the larger silver particles that were produced. With a 0.1 ng ml^{-1} detection limit, abrin-sensitivity a's was increased by 100 times. Kim *et al* used core–shell hybrid nanofibers and a silver staining technique to identify cTnI. Hydroquinone solutions containing $AgNO_3$ and the silver-reducing agent were electro spun separately. The test line's colour faded as a result of the silver ions becoming metallic silver in the vicinity of AuNPs. When compared to commercial LFA, the sensitivity of cTnI was up to ten times higher and the detection limit was 0.24 ng ml^{-1}. Anfossi *et al* [26] used this strategy to detect ochratoxin A (OTA) using competitive LFA, and the sensitivity was raised by a factor of ten. In comparison to the standard LFA, OTA detection takes a lot longer.

10.3.7 Sensitivity enhancement based on enzymatic amplification

Inspired by the ubiquitous use of enzymes as labels in bioassays, the nanocarrier enzyme probes have been used in LFA to improve the detection performance of various optical and electronic biosensing devices. AuNPs were used in the study as both enzyme carriers and labels for antibodies [27]. When employed as direct labels on LFA, AuNPs displayed red at the test and control lines. However, the insoluble chromogens generated when AuNPs are coupled with antibodies and inhibited with horseradish peroxidase (HRP) prevent the flow from moving them, darkening the colour of the lines. When compared to three substrates, TMB was found to be the best substrate for signal amplification (TMB for blue-violet, AEC for red, and DAB for grey-black). The signal amplification method described above was employed by Cho *et al* [28] to find *E. coli* O157:H7. The detection threshold that was attained was 100 CFU ml^{-1}, which was approximately 1000 times slower than the detection threshold of conventional AuNP-based LFA. Li *et al* created an all-encompassing 'add-on' technology called enzyme rapid signal amplification (EASE) In order to collect many signal molecules and achieve a 3-fold increase in sensitivity, EASE relies on the ultrafast and targeted deposition of polydopamine (PDA) at the test line [15]. When employing DAB as the substrate, LFA can detect p24 at a concentration of 10 ng ml^{-1}, whereas EASE can recognize p24 at a concentration of 10 pg ml^{-1}, allowing ultrasensitive HIV detection.

10.3.8 Sensitivity enhancement based on surface-enhanced Raman scattering

Surface roughness results in surface-enhanced Raman scattering, which increases the Raman signal in the excitation region of some suitably prepared metal conductor surfaces or solutions. Surface-enahnced Raman scattering (SERS) can outperform conventional Raman scattering by dix orders of magnitude or more [29]. Covian *et al* produced SERS-based LFA to detect pneumolysin using rhodamine B isothiocyanate as the Raman tag and gold-core–silver-shell nanoparticles as the plasmonic platform. SERS-based LFA's sensitivity was increased with a detection limit of 1 pg ml^{-1} in comparison to the electrochemical immunosensor's detection limit of 0.6 ng ml^{-1} and the chemiluminescence immunoassay's detection limit of 5.5 pg ml^{-1}. The ability of SERS nanotags to code by absorbing various Raman dyes on the metal surface enables a variety of detections [21]. Nile Blue A (NBA) Raman dye was encapsulated at the core–shell interface, and a novel LFA based on core–shell SERS nanotags was developed to realize rapid quantification of creatine kinase isoenzyme (CK-MB), cTnI, and myoglobin (Myo) on three test lines with detection limits of 0.55, 0.44, and 3.2 pg ml^{-1}, respectively. Methylene blue (MB), Nile blue A (NBA) and rhodamine 6G (R6G) Raman dye were encapsulated at the core shell contact in the follow up work. The stability of the Raman dye is essential for sensitive and precise detection. For the purpose of detecting neuron-specific enolase (NSE), a sign of traumatic brain injury, Gao *et al* [30] developed Au nanostar Raman dye silica sandwich nanoparticles with a LOD of 0.86 ng ml^{-1}. (TBI). Malachite green isothiocyanate (MGITC), a Raman dye, can be successfully stabilized by being sandwiched between AuNPs and thin silica. The SERS-based methodology outperformed well-established colorimetric techniques, especially in the plasma matrix [31]. Hollow gold nanospheres (HGN) and the Raman dye MGTTC were employed by Hwang *et al* [32] to identify staphylococcal enterotoxin B. (SEB) HGN augmentation of the SERS signal allowed for high-sensitivity detection with a LOD of 1 pg ml^{-1} and more than 30 times enhancement.

10.3.9 Sensitivity enhancement based on photothermal methods

For the detection of enrofloxacin, Li *et al* created a quantitative photothermal sensing LFA with a detection limit of 0.023 ng ml^{-1} [15]. Black phosphorus (BP)-Au nanosheets demonstrated good photothermal capabilities at an 808 nm wavelength, with a photothermal conversion efficiency that was 12.9% greater than black phosphorus nanosheets alone. A technique based on temperature contrast was developed [7, 9] to increase the sensitivity of LFA. The FDA-approved LFA for cryptococcal antigen (CrAg) detection can be replaced with one that has a 32-fold increase in sensitivity. A thermal contrast magnification (TCM) reader was developed by Wang, consisting of a laser emitter for various wavelengths, an infra-red camera for the heat reading produced, and data reading and processing software [14]. The reader can considerably increase the LFA antigen quantification's accuracy. Compared to the human eye or colorimetric readers, the TCA reader demonstrated an 8-fold higher sensitivity for the detection of malaria and *Clostridium difficile* (such as BD VeritorTM system readers). A high-contrast random granular pattern called a laser speckle is highly responsive to the refractive index and physical displacement of the medium [33, 34]. The NC membrane can be used as a diffusion medium to produce high-contrast speckle patterns since it is made up of randomly aligned nanofibers [35]. The sensitivity can be improved by 68 times in comparison to the FDA-approved LFA for CrAg detection. Using a US FDA-approved LFA to evaluate the developed PT-ability LSILFA's to detect CrAg, it was shown that PT-LSI exhibited a 68-fold increase in detection sensitivity.

10.3.9.1 Limitation

Even though the sensitivity of the technique is good and generates trustable results, there are a few limitations of the techniques that are yet to be overcome. Some of them are as follows:

- More work on the SERS tags is needed to generate a robust and appropriate amount of Raman's signal. To achieve better outcomes, the electromagnetic field of the tags must be improved.
- There has been a finding of low repeatability. There is a trade-off between the signal's intensity and the data acquisition parameters. A long acquisition time is required for a strong Raman signal. If we increase the sample area while decreasing the collection time, we will get a poor result.

10.4 Thermal contrast amplification

The heat created by GNPs has been extensively explored and applied to a variety of treatments, most notably cancer. This principle has been used in the LFA technique, and it has been discovered that the heat generated is proportional to both the laser energy used in the region to be detected and the GNPs present in the region [9]. Thermographic techniques are also utilized to ensure the effective application of the technology in diagnosis. The concentration of GNPs present in the test bands will be used to provide a quantitative result in the thermal analysis of the test bands. The cryptococcal antigen was tested to prove this technique. This is most commonly used to diagnose cryptococcal meningitis in immunocompromised people (Jarvis JN, Meintjes). Because the size and shape of the GNP are employed to improve the photothermal property of the particles, the diagnostic performance can be improved. The heat production property of nanorods and nanoshells of GNPs is ten times better than the spherical shape of the particle [4].

10.4.1 Limitation

Some of the limitations of the technique that should not be ignored are as follows:

- Presently, the data acquisition time is 10–15 min should be reduced to 3 min per test.
- The reproducibility of the technique is also to be taken care of as the concentration of GNPs on the test bands is not uniformly distributed.
- A portable reader is still a matter of research as the technique depends on the ambient temperature that can fluctuate thus hindering the result.

10.5 Thermophotonic lock-in imaging

If you are trying to do the industrial evaluation of materials then the thermographic technique is the most suitable and widely used. In this technique, a controlled thermal wave has to be created, to do so a continuous intensity-modulated laser is used with low power. The detected signal is then is evaluated by the lock-in demodulation with the help of the sample and the exciting light is used as a reference [36]. To put this simply, the different absorbers that are present at various locations in the depth of the feature have different absorption coefficients and optical scattering properties. This will accumulate to give an IR signal that can be used for detection. Recently it has been observed that this technique is widely used for the early detection of dental problems in humans [37]. This technique when combined with the LFA will improve its efficiency as now its property to inspect the depth of the particle/feature can be exploited. We are now able to find the GNPs that are present both on the surface and inside the membrane.

10.5.1 Limitation

- As this is a huge instrument it is therefore expensive; this has to be reduced significantly. Many parts are involved in the collection of the signal that can be later monitored and analyzed on the computer.
- Special importance has to be provided to the laser modulation frequency to improve the LOD of the instrument. Various types of thickness of the LFA have to be tested so that all types of LFA can be used with the technique.

10.6 Photothermal laser speckle imaging

If you are willing to measure the optical contrast which is generated by the moving sample, it can be done using this LSI technique. A specific pattern known as granular speckle is generated when the diffused matter is encountered by the laser [38]. A digital camera is also installed which can capture the pattern generated even when exposed for a short duration. This image can later be used to analyze the intensity pattern of the light. Fourier transformation can be used to study the collected intensity fluctuation profile so that ultimately the dynamics of the specimen can be mapped [39]. The incorporation of the pulse laser has improved the technique for the depth resolution of the specimen. When this technique was tested for the LFA, due to the multi-layer feature of LFA, the light of the probe was scattered resulting in the formation of the pattern. The light specifically excites the GNPs particles, at around 780 nm wavelength the heat generation takes place which results in the changing of the pattern. But in the LFA an optical sensor was used in the place of the digital camera so that the cost of the experiment can be reduced [40]. To minimize the external noise, an optical chopper is used in the experiment. Due to the presence of the GNPs, stronger signals can be generated so that a better analysis of the specimen can be conducted.

10.6.1 Limitation

Even though the intensity of the signal was increased the cost of the experiments was reduced, thanks to the GNPs and the optical sensors used. There are a few limitations that are still to be addressed, e.g.:

- The web camera and the laser pointers that are used need more testing, to ensure their robustness.
- The power stability of the laser is still a concern as it plays a crucial role in the long-term use of the technique.

Now that we know various types of modifications done to make the LFA more acceptable at a large range by increasing the sensitivity and specificity, let us have a look at the advantages of overall LFA over other types. These will be enough to make you believe the rising future of LFA on daily basis for diagnostic and other applications of LFA.

10.7 Advantages of LFA

Some of the advantages of using an LFA over other medical test methods are as follows:

- It has a single step assay and so is a rapid test.
- It can be performed easily and does not require much skill. Any good strip reader can diagnose the disease.
- It is cost-effective as large instruments are not involved.
- It has a comparatively greater shelf life under different environmental conditions.
- The sample volume required to carry out the process is small and yet it gives quite accurate results. Its sensitivity has been increasing with the certain modifications that have been done with the biosensors.
- The thermal sensor is better than the visual sensor as it has higher stability. The reason behind this is that the heat generated by the thermal sensor is all across the test strip whereas the visual sensor mainly relies on the colour regions.
- At the assay level, 'analytical sensitivity' is occasionally used as an alternative to limit-of-detection.
- The term 'specificity' for an assay refers to its capacity to distinguish only between a target molecule and its related compounds (i.e., analytical specificity). When applied to a population of samples, lab trials, in contrast hand, report 'diagnostic sensitivity' and 'diagnosing specificity' as percentage ratios (true positives detected/total positives, true negatives detected/total negatives) that accurately detect samples tested with the target molecule. A high-quality assay with high analytical sensitivity and specificity does not, however, ensure great clinical performance (high diagnostic sensitivity and specificity).
- Although the TCA reader improves LFA sensitivity and limit-of-detection, it is vital to consider how this boost influences diagnostic specificity.
- Indeed, utilizing the malaria first response LFA, we recorded many false positives with thermal contrast that did not occur with visual contrast.
- In one of the two false-positive cases, the blood (i.e., haemoglobin) staining on the nitrocellulose membrane was so black that the signal overpowered the membrane's natural background, resulting in a false-positive.
- It is possible that more false positives were caused by the test line's non-specific GNP binding. Since haemoglobin absorbs substantially in the visible region of the laser irradiation (532 nm), like gold, inadequate clearance of haemoglobin is a significant source of noise for malaria LFAs.
- Blood could result in false positives and potentially mask the thermal signal of GNPs if it is not washed off or otherwise removed from the test line after the test. This also applied to two more malaria LFAs (SD BIOLINE and ParaHIT).With both of these LFAs, the blood staining was so pervasive that it was impossible to obtain a reproducible signal above the background, much less an improvement with TCA. As a result, a reader's gain in analytical/

diagnostic sensitivity is probably going to result in a decrease in diagnostic specificity.
- The TCA reader would also increase the non-specific binding of GNPs on the test line, producing a heat signal. Uncertainty exists over the TCA's eventual limit-of-detection for GNPs on an LFA's test line. More investigation into heat transfer physics, optics, and molecular binding is therefore being done in order to identify this upper limit and use it as a resource for future TCA research.

10.8 Conclusion

The increased use of LFA has made it necessary to increase its sensitivity along with its specificity. As mentioned above serval experiments were conducted to achieve this, the use of green light was seen to have increased the sensitivity 32-fold. The use of gold particles to exploit its plasmonic property is also used. The GNPs that are used are easily excited by the laser which is then converted the energy into the electromagnetic field. This sensing mode can then be added to the LFA to increase its usage. The reader system was also modified for various LFA so that their proper use can be done. The duration of the technique is less and as not many heavy machines are used; they are cost-effective. Along with these, the advantages discussed in the chapter have given an upper edge to the use of LFA, and mainly the most effective thermal plasmonic LFA. The thermal plasmonic LFA along with the other types of LFA provides a great platform for detecting diseases at an early stage. When we combine the SERS along with the LFA they provide us with a speedy detection of the antigen/disease.

References

[1] Banerjee R and Jaiswal A 2018 Recent advances in nanoparticle-based lateral flow immunoassay as a point-of-care diagnostic tool for infectious agents and diseases *Analyst* **143** 1970–96

[2] Koczula K M and Gallotta A 2016 Lateral flow assays *Essays Bochem.* **60** 111–20

[3] Peng T *et al* 2020 Enhancing sensitivity of lateral flow assay with application to SARS-CoV-2 *Appl. Phys. Lett.* **117** 120601

[4] Qin W *et al* 2017 Carcinoembryonic antigen detection with 'Handing'-controlled fluorescence spectroscopy using a color matrix for point-of-care applications *Biosens. Bioelectron.* **90** 508–15

[5] Venkatraman V and Steckl A J 2015 Integrated OLED as excitation light source in fluorescent lateral flow immunoassays *Biosens. Bioelectron.* **74** 150–5

[6] Polo E *et al* 2013 Plasmonic-driven thermal sensing: ultralow detection of cancer markers *Chem. Commun.* **49** 3676–8

[7] Qin Z and Bischof J C 2012 Thermophysical and biological responses of gold nanoparticle laser heating *Chem. Soc. Rev.* **41** 1191–217

[8] Qin Z *et al* 2012 Significantly improved analytical sensitivity of lateral flow immunoassays by using thermal contrast *Angew. Chem. Int. Ed.* **51** 4358–61

[9] Qin Z *et al* 2016 Quantitative comparison of photothermal heat generation between gold nanospheres and nanorods *Sci. Rep.* **6** 1–13

[10] Jacques S L 2013 Optical properties of biological tissues: a review *Phys. Med. Biol.* **58** R37

[11] Govorov A O and Richardson H H 2007 Generating heat with metal nanoparticles *Nano Today* **2** 30–8

[12] Sánchez-Purrà M *et al* 2017 Design of SERS nanotags for multiplexed lateral flow immunoassays *Mol. Syst. Design Eng.* **2** 401–9

[13] Xi Z, Ye H and Xia X 2018 Engineered noble-metal nanostructures for *in vitro* diagnostics *Chem. Mater.* **30** 8391–414

[14] Wang X *et al* 2017 Simultaneous detection of dual nucleic acids using a SERS-based lateral flow assay biosensor *Anal. Chem.* **89** 1163–9

[15] Li J and Macdonald J 2016 Multiplex lateral flow detection and binary encoding enables a molecular colorimetric 7-segment display *Lab Chi* **16** 242–5

[16] You D J, San Park T and Yoon J-Y 2013 Cell-phone-based measurement of TSH using Mie scatter optimized lateral flow assays *Biosens. Bioelectron.* **40** 180–5

[17] Kor K *et al* 2016 Structurally responsive oligonucleotide-based single-probe lateral-flow test for detection of miRNA-21 mimics *Anal. Bioanal.Chem.* **408** 1475–85

[18] Kellner M J, Koob J G, Gootenberg J S, Abudayyeh O O and Zhang F 2019 Sherlock: nucleic acid detection with crispr nucleases *Nat. Protoc.* **14** 2986–3012

[19] Deng Y *et al* 2021 Recent advances in sensitivity enhancement for lateral flow assay *Microchim. Acta* **188** 1–15

[20] Chiu R Y *et al* 2014 Simultaneous concentration and detection of biomarkers on paper *Lab Chi* **14** 3021–8

[21] Zhang C *et al* 2019 Establishment and application of hyperbranched rolling circle amplification coupled with lateral flow dipstick for the sensitive detection of Karenia mikimotoi *Harmful Algae* **84** 151–60

[22] Alam N *et al* 2021 Improving the sensitivity of cellulose fiber-based lateral flow assay by incorporating a water-dissolvable polyvinyl alcohol dam *Cellulose (London, England)* **28** 8641–51

[23] Katis I N *et al* 2018 Improved sensitivity and limit-of-detection of lateral flow devices using spatial constrictions of the flow-path *Biosens. Bioelectron.* **113** 95–100

[24] Posthuma-Trumpie G A, Korf J and Van Amerongen A 2009 Lateral flow (immuno) assay: its strengths, weaknesses, opportunities and threats. A literature survey *Anal. Bioanal. Chem.* **393** 569–82

[25] Shen H, Song E and Wang Y *et al* 2022 In situ Raman enhancement strategy for highly sensitive and quantitative lateral flow assay *Anal. Bioanal. Chem.* **414** 507–13

[26] Anfossi L, Di Nardo F, Giovannoli C, Passini C and Baggiani C 2013 Increased sensitivity of lateral flow immunoassay for ochratoxin a through silver enhancement *Anal. Bioanal. Chem.* **405** 9859–67

[27] Parolo C, De La Escosura-Muniz A and Merkoci A 2013 Enhanced lateral flow immunoassay using gold nanoparticles loaded with enzymes *Biosens. Bioelectron.* **40** 412–6

[28] Cho I-H, Bhunia A and Irudayaraj J 2015 Rapid pathogen detection by lateral-flow immunochromatographic assay with gold nanoparticle-assisted enzyme signal amplification *Int. J. Food Microbiol.* **206** 60–6

[29] Blanco-Covian L, Montes-Garcia V, Girard A, Fernandez-Abedul M T, Perez-Juste J, Pastoriza-Santos I, Faulds K, Graham D and Blanco-Lopez M C 2017 Au@Ag SERRS tags coupled to a lateral flow immunoassay for the sensitive detection of pneumolysin *Nanoscale* **9** 2051–8

[30] Gao X *et al* 2021 A 'hot spot'-enhanced paper lateral flow assay for ultrasensitive detection of traumatic brain injury biomarker S-100β in blood plasma *Biosens. Bioelectron.* **177** 112967
[31] North S H, Shriver-Lake L C, Taitt C R and Ligler F S 2012 Rapid analytical methods for on-site triage for traumatic brain injury ed R G Cooks and E S Yeung *Annual Review of Analytical Chemistry* vol 5 (Palo Alto, CA: Annual Reviews) pp 35–56
[32] Hwang J, Lee S and Choo J 2016 Application of a sers-based lateral flow immunoassay strip for the rapid and sensitive detection of staphylococcal enterotoxin B *Nanoscale* **8** 11418–25
[33] Nguyen V T, Song S, Park S and Joo C 2020 Recent advances in high-sensitivity detection methods for paper-based lateral-flow assay *Biosens. Bioelectron.* **152** 17
[34] Zhao Y F, Huang Y, Zhao X W, Mcclelland J F and Lu M 2016 Nanoparticle-based photoacoustic analysis for highly sensitive lateral flow assays *Nanoscale* **8** 19204–10
[35] Song S, Choi S, Ryu S, Kim S, Kim T, Shin J, Jung H I and Joo C 2018 Highly sensitive paper-based immunoassay using photothermal laser speckle imaging *Biosens. Bioelectron.* **117** 385–91
[36] Tabatabaei N, Mandelis A and Amaechi B T 2011 Thermophotonic lock-in imaging of early demineralized and carious lesions in human teeth *J. Biomed. Opt.* **16** 071402
[37] Ojaghi A, Parkhimchyk A and Tabatabaei N 2016 First step toward translation of thermophotonic lock-in imaging to dentistry as an early caries detection technology *J. Biomed. Opt.* **21** 096003
[38] Völker A C *et al* 2005 Laser speckle imaging with an active noise reduction scheme *Opt. Express* **13** 9782–7
[39] Briers D *et al* 2013 Laser speckle contrast imaging: theoretical and practical limitations *J. Biomed. Opt.* **18** 066018
[40] Saisin L *et al* 2018 Significant sensitivity improvement for camera-based lateral flow immunoassay readers *Sensors* **18** 4026

Chapter 11

State-of-the-art of paper-based technology and challenges in its commercialization

Arun Sharma, Brijendra Kumar Kashyap and Nidhi Puranik

11.1 Introduction

Paper-based biosensor technology offers an incredible prospective for quick medical diagnosis and which is one of the best point-of-care (POC) biosensors. The main advantage of paper-based technology is that it is user-friendly, low-cost, simply and readily availabile (Hu *et al* 2017, Böhm *et al* 2018, Choi *et al* 2019). Many challenges are associated with these benefits in order to develop and commercialize it. Large scale manufacturing limitations and low performance are the main challenges connected with commercialization of paper-based biosensors (PBBs).

PBBs propose an economic foundation for rapid and trouble-free recognition of a biomarker in quantifiable diagnostics and supplementary areas such as foodstuffs and ecological scrutinization. In view of the fact that paper is a multipurpose substrate that facilitates reflexive solutions currently and is biocompatible, it is appropriate to exploit it as a biochemical sensing platform. In this chapter we will discuss the state-of-the-art of paper-based technology and challenges in its commercialization and also enlighten the existing inclination of PBBs in stipulations of invention and recognition practices in medical diagnostics. Key features and schemes to boost performance and amplify commercialization are projected in this chapter.

Today the Coronavirus disease 2019 (COVID-19) epidemic has grown to be a worldwide epidemic (Bedford *et al* 2020, Bernheim *et al* 2020, Chen *et al* 2020, Zheng *et al* 2020). Besides COVID-19 many other pathogen outbreaks may occur in a community or geographical region, and affect numerous countries. These pathogens mainly include novel H1N1 influenza, Botulinum neurotoxins (BoNTs), anthrax, tularaemia, viral haemorrhagic fevers and many more. Outbreaks may last for a few days or weeks, or even for several months or years. These pathogens are capable of infecting a significant number of people. Human beings generally have little to no immunity against such pathogens. These viruses spread rapidly from person to person

doi:10.1088/978-0-7503-5820-0ch11

© IOP Publishing Ltd 2023

globally. This causes a large number of deaths and builds social disorder, financial failure and general hardship.

It is necessary for communities to prepare so that they are ready for the next flu pandemic. The deadly effects of pathogens have provoked the advancement of diagnostic instruments to control the spread of infection. Although cautious technologies such as quantitative real time polymerase chain reaction (qRT-PCR) have been mostly used to detect COVID-19, they are time-consuming, labour-intensive and not available in isolated regions (He *et al* 2020). Therefore, point-of-care (POC) biosensors, including PBBs and chip-based biosensors, are required.

Paper-based biosensors are reliable and can produce excellent results particularly in rapid clinical diagnosis. Electrochemical PBBs have potential for miniaturization, require a comparatively small quantity of samples, and are cost-effective for extensive fabrication. These portable and hand-held biosensors are well-suited for on-site and off-site detection of pathogens. In this framework, PBBs mechanisms come together with key aspects of paper substrates (low cost, trouble-free management and compatibility with biomarkers, proteins and biomolecules), with enhanced selectivity and specificity of biorecognition events on the surface. Other than health diagnosis there are many more applications of paper-based devices in various fields such as water analysis, environmental and foodstuff monitoring.

Paper is a porous and highly versatile material which exhibits flexibility and biocompatibility with eco-friendly substrates that can be utilized in the production of efficient and cost-effective biosensors and devices for reliable, fast and sensitive detection of targeted antigens of interest (Amrita *et al* 2018). Paper is a multifarious substance capable of improving biosensor analytical devices that use a small amount of reagent and little sample use in the range of microliters (μl). Paper is mostly composed of fibrous cellulose material. Cellulose is a hydrophilic polymer that constructs paper substrate that is permeable to aqueous liquids. Recently, the functions of cellulose have been extending into the promising areas of nanomedicine, nanotechnology and bionanotechnology (Eichhorn *et al* 2018, Morais and Curto *et al* 2018, Xu *et al* 2018).

There are many varieties of paper such as nitrocellulose functional membrane, bioactive printing paper, cellulose chromatographic paper, Whatman® filter paper grade 1 and grade 2 that can be used for the design of paper-based biosensors. Even filter papers have been generally used as substrate materials for paper-based immunosensing applications. These papers can be categorized according to diverse assets such as thickness, pore size, flow rate and particle retention. The outstanding properties of cellulose fibre-based papers and novel characteristics of nanocellulose, formulate the cellulose polymer which is one of the most attractive and pioneering substance with various functions (Mroz *et al* 2018). Nowadays, it is utilized in the progress of PBBs and paper-based analytical detection equipment (Zhu *et al* 2019). Nanocellulose fibre-based papers, consist of outstanding optical properties, adequate thermal stability for field use, low-cost, optical transparency, biocompatibility, hydrophilicity, ease of surface functionalization, high porosity for immobilization, good mechanical strength and flexibility for biosensing applications (Pourreza *et al* 2015).

Nanoparticles can also be used to modify a paper surface for enhanced biosensing performance. In previous reports, gold nanoparticles (Au NPs), bimetallic nanoparticles, silver nanoparticles (Ag NPs), carbon nanotubes (CNTs) and nanosheets have been used in the fabrication of PBBs. New and quickly growing interest in paper-based analytical detection devices has been observed in last decade (Zhu *et al* 2019). Finally, the existing challenges in commercialization of PBBs and upcoming perception of mounting vigorous point-of-care biosensors to quickly detect pathogens in various materials are briefly highlighted.

11.2 State-of-the-art of paper-based biosensors

Paper-based biosensors (PBBs) have attracted interest in the last 10 years from the scientific research community because of their exceptional benefits and practical use. Papers as used in analytical devices impart numerous fascinating attributes such as manufacturing of reagent-free equipment, extraordinary potential to identify the target antigen in gaseous and liquid medium without any complicated tools. The porous nature of the surface of paper is responsible for immobilizing reagents and sample of interest that manage appropriate solution flow without the need for external things. In this context, the development of highly sensitive, selective, and user-friendly smart and sustainable analytical PBBs are concisely interpreted.

11.2.1 Recent trends in PBBs

The more recent trends in PBBs are systemically discussed in this context. Infectious disease monitoring is explored in PBBs using both antibodies and nucleic acids. This strategy in more promising than single antibody based immunoassays. A 'Lab-on-a-disc' biosensor has been developed with this view (Loo *et al* 2017). Multiple channel PDMS-based biosensors offer real time signal recognition with simultaneous extraction and amplification process (Nayak *et al* 2017). It takes about two hours for completion of analysis and getting results (Darwish *et al* 2018). PPB commercial production for COVID-19 detection is available which requires 20 μl sample volume with 91.54% clinical sensitivity and 97.02% clinical specificity. The most popular screening option used in this detection is where fabrication of lateral flow test strip on high-scale is permitted (Li *et al* 2020, Sheridan 2020). Several PBBs use microfluidic 3D-printing technology; metal ions, for example silver, magnesium, calcium etc for colorimetric approach for multiplex detection at the same time (Xia *et al* 2016, Lam *et al* 2017). It creates partition in the detection zone and reaction zone on the paper to simplify the procedure.

More promising rapid detection of viral pathogens by the naked eye is possible which produces colour signals on the surface of the paper (Mello and de Campos Vidal 2017, Trinh and Lee 2019). Briefly, the proposed paper-based biosensor is composed of three zones, i.e., the sample zone, reaction zone and detection zone. PBBs have remarkable potential for recognizing and controlling the reach of COVID-19 and many more pathogens. PBBs can make use of smartphones for suitable health administration which is needed for fast on-site and off-site analysis (Li *et al* 2020). Automation and completely disposable integrated PBBs may explore the new era of clinical diagnosis (Yin *et al* 2020). This technology can be suitable for the rapid detection of many pathogens using a wide range of samples. In the early stages of disease, PBBs have the potential to track patient health conditions to observe signals with the naked eye without requiring additional tools. In short, the trending PBBs with aforementioned capabilities could play a key role in managing outbreaks.

11.2.2 Fabrication and printing procedures

In this context, various forms of paper that are presently employed in the production of PBBs, and widespread manufacturing techniques encompassing wax printing to origami and kirigami-based methods. Microfluidic paper-based analytical devices (μPADs) and PBBs can be simply fabricated economically utilizing convenient fabrication approaches like wax printing (Lu *et al* 2009). The journey of PBBs is briefly discussed from the development of dipstick techniques in 1956 for the detection of glucose in urine which was time consuming and imprecise and the obtained results were not satisfactory (Free *et al* 1957). In 1980s pregnancy test strips were becoming popular and associated with enhanced performance (Yetisen *et al* 2013). Furthermore, it has been developed for the exposure of pathogenic micro-organisms (e.g., *Staphylococcus aureus* and *Pseudomonas aeruginosa*) and identification of small amounts of pesticides in meal samples and beverages as well as viewing blood coagulation (Hossain *et al* 2009, Li *et al* 2011, Li *et al* 2014).

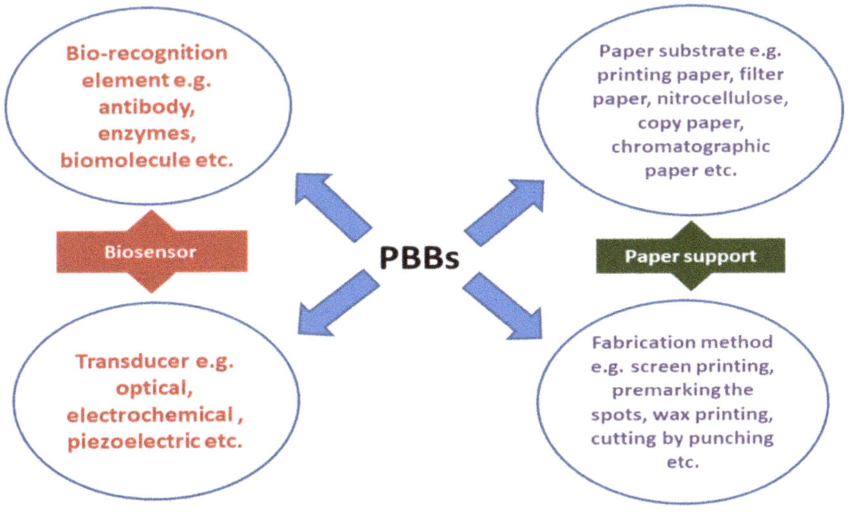

1D, 2D and 3D microfabrication techniques are used for manufacturing of PBBs. These techniques mainly include etching, hot embossing, plasma etching, cutting, photolithography, inkjet printing, alkyl ketene dimer (AKD) printing, laser-assisted cutting, wax printing, flexographic printing, PDMS (polydimethylsiloxane), plotting wax patterning, shaping, hydrophobic silanization, pore sealing and origami- and kirigami-based approaches (Martinez *et al* 2008, Carrilho *et al* 2009, Dungchai *et al*

2011, Songjaroen *et al* 2012, Kumar *et al* 2015, Shamkhalichenar *et al* 2017, Bernasconi *et al* 2018, Tortorich *et al* 2018). In brief several pros and cons of each method are listed in table 11.1.

Furthermore, the piezoelectric inkjet printing method is utilized for production of a bioactive paper-based device that is modified with enzymes supported on the paper surface via biocompatible sol–gel silica layers (Hossain *et al* 2009). Graft copolymerization is one of the most commonly used methods that can allocate immobilization of biomolecules on cellulose filter paper (Tyagi *et al* 2008). Wax printing followed by carbon black ink is utilized for the fabrication of conventional printing paper (Cinti *et al* 2017). This will produce high porosity and good absorbance for the reagents on the paper surface which is essential for the analysis of a large array of analytes (Ostrov *et al* 2017). Furthermore, various immobilization techniques such as encapsulation, cross-linking, physical adsorption, covalent binding, hydrophobic attraction, silanization, entrapment, electrostatic attraction, sol-gel entrapment, nanobeads etc are used for biomolecules (Geffroy *et al* 2000, Karra-Châabouni *et al* 2008, Hossain *et al* 2011, Ibrahim *et al* 2013, Credou *et al* 2014).

Table 11.1. Key benefits and limitations of fabrication methods

S. No.	Method used for fabrication and printing	Use and benefits	Drawbacks and limitations
1.	Inkjet printing	Well organized, lessens cross-contamination high-speed production and fine resolution	Costly bio-ink printer, ink bleeding and not good for high volume printing
2.	Wax printing	Economical, simple process and short fabrication time	Poor resolution, unstable at high temperatures
3.	Laser cutting	Easy to handle and low-cost	Dedicated apparatus is required
4.	Photolithography	Superb resolution and appropriate for extensive fabrication	Pricey and complicated equipment, unsettled against twisting or breakdown
5.	Hot embossing	Little fabrication time and proficient	Customized equipment
6.	Polydimethylsiloxane (PDMS)	Inexpensive and workable	Bad resolution, advanced equipment for patterning and fabrication of moulds
7.	Origami and kirigami	Complex and modern designs, easy fabrication	Operational mechanism
8.	Hydrophobic silanization	Economical and quick fabrication	Wet adhesion and hydrolytic stability

11.2.3 Utilize nanoparticles and nanomaterials in PBBs

Incorporation of nanoparticles, nanomaterials, nanocomposites and quantum dots provide selectivity, wide dynamic range and excellent limit of detection for the targeted antigens because of their unique chemical and physical properties (Sharma *et al* 2015). Carbon nanotubes (CNTs) and graphene nanosheets can generate high electrical conductivity (Sharma *et al* 2016). Nanoparticles of metallic gold and silver enable immobilization in order to show excellent biocompatibility, high active surface area that is suitable for variety of biomarkers in clinical diagnosis.

Moreover, nanomaterials of oxides of tungsten and molybdenum exhibit good electrochromic properties. Semiconductor metallic oxide nanoparticles provide excellent chemiresistive properties. All of these properties are responsible for facilitating multi-stage chemical magnification of the biosensor diagnostic signal to attain low limit of detection (LOD) and ultra-high sensitivity (Sharma *et al* 2014). Some nanomaterials, such as the graphene nanosheets and Au NPs in combination offer excellent functionalization of biomolecules in immunosensing for attaching on the surface (Sharma *et al* 2016).

The use of nanoparticles and nanomaterials in PBBs enhance the biosensing performance and provoke researchers to develop novel simplified tools for achieving high sensitivity. Silver nanoparticles (Ag NPs) are utilized in electrochemical PBBs with a detection limit of 767 fM (Scida *et al* 2014). Paper modified with carbon nanotubes (CNTs) bundles has revealed an outstanding biotin–avidin interface with a limit of detection of 25 ng ml^{-1} (Cao *et al* 2017). Reduced graphene oxide (rGOx) and quantum dots (QDs) can be used for the functionalization in PBBs to amplify signal strength (Sharma *et al* 2014, Katarzyna *et al* 2020). In one of the most popular glucose biosensors, tin(IV) oxide (SnO2) nanoparticles are attached to nanocellulose fibres using the liquid phase deposition technique. This combination reduces storage time and reveals superb morphology which provides a 0.5–12 mM wide dynamic range with 0.96 correlation coefficient (Mahadeva *et al* 2011).

MicroRNA-141 (miR-141) and microRNA-21 (miR-21) biomarkers have been detected by means of gold nanoparticles (Au NPs) embellished 2D molybdenum sulphide (MoS2) with silver nanowires (Ag NWs) composites. Inclusion of copper metal organic frameworks (Cu-MOFs) with Pt NPs (PtCuMOFs) modification is responsible for producing high sensitivity by means of electrochemical signals (Tian *et al* 2019, Ratajczak *et al* 2020). Pure cellulose paper is utilized for the recognition of cancer antigen 125 (CA125) based on the electrochemical approach. In this work, a CA125 antibody was immobilized on screen-printed carbon electrode, tailored by reduced graphene oxide/thionine/gold nanoparticles (rGOx/Thi/Au NPs) nanocomposites.

Poly(3,4-ethylenedioxythiophene):poly(styrenesulfonate) and nano-dimensional iron oxide doped (nFe_2O_3@PEDOT:PSS) nanocomposite reformed conducting PBBs has been used for the detection of a cancer biomarker, carcinoembryonic antigen (CEA) (Kumar *et al* 2019). In numerous paper-based immunosensor blueprints electrocatalytic properties and electrical conductivity of biosensor were improved by putting extremely conductive carbon nanomaterials such as graphene nanosheets or carbon nanotubes (CNTs). A prostate cancer biosensor was found on micro-pore filter paper in which multi-walled carbon nanotubes (MWCNTs) were placed (carbon nanotube@paper biosensor) which is useful for the early stage detection (Ji *et al* 2018).

Mesoporous silica nanoparticles (MSNs) covered with cadmium telluride quantum dots (CdTe QDs) were conjugated with DNA aptamers to achieve the elevated affinity and sensitivity for the concurring detection of MCF-7, HL-60 and K562 tumour cells in a microfluidic paper-based analytical device. The QDs are responsible for boosting the fluorescence intensity which helps for multiplexed screening of cancer cells. In this study, exceptionally low detection limits have been attained for MCF-7, HL-60, and K562 cells of 62, 70 and 65 cells ml^{-1} respectively. The developed μPAD can be employed for the recognition of transmitting cancer cells to inhibit metastasis (Liang *et al* 2016).

11.2.4 Detection of target antigen using PBBs

The paper surface is modified to detect various pathogens. Researchers found that electrochemical PBBs have excellent prospects for the sensitive detection of different antigens as shown in table 11.2.

3D paper-based electrochemiluminescence (ECL) immunodevice has been developed for the simultaneous detection of tumour markers, e.g., carcinoma antigen 125 (CA125), α-fetoprotein (AFP), carcinoembryonic antigen (CEA) and carcinoma antigen 199 (CA199) (Ge *et al* 2012). Under optimized conditions, 0.15 ng ml^{-1}, 0.6 U ml^{-1}, 0.17 U ml^{-1} and 0.5 ng ml^{-1} limit of detection is found for AFP, CA125, CA199 and CEA, respectively. In the near future, PBBs, portable chips of screen-printed sensors and low-cost μPAD technology are expected to grow significantly in clinical research and medical sciences (Katarzyna *et al* 2020).

11.2.5 Application of PBBs for clinical diagnostics

PBBs symbolize a promising tool for disease diagnostics having the capability to sense multiple antigens simultaneously, so-called multiplexed analysis. Concurrent recognition of microRNA-141 (miR-141) and microRNA-21 (miR-21) biomarkers have been done using cyclic voltammetry (CV), electrochemical impedance spectroscopy (EIS) and square wave voltammetry (SWV) techniques (Tian *et al* 2019). Newly challenging task are for the identification of cancer biomarkers at very low concentrations. *In situ* screening for anticancer drugs such as fluorouracil, cisplatin or paclitaxel and cancer cells is detected by disposable paper-based aptasensor (Wu *et al* 2016). Cancer cells release exosomes with sizes of approximately 100 nm in diameter which give information about cell condition, genomic codes, effects other cells and provoke healthy cell to spread disease, etc. Effective paper-based aptasensors have been developed for the recognition of exosomes that are helpful for the early diagnosis of cancer (Chen *et al* 2018).

Table 11.2. Detection of different antigens with their LOD using electrochemical paper-based biosensors (PBBs)

S. No.	Type of modified paper matrices used in detection	Target antigen	Limit of detection (LOD)	References
1.	Reduced graphene modified electrochemical PPBs	Carcinoembryonic antigen (CEA)	25.8 μA ng^{-1} ml cm^{-2}	Kumar *et al* (2015)
2.	Permanent board marker plotting electrochemical PBBs	Prostate-specific antigen (PSA)	360.2 ng l^{-1}	Ruecha *et al* (2014)
3.	PDMS/paper/glass hybrid microfluidic PBBs	Lactobacillus acidophilus	11.0 CFU ml^{-1}	Nie, *et al* (2012)
4.	Origami-based 3D-PBBs (horseradish peroxidase (HRP)-mediated enzymatic detection)	Carcinoma antigen 199 (CA199)	8.0 mU ml^{-1}	Zang *et al* (2012)
		Carcinoma antigen 125 (CA125)	6.0 mU ml^{-1}	
		Carcinoembryonic antigen (CEA)	5.0 pg ml^{-1}	
		σ-fetoprotein (AFP)	0.01 ng ml^{-1}	
5.	Graphene oxide (GOx)-PBBs	Prostate-specific antigen (PSA)	0.0012 ng ml^{-1}	Li *et al* (2014)
6.	Cerium dioxide, gold nanorods, and glucose oxidase (CeO_2-Au@GOx)	MicroRNA-21 (miR-21)	0.434 fM	Sun *et al* (2018)
7.	$Co_2(OH)_2CO_3$-CeO_2 peroxidase-mimics nanocomposites with antibodies based PBBs	Carcinoembryonic antigen (CEA)	0.51 pg ml^{-1}	Alizadeh *et al* (2018)
8.	Amino-functionalized graphene (NH_2-G), thionine (Thi) and gold nanoparticles (Au NPs)	Neuron-specific enolase (NSE)	10 pg ml^{-1}	Fan *et al* (2017)
9.	Cadmium telluride quantum dots (CdTe QDs) coated with mesoporous silica nanoparticles (MSNs) modified with DNA aptamers	MCF-7 tumour cells	62 cells ml^{-1}	Liang *et al* (2016)
		HL-60 tumour cells	70 cells ml^{-1}	
		K562 tumour cells	65 cells ml^{-1}	
10.	Graphene oxide nanosheets and chitosan modified screen-printed carbon ink nanobioprobes consisting of silica nanoparticles (SiO_2)-horseradish peroxidase (HRP) and antibodies based PBBs	alpha-fetoprotein (AFP)	–	Wu *et al* (2013)
		Carcinoembryonic antigen (CEA)		
		Cancer antigen 125 (CA125)		
		Carbohydrate antigen 153 (CA153)		

11.	Amino-functionalized graphene (NG)-thionin (THI)-gold nanoparticles (Au NPs) (NG-THIAuNPs) and Prussian blue (PB)-poly (3,4-ethylenedioxythiophene) (PEDOT)-Au NPs (PEDOT-PB-Au NPs) nanocomposites	Carcinoembryonic antigen (CEA) Neuron-specific enolase (NSE)	2 pg ml^{-1} 10 pg ml^{-1}	Wang *et al* (2019)
12.	Colorimetric vertical-flow DNA microarray (DNA-VFM) based PBBs	*Neisseria meningitidis*	4.4 nM	Rivas *et al* (2018)

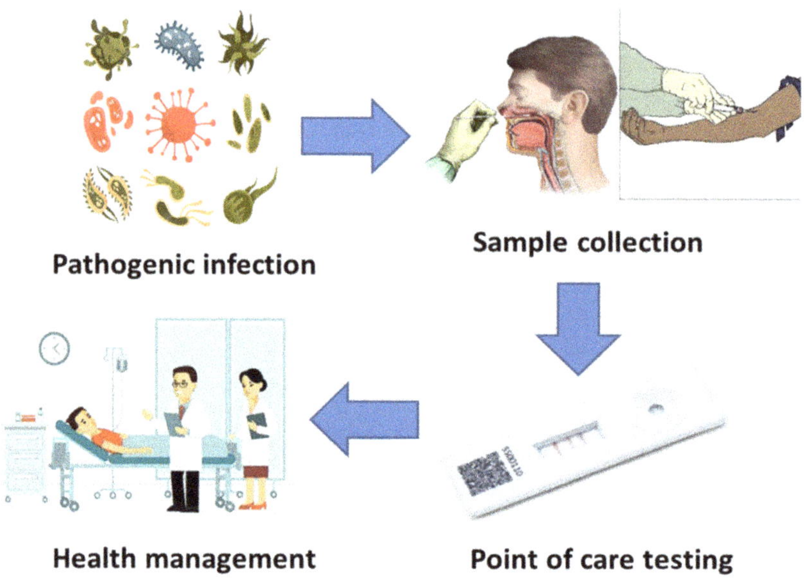

Moreover, paper-based biosensing provides straightforward and convenient detection approaches as offered in this chapter. Many benefits such as that they are user-friendly, portable, equipment-free, easy to dispose of, small sample volume (in μl range) is required for the analysis, visible colour alteration, which eradicates the requirement of well-trained therapeutic personnel to carry out and assess the outcomes of the analytical clinical investigations. μPADs and PBBs cut unwanted expenses and allow diseases to be quickly diagnosed in remote settings. These procedures are substitutes for typical laboratory experiments and have been extensively considered because of their reliability and high sensitivity (Ahmed *et al* 2016). Disease analytics can be successfully done using diverse natural fluids such as urine, blood, saliva, tears and sweat by the application of μPADs and PBBs (Lopez *et al* 2016).

Furthermore, clinical functions of PBBs for diagnosis and detection of biomarkers associated with diabetes, kidney and liver complications, low-cost and handy point-of care equipment can be practical devices in other fields such as monitoring the quality of foodstuff and in farming applications. PBBs are also able to examine heavy metals and toxins in environmental specimens, including polluted water sources and waste analysis. Paper microfluidics (μPADs) has not only prepared effortless analytical tools which are readily accessible worldwide, but also became a pivotal accredit expertise for biomedical investigation and multimodel applications.

11.2.6 Complementary use of paper-based devices

Environmental pollutants, insecticides, toxins, and heavy metals are the foremost constituents that contribute to water contamination, and are dangerous to individuals health as well as to the environment (Almeida *et al* 2018). Accurate detection of such pollutants is essential for supplying access to pure water. Various methods such as traditional ELISA, spectrophotometry, electrochemical approach etc are being used for analysis of impurities in water. But, these techniques are expensive, time-consuming, require complicated devices and well-trained human resources (Hu *et al* 2014, 2017). Hence, there is a demand for trouble-free, low-cost, and well-organized policies for exploring environmental resources including water. The use of PBBs and μPADs is one of the best approaches to test for the exstence and volume of water pollutants.

Paper-based appliances can be worn for alcohol detection with a LOD of 0.52 mM (Cinti *et al* 2017). Glossy paper printed with ITO nanopowder discreted in poly-diallyldimethylammonium chloride (PDDAC) is utilized for exposure of ethanol at room temperature (Arena *et al* 2010). Portable PBBs utilize immobilization of antibodies on the paper surface that has been applied particularly for pregnancy tests and glucose detection. μPADs employ manifold pathways for reagent and sample liberation by lateral flow to the reaction zone with more multifaceted structural design. However, the working idea of μPADs is similar to the PBBs. Generally, μPADs incorporate multiplex sensors or multiple electrodes fabricated in electrochemical cells on the paper matrix.

Industrial wastewater consisting of heavy metal ions are also dangerous to the environment once their concentrations surpass the normal boundary. A fluorometric paper-based sensor has been developed to screen heavy metal (Co^{2+}, Zn^{2+}, Hg^{2+} and Ag^{2+}) cations from polluted water (Feng *et al* 2013). Likewise, a paper-based 3D vertical assay device was made for colorimetric identification of metallic pollutants in aqueous systems, allowing multiple examinations to be accomplished simultaneously (Wang *et al* 2014). This device contains three layers of tape and four layers of paper. Hydrophobic patterns were generated using a wax printer. Sample testing was performed at the hydrophilic zone where liquid is allowed to flow. Chromogenic reagents are specific to metal and reserved in each sample zone for the targeted metal ion that is going to be detect (Cr^{4+}, Cu^{2+}, Ni^{2+}, Cd^{3+}). Colour alteration and colour intensity can be easily determined using a mobile phone camera.

Hydrogen sulfide is one of the toxic gases that has hazardous characteristics which may appear in individuals health if present in minute concentrations in the blood (Songjaroen *et al* 2012, Vella *et al* 2012). To identify hydrogen sulfide gas at low concentrations a paper-based sensor was developed. The sensor used palladium (II) and ethylene glycol based filter paper. Palladium (II) can be efficiently linked with sulfide groups and formed palladium (II) sulfide (PdS). The fluorescence spectra are recorded with the help of spectrophotometer and the obtained results are quantified.

Consequently, μPADs have the benefit of analogous controls as PBBs except they usually consume a smaller quantity of sample (a drop) and hence involve fewer reagents. The efficiency of the measurement scheme results in the improvement of the recognition throughput, miniaturization as per requirement and lowering of the detection charges. Special detection of working mechanisms is used by PBBs and their functions in a range of areas from clinical indicatives to investigation of ecological particulates, immunosensing of antigens, monitoring sun exposure and for sensing targeted analytes in cell cultures. Sun exposure due to UV radiation causes damage to epithelial skin cells which produces toxic outcomes on the body including melanoma, carcinoma and many other types of skin cancer. In this way, paper-based sensors are contributing to identifying sun exposure for early diagnosis of skin cancer without using hi-tech facilities.

The sun exposure paper-based sensor mechanisms by photo-reactive chemicals those are susceptible to sunlight. Some halogenic compounds are capable of altering pH levels subsequent to UV exposure. Particularly, the device encloses several layers of such types of halogenic compounds that transform their pH levels. A single layer paper-based sensor was developed which combines with titanium dioxide (TiO_2) as a good photo-catalyst and brilliant blue FCF (food dye) (Khiabani *et al* 2016). The colour intensity would be decreased during the exposure of UV light on TiO_2 layer. Discoloration on the TiO_2 film indicaties exposure to UV radiation. The thickness of the TiO_2 layer and the proportion of TiO_2 to brilliant blue FCF and the rate of discoloration are attuned to diverse skin forms (Khiabani *et al* 2016). The sun exposure paper-based sensor is economical and convenient for all kinds of body skin, and has the potential to be useful.

11.3 Challenges in commercialization of PPBs

In the last decades, the number of biomarkers and their detection modes have increased significantly. At present PPBs are capable to executing the critical needs of speedy and trouble-free clinical investigations in remote areas or resource-limited settings. These paper-based tools present a sensing platform for various biomarkers with several capacities to detect them in ultra-trace of concentrations in clinical samples (López-Marzo *et al* 2016). In this modern era there is an urgent need to improve the performance of PBBs in terms of high efficacy and efficiency.

In spite of the favourable exertions of paper-based sensors and devices, there are several barriers concerning sensitivity, perfection, vulnerability, and simultaneous exposure of numerous antigens. In current trends, PBBs have been tried to engineer by means of shaping to deal with these problems. Moreover additional revealing applications such as electrochemistry, chemiluminescence, fluorescence, and electrochemiluminescence are currently being utilized for tracking analytes in addition to colorimetric techniques. However, these approaches also demonstrate pitfalls related to price, lucidity and sensitivity (Liana *et al* 2012).

11.3.1 Current status of paper-based biosensing devices

Presently, many PBB products and detection kits are available in the market for the medical diagnosis of various target analytes including HIV, malaria, typhoid, cancer etc. Commercially, pregnancy tests (Accu-Tell Rapid hCG, Accu BioTech Co. Ltd, USA), typhoid kits (TyphiDot, Malaysian Biodiagnostic Research SDN BHD; TUBEX, IDL Biotech; Multi-Test Dip-S-Ticks, PANBIO INDX, Inc.). HIV (Uni-Gold HIV, Trinity biotech manufacturing Ltd Co., Ireland), and malaria testing kit (IMMUNOQUICK Malaria falciparum, Biosynex Strasbourg, France; SD BIOLINE Malaria Ag P.f/Pan, Standard Diagnostics Inc. Giheung-gu, Korea) kits are successfully available worldwide.

Moreover, research groups are working on multiplex detection on a single test strip to quantify the various specific antigens present in the sample (Wu *et al* 2015). Recent advances in the multiplexed mode is achieved for the synchronized detection of glucose, lactate and uric acid (Zhao *et al* 2013). Some other groups have identified differential glycated haemoglobin and CEA (carcinoembryonic antigen) using photo-electrochemical approach (Boonyasit *et al* 2016, Ma *et al* 2016). Recently, a paper-based electrochemical immunosensor hs been developed for the finding of a tumour biomarker popularly known as a carcinoembryonic antigen (CEA) (Kumar *et al* 2019).

11.3.2 Assessment of performance of paper-based biosensing devices

Dextran based protectants can be applied on paper matrix to improve the self-life of PBBs up to 4 months (Cao *et al* 2017). Thermal stability can be achieved by aptamers which can replace moieties sensitive towards temperature (Kuswandi *et al* 2019). Scrupulous efforts have been performed to widen PBBs performances in which detection limit and linear range are the most important factors.

11.3.3 Manufacturing and commercial issues

PBBs have tremendous potential in highly sensitive detection which requires very low amounts of sample. Some negative aspects such as shipping practicability and stabilities are also associated (Ahmed *et al* 2016) and to resolve these many research groups are working on various internal and external factors to achieve commercially beneficial PBBs as required and expected by users. These factors mainly incorporate tools for accuracy and precision in disease diagnosis, multiplexing issues, automation with miniaturization, false positive and negative results, better shelf-life, fit for POC-analysis, prolong thermal stability, no requirement for special reagents for sample pre-treatment and lowere sample volume to obtain quantitative results (Kuswandi *et al* 2020).

Besides this cellulose PBBs have a tendency to absorb contaminants on the paper matrices and condensing moisture which may alter the results. Design issues such as uniformity in pore size and distribution, purity of paper, composition, paper quality, surface hydrophilicity, filtration speed and various physicochemical properties are responsible for unpredicted effects (Liana *et al* 2012). In absence of desired physical properties such as stiffness, porosity, hydrophilicity, lateral fluid flow rate and others are not fit for the development of PBBs. In manufacturing the development of a new generation of PBBs to overcome these factors are added values and make them successful for commercial uses.

The most common issue is to maintain the activity of biomolecules particularly used for biorecognition of targeted antigens. This mainly concerns the aptamers, enzymes, redox probe molecules and antibodies which are susceptible to getting oxidized in open conditions in the presence of reagents. It is necessary to maintain dry conditions on the paper matrices in order to protect these antibodies and enzymes from environmental oxidation in air. Pores (channels) of the paper matrix provide stability to biomolecules against their self-degradation in the freeze drying state which is required for the prolonged biological activity of recognition elements. It is recommended to store PBBs in dry sealed containers which is difficult to maintain for their practical utility (Katarzyna *et al* 2020).

It is a time of need to remove interferents and moisture from paper surface which may alter the results and affects sensitivity. To build PBBs for commercial use it is necessary to focus more on mechanical strength, paper porosity, moisture absorbents, temperature stability, functionality and reusability of biological elements.

11.3.4 Future perspectives to improve paper, design and biosensing

It is a challenge to eliminate real problems associated with PBBs. These are mainly inappropriate flow of sample, improper fabrication practices and insufficient characteristics of biosensing performance. In order to obtain well-functioning and sophisticated PBBs, it is essential to improve paper material, design and biosensing quality. The material chosen for paper matrices plays a crucial role to obtaine a high signal to noise ratio. Accuracy in the results and reproducibility can be achieved by amplifying the signal strengths and minimizing environmental noise factors.

Many research groups are working on designing high-quality paper substrates with uniform spatial arrangements. Cellulose and hemicelluloses based paper substrates are not good for electrochemical detection of pathogens because of their poor conductivity. Due to this many PBBs are worked on optical methods of biosensing in which a colorimetric approach is used. Comparatively low sensitivity is obtained in the case of colorimetric modes due to a number of limitations such as inconsistent lighting conditions and difficult to produce measurable signals into colour readout. To overcome this problem, electrochemical PBBs come into the picture to allow better signal amplification using conducting polymers and nano-materials at modified paper matrices.

Reagent flow rates on the patterned surface of PBBs needs to be optimized to achieve high sensitivity and better analytical performance. Signal amplification has been increased many times using improved design under optimized conditions for fluidic substances. Previously published reports on malaria and salmonella revealed accurate outcomes using pre-processing reagents compositions and experimental conditions (Fridley *et al* 2014, Jin *et al* 2015). Hybrid systems and advanced nanomaterials are more promising tools to get high performance PBBs and excellent detection limits in medical diagnostics.

Quality of biosensors, use of biorecognition elements and many environmental factors significantly affect signal to noise ratio in colorimetric assay. In order to get high sensitivity electrochemical PBBs is one of the most promising analytical systems for better signal amplification and reproducibility. Additionally, due to poor thermal stability and lower shelf-life, enzymatic PBBs are not suitable for practical applications in remote settings. For commercial purposes, long shelf-life is required that can be achieved by incorporation of nanomaterials. Such enzymatic nanocomposites exhibit thermal stability, outstanding catalytic and electrochemical properties which can be useful for getting improved biosensing immunoassays.

11.3.5 Challenges and visualization

Lack of quantification is attained in commercial production of COVID-19 detection kits (Biolidics) which is one of the most popular PBBs (Choi *et al* 2020). Moreover, where nanomaterials are used in the fabrication of PBBs complex synthetic procedures are required and consist of lengthy fabrication processes (Choi *et al* 2016a). Storing the nanomaterials and reagents on the paper surface is very challenging to formulate and it is additionally relevant in remote settings (Tang *et al* 2017b). Integrated PBBs require external heat blocks or heaters for signal amplification.

Development of low-cost PBBs is the most challenging task. These challenges consist of insufficient fabrication technologies, wasteful sample flow and inadequate diagnostic performances, that are elevated detection limits, poor specificity, low stability and reproducibility, confused multiplexing and subjective figure elucidation. Nowadays, many PBBs have responded effectively to most of above mentioned challenges. However, to respond to a number of the challenges more study is needed. However, it is very difficult to develop a paper-based biosensor which can tackle all the challenges at the same time.

While different restrictive factors such as pore volume distribution, sample run properties, substrate spatial distribution, etc have been broadly enhanced for PBBs platform; several viable promising models are still rising (Ahmed *et al* 2016). That shows additional perfections in such prototypes to reduce the detection time and elevate signal to noise ratio in the entire paper-based biosensing arrangements of experimental analysis to contend with conventional analytical means. Worldwide these challenges are being worked on by many active researchers from various academic and commercial organizations.

Their main focus is to develop robust, field usable, more versatile and user-friendly PBBs that will be appropriate for gaining computerized application with smart detection in upcoming technologies (Mukundan *et al* 2018). Such evolution, and progress, as well as commercialization of PBBs present benefits to the scientific community and developed countries which can be useful for millions of citizens who live in remote areas or resource-limited regions globally.

On the other hand it is essential to communicate that there are several restrictions of PBBs that must be remitted prior to their commercialization. PBBs can cause problems concerning the accuracy and sensitivity of antigens (Gosselin *et al* 2017). These weaknesses must be removed before the biosensors can be relied on for perfect infection identification. In summary, the effectiveness of the manufacturing of PBBs must be enhanced by bulk production of these tools. At present a number of these tools involve complex fabrication approaches that must be rationalized before commercialization (Dungchai *et al* 2010, Klasner *et al* 2010, Yang *et al* 2014). The most important is that the price of these tools must be reduced in order to really have an effect on resource-limited environments.

11.4 Conclusion

Currently, PBBs have attraced more interest because they facilitate the requirement to offer a choice of biomarker identifications in medical diagnostics. Many attempts have been made to obtain them in commercialized form. Moreover, great efforts have been made to attain highly sensitive detection at low cost. To reduce the assay time and overall cost, researchers are aiming for multiplexing biosensing designs. The careful efforts regarding PBBs devices, regrettably, result in answers that have mostly qualitative or semi-quantitative outcomes, which still require advance up gradation. Hence, these can be griped by concerning matchless engineering technologies and advanced manufacturing. In order to get a prosperous outcome, μPADs comprising some critical points of modern technologies for large mass production of paper-based matrices and eco-friendly PBBs application is more vital decisive step.

PBBs present an economical opportunity for the production of a trouble-free and convenient analytical arrangement that can be enormously valuable in resource-constrained sites, such as in emerging countries or difficult settings where fully-furnished equipment and well trained therapeutic personnel are not available. In future, it is presumed that new progressive efforts on paper-based devices will provide a path for their viable accomplishment as quantifiable diagnostics, which might significantly boost the physical supervision and infection detection. Since, PBBs offer reasonable platforms for trouble-free, precise and speedy detection of diseases, in accumulation to check foodstuff quality and coverage with detection and identification of pathogens.

Conflicts of interest

The authors affirm no inconsistency of attention.

References

Ahmed S, Bui M and Abbas A 2016 *Biosens. Bioelectron.* **77** 249

Ahmed S, Bui M P and Abbas A 2016 Paper-based chemical and biological sensors: engineering aspects *Biosens. Bioelectron.* **77** 249–63

Almeida M I G S, Jayawardane B M, Kolev S D and McKelvie I D 2018 Developments of microfluidic paper-based analytical devices (μpads) for water analysis: a review *Talanta* **177** 176–90

Arena A, Donato N, Saitta G, Bonavita A, Rizzo G and Neri G 2010 Flexible ethanol sensors on glossy paper substrates operating at room temperature *Sensors Actuators* B **145** 488–94

Bedford J, Enria D, Giesecke J, Heymann D L, Ihekweazu C and Kobinger G *et al* 2020 COVID-19: towards controlling of a pandemic *Lancet* **395** 1015–8

Bernasconi R, Mangogna A and Magagnin L 2018 *J. Electrochem. Soc.* **165** B3176

Bernheim A, Mei X, Huang M, Yang Y, Fayad Z A and Zhang N *et al* 2020 Chest CT findings in coronavirus disease-19 (COVID-19): relationship to duration of infection *Radiology* **295** 685–91

Böhm A, Trosien S, Avrutina O, Kolmar H and Biesalski M 2018 Covalent attachment of enzymes to paper fibers for paper-based analytical devices *Front. Chem.* **6** 214

Boonyasit Y, Chailapakul O and Laiwattanapaisal W 2016 A multiplexed three-dimensional paper-based electrochemical impedance device for simultaneous label-free affinity sensing of total and glycated haemoglobin: The potential of using a specific single-frequency value for analysis. *Anal. Chim. Acta* **936** 1–11

Cao R, Tian W and Shen W 2017 Polysaccharides as protectants for paper-based analytical devices with antibody. *Talanta* **165** 357–63

Carrilho E, Martinez A W and Whitesides G M 2009 Understanding Wax Printing: A Simple Micropatterning Process for Paper-Based Microfluidics. *In Anal. Chem.* **81** 7091–5

Chen L, Xiong J, Bao L and Shi Y 2020 Convalescent plasma as a potential therapy for COVID-19 *Lancet Infect. Dis.* **20** 398–400

Chen X, Lan J, Liu Y, Li L, Yan L and Xia Y *et al* 2018 A paper-supported aptasensor based on upconversion luminescence resonance energy transfer for the accessible determination of exosomes *Biosens. Bioelectron.* **102** 582–8

Choi J R 2020 Development of point-of-care biosensors for COVID-19 *Front. Chem.* **8** 2296–646

Choi J R, Hu J, Tang R, Gong Y, Feng S and Ren H *et al* 2016a An integrated paper-based sample-to-answer biosensor for nucleic acid testing at the point of care *Lab Chip* **16** 611–21

Choi J R, Yong K W, Choi J Y and Cowie A C 2019 Emerging point-of-care technologies for food safety analysis *Sensors* **19** 817

Cinti S, Basso M, Moscone D and Arduini F 2017 *Anal. Chim. Acta.* **960** 123

Cinti S, Mazzaracchio V, Cacciotti I, Moscone D and Arduini F 2017 Carbon black-modified electrodes screen-printed onto paper towel, waxed paper and parafilm M® *Sensors* **17** 2267

Credou J and Berthelot T 2014 *J. Mater. Chem.* B **2** 4767

Darwish N T, Sekaran S D and Khor S M 2018 Point-of-care tests: a review of advances in the emerging diagnostic tools for dengue virus infection *Sensors Actuators* B **255** 3316–31

Dungchai W, Chailapakul O and Henry C S 2010 Use of multiple colorimetric indicators for paper-based microfluidic devices *Anal. Chim. Acta* **674** 227–33

Dungchai W, Chailapakul O and Henry C S 2011 *Analyst* **136** 77

Eichhorn S, Rahatekar S, Vignolini S and Windle A 2018 New horizons for cellulose nanotechnology *Philos. Trans. R. Soc.* A **376** 20170200

Fan Y, Liu J, Wang Y, Luo J, Xu H and Xu S *et al* 2017 A wireless point-of-care testing system for the detection of neuron-specific enolase with microfluidic paper-based analytical devices *Biosens. Bioelectron.* **95** 60–6

Feng L, Li H, Niu L-Y, Guan Y-S, Duan C-F, Guan Y-F, Tung C-H and Yang Q-Z 2013 A fluorometric paper-based sensor array for the discrimination of heavy-metal ions *Talanta* **108** 103–8

Free A H, Adams E C, Kercher M L, Free H M and Cook M H 1957 Simple specific test for urine glucose *Clin. Chem.* **3** 163–8

Fridley G E, Le H and Yager P 2014 *Anal. Chem.* **86** 6447

Ge L, Yan J, Song X, Yan M, Ge S and Yu J 2012 Three-dimensional paper-based electrochemiluminescence immunodevice for multiplexed measurement of biomarkers and point-of-care testing *Biomaterials* **33** 1024–31

Geffroy C, Labeau M, Wong K, Cabane B and Cohen Stuart M 2000 *Colloids Surf.* A **172** 47

Gosselin D, Belgacem M N, Joyard-Pitiot B, Baumlin J M, Navarro F, Chaussy D and Berthier J 2017 Low-cost embossed-paper micro-channels for spontaneous capillary flow *Sensors Actuators* B **248** 395–401

He J-L, Luo L, Luo Z-D, Lyu J-X, Ng M-Y and Shen X-P *et al* 2020 Diagnostic performance between CT and initial real-time RT-PCR for clinically suspected 2019 coronavirus disease (COVID-19) patients outside Wuhan, China *Respir. Med.* **168** 105980

Hossain S and Brennan J 2011 *Anal. Chem.* **83** 8772

Hossain S M, Luckham R E, McFadden M J and Brennan J D 2009 Reagentless bidirectional lateral flow bioactive paper sensors for detection of pesticides in beverage and food samples *Anal. Chem.* **81** 9055–64

Hu J, Choi J R, Wang S, Gong Y, Feng S and Pingguan-Murphy B *et al* 2017 Multiple test zones for improved detection performance in lateral flow assays *Sensors Actuators* B **243** 484–8

Hu J, Wang S, Wang L, Li F, Pingguan-Murphy B, Lu T J and Xu F 2014 Advances in paper-based point-of-care diagnostics *Biosens. Bioelectron.* **54** 585–97

Hu J, Yew C-H T, Chen X, Feng S, Yang Q, Wang S, Wee W-H, Pingguan-Murphy B, Lu T J and Xu F 2017 Paper-based capacitive sensors for identification and quantification of chemicals at the point of care *Talanta* **165** 419–28

Ibrahim M, Koschella A, Kadry G and Henze T 2013 *Carbohydr. Polym.* **95** 414

Ji S, Lee M and Kim D 2018 Detection of early stage prostate cancer by using a simple carbon nanotube@paper biosensor *Biosens. Bioelectron.* **102** 345–50

Jin S-Q, Guo S-M, Zuo P and Ye B-C 2015 *Biosens. Bioelectron.* **63** 379

Karra-Châabouni M, Bouaziz I, Boufi S, Botelho, do Rego A M and Gargouri Y 2008 *Colloids Surf. B Biointerfaces* **66** 168

Khiabani P S, Soeriyadi A H, Reece P J and Gooding J J 2016 Paper-based sensor for monitoring Sun exposure *ACS Sens.* **1** 775–80

Klasner S A, Price A K, Hoeman K W, Wilson R S, Bell K J and Culbertson C T 2010 Paper-based microfluidic devices for analysis of clinically relevant analytes present in urine and saliva *Anal. Bioanal. Chem.* **397** 1821–9

Kumar S, Kumar S, Srivastava S, Yadav B K, Lee S H, Sharma J G, Doval D C and Malhotra B D 2015 *Biosens. Bioelectron.* **73** 114

Kumar S, Umar M, Saifi A, Kumar S, Augustine S and Srivastava S *et al* 2019 Electrochemical paper based cancer biosensor using iron oxide nanoparticles decorated PEDOT:PSS *Anal. Chim. Acta* **1056** 135–45

Kuswandi B. and Ensafi A. A. 2019 Perspective—Paper-Based Biosensors: Trending Topic in Clinical Diagnostics Developments and Commercialization. *J. Electrochem. Soc.* **167** 037509

Kuswandi B and Ensafi A A 2020 *J. Electrochem. Soc.* **167** 037509

Lam T, Devadhasan J P, Howse R and Kim J 2017 A chemically patterned microfluidic paper-based analytical device (C-μPAD) for point-of-care diagnostics *Sci. Rep.* **7** 1–10

Li C-Z, Vandenberg K, Prabhulkar S, Zhu X, Schneper L, Methee K, Rosser C J and Almeide E 2011 Paper based point-of-care testing disc for multiplex whole cell bacteria analysis *Biosens. Bioelectron.* **26** 4342–8

Li H, Han D, Pauletti G M and Steckl A J 2014 Blood coagulation screening using a paper-based microfluidic lateral flow device *Lab Chip* **14** 4035–41

Li L, Xu J, Zheng X, Ma C, Song X, Ge S, Yu J and Yan M 2014 *Biosens. Bioelectron.* **61** 76

Li Z. *et al* 2020 Development and clinical application of a rapid IgM-IgG combined antibody test for SARS-CoV-2 infection diagnosis. *J. Med. Virol.* **92** 1518–24

Liana D D, Raguse B, Gooding J J and Chow E 2012 Recent advances in paper-based sensors *Sensors* **12** 11505–26

Liana D D, Raguse B, Gooding J J and Chow E 2012 Recent advances in paper-based sensors *Sensors* **12** 11505–26

Liang L, Su M, Li L, Lan F, Yang G and Ge S *et al* 2016 Aptamer-based fluorescent and visual biosensor for multiplexed monitoring of cancer cells in microfluidic paper-based analytical devices *Sensors Actuators* B **229** 347–54

Loo J, Kwok H, Leung C, Wu S, Law I and Cheung Y *et al* 2017 Sample-to-answer on molecular diagnosis of bacterial infection using integrated lab-on-a-disc *Biosens. Bioelectr.* **93** 212–9

Lopez-Marzo A M and Merkoci A 2016 Paper-based sensors and assays: a success of the engineering design and the convergence of knowledge areas *Lab Chip* **16** 3150–76

Lu Y, Shi W, Qin J and Lin B 2009 Fabrication and characterization of paper-based microfluidics prepared in nitrocellulose membrane by wax printing *Anal. Chem.* **82** 329–35

Ma X, Chen Z, Kannan P, Lin Z, Qiu B and Guo L 2016 *Anal. Chem.* **88** 3227

Mahadeva K and Kim J 2011 Conductometric glucose biosensor made with cellulose and tin oxide hybrid nanocomposites *Sensors Actuators* B **157** 177–82

Martinez A W, Phillips S T, Wiley B J, Gupta M and Whitesides G M 2008 *Lab Chip.* **8** 2146

Mello M L S and de Campos Vidal B 2017 The Feulgen reaction: a brief review and new perspectives *Acta Histochem.* **119** 603–9

Morais F and Curto J 2018 Design of porous nano cellulose based biopolymers for nanomedicine applications *Curr. Sci. Res. Biomed. Sci.* **1** Article 180003

Mroz A, Ratajczak K, Zaton P and Krajewski K 2018 Cellulose diversity in trees and its impact on properties of wood-state of the art *Ann. WULS -SGGW, Forest. Wood Technol.* **102** 90–6

Mukundan R, Khosla A, Sekhar P K, Hesketh P, Henry C and Magagnin L 2018 *J. Electrochem. Soc.* **165** Y9

Nayak S, Blumenfeld N R, Laksanasopin T and Sia S K 2017 Point-of-care diagnostics: recent developments in a connected age *Anal. Chem.* **89** 102–23

Nie J, Zhang Y, Lin L, Zhou C, Li S, Zhang L and Li J 2012 *Anal. Chem.* **84** 6331

Ostrov N, Jimenez M, Billerbeck S, Brisbois J, Matragrano J, Ager A and Cornish V W 2017 A modular yeast biosensor for low-cost point-of-care pathogen detection *Sci. Adv.* **3** e1603221

OuYang L, Wang C, Du F, Zheng T and Liang H 2014 Electrochromatographic separations of multi-component metal complexes on a microfluidic paper-based device with a simplified photolithography *RSC Adv.* **4** 1093–101

Pourreza N, Golmohammadi H, Naghdi T and Yousefi H 2015 Green *in situ* synthesized silver nanoparticles embedded in bacterial cellulose nanopaper as a bionanocomposite plasmonic sensor *Biosens. Bioelectron.* **74** 353–9

Ratajczak K and Stobieck M 2020 High-performance modified cellulose paper-based biosensors for medical diagnostics and early cancer screening: a concise review *Carbohydr. Polym.* **229** 115463

Rivas L, Reuterswärd P, Rasti R, Herrmann B, Mårtensson A, Alfvén T, Gantelius J and Andersson-Svahn H 2018 A vertical flow paper-microarray assay with isothermal DNA amplification for detection of *Neisseria meningitidis* *Talanta* **183** 192–200

Ruecha N, Rangkupan R, Rodthongkum N and Chailapakul O 2014 *Biosens. Bioelectron.* **52** 13

Scida K, Cunningham J C, Renault C, Richards I and Crooks R M 2014 *Anal. Chem.* **86** 6501

Shamkhalichenar H and Choi J W 2017 *J. Electrochem. Soc.* **164** B3101

Sharma A, Rao* V K, Kamboj D V, Gaur R, Shaik M and Shrivastava A R 2016 Enzyme free detection of staphylococcal enterotoxin B (SEB) using ferrocene carboxylic acid labeled monoclonal antibodies: an electrochemical approach *New J. Chem.* **40** 8334–41

Sharma A, Rao* V K, Kamboj D V, Gaur R, Upadhyay S and Shaik M 2015 Relative efficiency of zinc sulfide (ZnS) quantum dots (QDs) based electrochemical and fluorescence immunoassay for the detection of staphylococcal enterotoxin B (SEB) *Biotechnol. Rep.* **6** 129–36

Sharma A, Rao* V K, Kamboj D V and Jain R 2014 Electrochemical immunosensor for staphylococcal enterotoxin B (SEB) based on platinum nanoparticles-modified electrode using hydrogen evolution inhibition approach *Electroanalysis* **26** 2320–7

Sharma A, Rao* V K, Kamboj D V, Upadhyay S, Shaik M, Shrivastava A R and Jain R 2014 Sensitive detection of staphylococcal enterotoxin B (SEB) using quantum dots by various methods with special emphasis on an electrochemical immunoassay approach *RSC Adv.* **4** 34089–95

Sheridan C 2020 Fast, portable tests come online to curb coronavirus pandemic *Nat. Biotechnol.* **38** 515–8

Singh A T, Lantigua D, Meka A, Taing S, Pandher M and Camci-Unal G 2018 Paper-Based Sensors: Emerging Themes and Applications *Sensors* **18** 2838

Songjaroen T, Dungchai W, Chailapakul O, Henry C S and Laiwattanapaisal W 2012 Blood separation on microfluidic paper-based analytical devices *Lab Chip* **12** 3392–8

Sun X, Wang H, Jian Y, Lan F, Zhang L and Liu H *et al* 2018 Ultrasensitive microfluidic paper-based electrochemical/visual biosensor based on spherical-like cerium dioxide catalyst for miR-21 detection *Biosens. Bioelectron.* **105** 218–25

Tang R, Yang H, Choi J R, Gong Y, You M and Wen T *et al* 2017b Capillary blood for point-of-care testing *Crit. Rev. Clin. Lab. Sci.* **54** 294–308

Tortorich R, Shamkhalichenar H and Choi J-W 2018 *Appl. Sci.* **8** 288

Trinh T N D and Lee N Y 2019 A foldable isothermal amplification microdevice for fuchsin-based colorimetric detection of multiple foodborne pathogens *Lab Chip* **19** 1397–405

Tyagi C, Tomar Lomas K and Singh H 2008 Surface modification of cellulose filter paper by glycidyl methacrylate grafting for biomolecule immobilization: influence of grafting parameters and urease immobilization *J. Appl. Polym. Sci.* **111** 1381–90

Vella S J, Beattie P, Cademartiri R, Laromaine A, Martinez A W, Phillips S T, Mirica K A and Whitesides G M 2012 Measuring markers of liver function using a micropatterned paper device designed for blood from a fingerstick *Anal. Chem.* **84** 2883–91

Wang H, Li Y-J, Wei J-F, Xu J-R, Wang Y-H and Zheng G-X 2014 Paper-based three-dimensional microfluidic device for monitoring of heavy metals with a camera cell phone *Anal. Bioanal. Chem.* **406** 2799–807

Wu L, Ma C, Zheng X, Liu H and Yu J 2015 *Biosens. Bioelectron.* **68** 413

Wu L, Zhang Y, Wang Y, Ge S, Liu H and Yan M *et al* 2016 A paper-based electrochemiluminescence electrode as an aptamer-based cytosensor using PtNi@carbon dots as nanolabels for detection of cancer cells and for *in situ* screening of anticancer drugs *Microchim. Acta* **183** 1873–80

Xia Y, Si J and Li Z 2016 Fabrication techniques for microfluidic paper-based analytical devices and their applications for biological testing: a review *Biosens. Bioelectron* **77** 774–89

Xu X, Li R, Tang C, Wang H, Zhuang X and Liu Y *et al* 2018 Cellulose nanofiber-embedded sulfonated poly (ether sulfone) membranes for proton exchange membrane fuel cells *Carbohydr. Polym.* **184** 299–306

Yetisen A K, Akram M S and Lowe C R 2013 Paper-based microfluidic point-of-care diagnostic devices *Lab Chip* **13** 2210–51

Yin J, Zou Z, Hu Z, Zhang S, Zhang F and Wang B *et al* 2020 A 'sample-in-multiplex-digital-answer-out' chip for fast detection of pathogens *Lab Chip* **20** 979–86

Zang D., Ge L., Yan M., Song X. and Yu J. 2012 Electrochemical immunoassay on a 3D microfluidic paper-based device. *Chem. Commun.* **48** 4683

Zhao C., Thuo M. M. and Liu X. 2013 A microfluidic paper-based electrochemical biosensor array for multiplexed detection of metabolic biomarkers. *Sci. Technol. Adv. Mater.* **14** 054402

Zheng Y-Y, Ma Y-T, Zhang J-Y and Xie X 2020 COVID-19 and the cardiovascular system *Nat. Rev. Cardiol.* **17** 259–60

Zhu G, Yin X, Jin D, Zhang B, Gu Y and An Y 2019 Paper-based immunosensors: current trends in the types and applied detection techniques *TrAC Trends Anal. Chem.* **111** 100–17

Chapter 12

Sensing technologies used in microfluidic paper-based analytical devices (μPADs)

Pallavi Singh Chauhan, Neha Sharma and Rajesh Singh Tomar

There is great interest in developing low-cost portable biosensor platforms for a variety of applications, including disease diagnosis in point-of-care (POC) settings. Modern diagnostic tests available in developed countries require complex laboratory infrastructure. Therefore, they are not suitable for environments with limited financial resources, basic health facilities and few skilled technicians. Cellulose and flexible tracing paper-based sensors have shown great potential in developing reliable, affordable and portable devices for diagnosing diseases. These units offer promising solutions for disease management in resource-constrained settings. With the advent of analytical techniques, micro-devices have brought compelling benefits, including highly sensitive detection and analysis. In the past decade, a new generation of paper microfluidic analyzers has emerged, an area that will change the way diseases are diagnosed and detected.

12.1 Introduction

Paper-based microfluidic devices are created by modelling paper with hydrophobic barriers to identify hydrophilic channels and regions. Conventional microfluidic devices are made of silicon, glass or polymer. For example, polydimethylsiloxane (PDMS) or poly methyl methacrylate (PMMA), paper microflow devices can be supplied in small quantities (Wang *et al* 2013, Busek *et al* 2021). Unlike conventional microflow devices, paper devices can be easily manufactured without a clean room. It is made of inexpensive and readily available materials and does not require computer controlled pumps to make paper microflows, more accessible to researchers of all disciplines for bedside diagnostic testing. It provides an ideal platform for development of point-of-care. This technique can be used to analyze analytes of clinical relevance in developed countries. It will meet these challenges while being simple, economical and meeting guaranteed laboratory standards (cheap, accurate,

doi:10.1088/978-0-7503-5820-0ch12 © IOP Publishing Ltd 2023

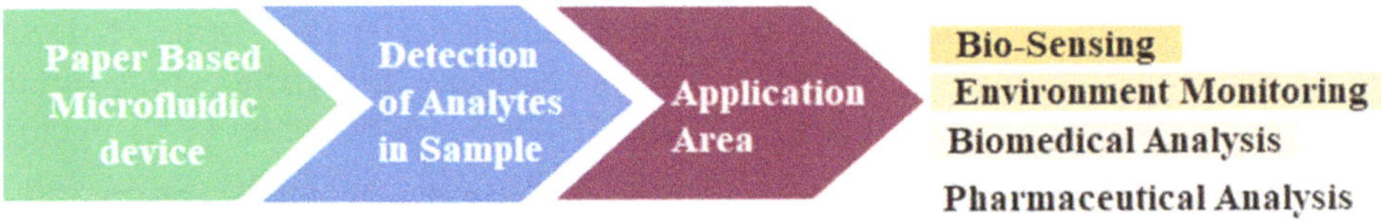
Paper Based Microfluidic device
Detection of Analytes in Sample
Application Area
Bio-Sensing
Environment Monitoring
Biomedical Analysis
Pharmaceutical Analysis

Figure 12.1. Applications of paper-based microfluidic device.

specific, easy to use, fast and robust, no equipment or shipping required). Paper microfluidic analyzers (microPAD or μPAD) increase the need for accurate diagnosis of infectious diseases and non-communicable diseases (Chowdury *et al* 2021) and developed to support fast diagnosis of infectious diseases. The widespread use of paper microflows is driving the exponential growth of this field, as evidenced by the recent trend in the number of publications in this field. A recent PubMed literature search found the topic 'paper microfluidics' or 'paper microfluidics', in 2979 articles published between 2007 and 2020 (Charbaji *et al* 2021). Many articles on biosensors, biomedical applications, flow control and electrochemical analysis have also been published in microPAD journals. The purpose of this review is to provide a complete overview of modern paper microfluidic device manufacturing techniques, as seen in figure 12.1 (Escobar *et al* 2021).

12.2 Components of microfluidic devices

Components of microfluidic devices are often clearly divided into two groups. The first micro total analysis systems (μTAS) include microfluidic devices made of different processes and materials which is connected to external units such as sampling units, sensor units, and electronic units (Scott *et al* 2021). Another type of microfluidic device is an inexpensive, lightweight paper lab chip with a fully equipped lab unit that performs a specific task primarily for the detection of a variety of materials. The main elements of the first group of microflow units are syringes, tubes, pumps, valves, tanks, actuators, electromagnets, microwave ovens, droplet generators and bubbles (Azimi-Boulali *et al* 2020). In the semiconductor industry, a method is being developed for the production of LOC elements. The first microfluidic components are silicon and glass, quartz, and soft or hard polymers are used in production (Niculescu *et al* 2021). In addition, various biomaterials such as calcium alginate, cross-linked gelatine and hydrogel were used. They have been shown to be useful in providing a physiologically relevant cellular microenvironment for cell growth and tissue culture. Glass is the main alternative to silicon because it is cheap, transparent, negatively charged, and a good current carrier (Świontek *et al* 2021). Due to the use of polymers, it is possible to make inexpensive and disposable devices. They also provide interesting properties for microfluidic devices. The flexible material has excellent structural rigidity, allowing the construction of small and rigid microfluidic devices. Channels can be formed by polymer moulding and a variety of soft lithography and stamping methods, and each part can be thermo-formed or glued. But their surface chemistry is more complex than that of silicon and glass. They are generally incompatible with organic solvents and cannot be used at high temperatures. Quartz and glass sculptures are heavier than other materials, such as polymers, lightweight flexible silicone rubber, thermostat, poly methyl methacrylate (PMMA), poly(dimethylsiloxane) (PDMS), polyamides (PA), cyclulfin (COC) copolymers and SU-8 (passive photoresist). Microstructure costs can be reduced by using these materials in microfluidics, which are the most widely used materials today (Männel *et al* 2021).

12.3 Detection techniques, separation methods and applications of microfluidic devices

They are widely used in biological, chemical and biomedical analysers. There are various detection methods in the field of chemical and biological diagnostics or analysis on microfluidic platforms. Microflow detection methods can be divided into three main types: optical methods, electrochemical methods, and mass spectroscopy (Ochoa *et al* 2021, Zhang *et al* 2021). Among these methods, optical and electrochemical methods are most commonly used because of their selectivity and sensitivity. In addition to the above basic techniques, techniques such as nuclear magnetic resonance (NMR), magneto-resistance and acoustic spectroscopy are combined with microfluidics for sensing applications (Plata *et al* 2021). Common optical detection methods include direct detection to track the properties of light, including methods based on fluorescence, absorption and luminescence, and detection to modulate the properties of light, such as surface plasmon resonance (SPR) detection. In addition, it was reported that various optical technologies of photonic crystals, photocavity structures and detection are integrated into microfluidic systems using one and two-dimensional PC surfaces or three-dimensional photonic crystals, optical resonators (Zaky *et al* 2021). The resonator performs cell monitoring or rheological measurements of the fluid using a whisper corridor and optical tweezers.

Electrochemical measurements are based on the modification of the electrical properties of the types of analytes that have undergone redox reactions and are commonly used to detect electrically active species (Caizán-Juanarena *et al* 2020). Accurate detection of analytes can be achieved using cyclic voltammetry curves and electric current time curves (Paut *et al* 2021). When selective ions pass through the membrane and a local equilibrium is established at the sensor interface, the resulting charge distribution creates a potential between the working electrode and the reference electrode, depending on the type and concentration. Different species have unique conductivity reactions depending on their concentration. This is, in principle, the most widely used method in electrochemical measurements because it can be handled with any charge of interest. The discovery includes frequency-band conductivity measurements on the conventional contact-based conductance sensor and capacitive-coupled non-contact conductance (C4D) sensor methods such as potential gradient sensing (He *et al* 2021). Electrochemical proofs are often used in electrochemical (capillary) processes (e.g., capillary electrophoresis separation) or in electrophoresis systems. In this sense, the 'electrochemical process' in this review actually includes studies on electrophoresis (Przybylska *et al* 2021).

The main application is the study of proteomic bodies for further identification in models for protein separation and fragmentation. Identification after separation takes place in two ways. A method for direct detection is achieved by searching the database for each type of protein. To date, several MS configurations have been developed integrated with microfluidic devices for this application, such as MS ionization electrospray (ESI) and laser matrixing matrix (MALDI)—MS (Maccarrone *et al* 2017). In the future, when NEMS-MS encounters a microfluidic, it is expected to enable us to provide a highly efficient microfluidic platform for the analysis of biological or chemical species (B. Proteins or Make Nanoparticles). In addition to isolating and identifying proteins, MS is also used to quantify protein expression under different conditions (especially in disease states). However, reduction requirements and high sensitivity are currently one of the most important technical obstacles. However, microcurrents look promising for technological progress in this area. The multichannel microfluidic architecture enables high-power processing and multiplexing (Yue *et al* 2021). Given these factors, their combination with microfluids may be the best laboratory solution on the MS chip for quantitative proteomic applications. As far as we know, there are no other reports of microfluidic diagnostics based on multiple sclerosis, but much remains to be done to do interesting research.

Nuclear magnetic resonance spectroscopy can reveal a variety of biological and chemical analyses such as proteins and nucleic acids (Muniyappan *et al* 2021). However, their use in microscopic systems is limited due to the low sensitivity of current NMR detection techniques. More recently, this problem has been solved by the hyperpolarization technique (for example, by adding high-polarity para hydrogen signal amplifiers). The finite response time/polarization meter is a major technical bottleneck for the detection of NMR-based microfluidic assays (Kiss *et al* 2021). As with MS spectroscopy, another major obstacle is system shrinkage. Despite technical challenges, NMR remains a competitive technology for microfluidic applications compared to photonic or electrochemical processes. This process is time-consuming as there is no problem in getting light for ROI and acquisition time is much shorter. Solving the problem of weak NMR signals in microsystems by amplifying additional signals or better detection tools will unlock a wider range of NMR applications in the laboratory (Nassar *et al* 2021).

12.4 Customization of devices for specific applications

Paper-based microfluidics provides a completely unique possibility for analysis of diverse diseases because of their ease of fabrication, affordability, reproducibility, sensitivity and low limits of detection. The technique is used for the detection of a number of analytes in present in urine, blood and saliva (Sher *et al* 2017). The discipline of PADs has continued to grow at an exponential rate, with significant implications for academic and industrial groups. Paper-based analytical devices (PADs) are devices that employ cellulose as a substrate for point-of-care diagnostics, biosensing, environmental monitoring, biomedical and pharmaceutical analysis, clinical diagnosis, and forensic investigations (Lisowski *et al* 2013). Paper has also been used in chemical/biochemical analysis, such as home pregnancy tests (Gong *et al* 2017), paper chromatography (Meredith *et al* 2016), paper-based colorimetry, paper-based filtration and purification, pH test, and so on.

Some specific applications are given below.

12.4.1 For cancer

Recently, graphene/gold nanocomposite based paper dot immune-graphene-gold filtration assay has been constructed for the specific detection of MCF-7 and has been used in cancer diagnosis due to specific photothermal properties. It is a simple and quick method which has a comparatively low detection limit of 600 MCF-7 cells (Zhou *et al* 2016). In addition, glucose is the most powerful and unique analyte to monitor and diagnosis of diabetes and has been found to be a cancer biomarker, and has been used in POC diagnostics. A thread/paper-based analytical device has been developed in both flat- and cone-shape platforms and used to detect glucose (Gonzalez *et al* 2016).

12.4.2 C-reactive protein

A simple, rapid and less expensive paper-based tool was developed in 2016 for the detection and evaluation of C-reactive protein (CRP). This test was based on a latex agglutination test. The paper was firstly coated through the wax-printing technique and three fluidic channels were created. Subsequently, CRP ranges had were decided via serum stain length in the channel (Lin *et al* 2016).

12.4.3 For virus detection

The major infectious diseases including HIV, dengue, malaria, tuberculosis and hepatitis C virus are particularly attractive in the context of healthcare POC diagnostics. Dengue is the fastest spreading mosquito-borne disease. A paper-based test strip was constructed for the detection of a dengue virus. It was based on an agarose-incorporated lateral flow method. This method improved the sensitivity of a modified test strip by approximately tenfold compared with an unmodified strip due to the increased interaction between gold nanoparticle-detector probes and target (Han *et al* 2016, Choi *et al* 2017).

12.4.4 For liver function

Vella *et al* published a paper-based technique for liver function analysis using fingerstick blood that simultaneously evaluated two enzymatic markers, alkaline phosphate (ALP) and aspartate aminotransferase (AST), as well as total serum protein. ALP and AST are primarily produced by liver cells and are frequently seen in amazingly low amounts in the bloodstream. ALP and AST concentrations rise quickly as a result of a damaged or diseased liver, making them suitable markers for diagnosis of liver diseases (Vella *et al* 2012).

12.4.5 For immune sensor

In this study, a paper-based lateral flow immunosensor with a unique microfluidic valve technology was developed as a point-of-care (POC) device. To make the fluidic network, layers of paper and tape were employed to create a three-dimensional structure. Multiple directional valves are implanted in the test strip layers, unlike conventional LFIAs, to manage the sequence and time of mixing for the sample and multiple reagents. We present a four-valve mechanism (table 12.1) that automatically directs three distinct fluids to flow consecutively over the sensing region in this work. A three-step alkaline phosphatase-based enzyme-linked immuno sorbent assay (ELISA) technique with rabbit IgG as the model analyte was used to demonstrate the device's potential for immunoassays as proof of concept. The detection limit of about 4.8 fm was obtained (Roman *et al* 2014).

PADs are popular for a range of reasons, including (i) low cost, (ii) power free due to cellulose fibre networks, (iii) compatibility with smaller sample volumes, (iv) the ability

Table 12.1. Customized applications of microfluidic paper-based analytical devices (μPADs).

S. No.	Application	Principle	Mechanism	References
1	Cancer	Based on paper dot immune-graphene-gold filtration assay and colorimetric based assay	Solutions of different enzyme, substrate and chemical were transported or immobilized at the analysis sites.	Gonzalez *et al* (2016), Zhou *et al* (2016)
2	C-reactive protein (CRP)	Based on latex agglutination test	The paper was coated with wax-printing technique and created three fluidic channels.	Lin *et al* (2016)
3	Virus detection	Based on agarose-incorporated lateral flow method	A three-dimensional fluidic network is designed by a layered construction of wax-patterned papers, resulting in the attainment of variable fluidic paths.	Han *et al* (2016), Choi *et al* (2017)
4	For liver function	Paper-based technique	Using fingerstick blood that simultaneously evaluates two enzymatic markers, alkaline phosphate (ALP) and aspartate aminotransferase (AST), as well as total serum protein.	Vella *et al* (2012)
5	For immune sensor	Based on lateral flow immunoassays	To make the fluidic network, layers of paper and tape were employed to create a three-dimensional structure. A three-step alkaline phosphatase-based ELISA)technique with rabbit IgG as the model analyte was used to demonstrate the device's potential for immunoassays as proof of concept.	Roman *et al* (2014)

Table 12.2. Advantages of microfluidic paper-based analytical devices (μPADs).

S. No.	Advantages
1.	Low cost
2.	Power free
3.	Ability to evaluate small sample
4.	Ability to store reagents
5.	Ease of use and assembly
6.	Easy accessibility and processability
7.	Durable
8.	Lightweight and portable
9.	Need less storage space
10.	Capable of giving fast results

to store reagents, (v) ease of use and assembly, and (vi) accessibile and processabile. The combination of microfabrication techniques and paper has resulted in the establishment of *de novo* cost-effective electrochemical sensors with durable, easy, and quick applications (table 12.2) in a variety of sectors (Colozza *et al* 2021).

12.5 Paper as a platform for POC diagnostics

PADs have been initially designed for point-of-care diagnostic applications in developing countries, but they are set to shift the direction of clinical diagnosis of numerous diseases mechanistically, because of their quick, cost-effective, portable, and stable features. These systems have been used to detect a variety of biological components, such as DNA, proteins, and cancer cells. Their ability to detect harmful pathogens such as viruses and bacteria makes them useful monitoring tools in biosafety (Lu *et al* 2012, Su *et al* 2014, Tang *et al* 2014).

12.5.1 Paper and other porous membranes

Hemp, linen, jute, bamboo, sisal, grass, wood, cotton, and straw are some of the raw materials used to make paper (Yetisen *et al* 2013). Paper is a fibrous and porous substance having a variety of qualities, including strong absorbency, air permeability, and a high surface-to-volume ratio (Wang *et al* 2012, Akyazi *et al* 2018). Müller and Clegg were the first to introduce the concept of paper-based microfluidic channels in 1949. In 2007, Harvard University's Whitesides Group created the first functioning paper-based device capable of detecting a protein glucose assay (Martinez *et al* 2007). Due to its light weight, low cost, easy availability, biocompatibility with various substrates, flexibility, and hydrophilic nature, paper is becoming increasingly popular. Microfluidic applications such as dipstick tests, lateral flow assays (LFAs), and microfluidic analytical devices (μPADs) have all benefited from the use of filter paper as a basis (Akyazi *et al* 2018).

Cellulose and nitrocellulose are two of the most common types of paper used in the fabrication of point-of-care testing devices that wick fluids by capillary action. Aside from cellulose-based paper and nitrocellulose, there are a variety of porous membranes with varying physical and chemical properties that might be employed to construct paper-based microfluidic devices. Cellulose fibres with a high density of hydroxyl functional groups (single bond OH) and few carboxylic acid groups are hydrophilic in nature (single bond COOH). The process of nitrating cellulose yields nitrocellulose (i.e., by replacing hydroxyl groups with nitrate groups). Nitrocellulose membranes have a high affinity for protein binding and are commonly employed in lateral flow tests and western blots. Filter and chromatography papers are made of cellulose, which is also used to manufacture dipsticks and PADS, whereas LFAs are made of nitrocellulose paper (Yetisen *et al* 2013). After that, the polymer is cast into membranes with regulated porosity (Costa *et al* 2014, Gong *et al* 2017).

As a material for creating POC diagnostic devices, paper, which is defined broadly as any hydrophilic porous membrane, has several distinct advantages. It's low-cost, readily available, and compatible with a variety of printing and processing methods. It can be easily stored, stacked, and transported, and there is already a large-scale manufacturing activity for paper products that will be used to make paper-based products. Different thicknesses and porosities of paper are available (Martinez *et al* 2008, Camplisson *et al* 2015).

12.5.2 Conventional paper-based point-of-care assays: dipsticks and lateral flow assays

Conventional paper-based POC assays have two most common POC diagnostic technologies, i.e., dipstick assays and LFAs. These porous membrane-based technologies were developed long before paper-based microfluidic devices, and they demonstrate many of the advantages of paper-based assays.

12.5.2.1 Dipstick assays

Dipsticks or test strips are made up of paper pads that are glued to a plastic strip and contain dried reagents. The strip is temporarily dipped into a liquid sample, analytes in the sample react with reagents on the pads to cause colour changes, and the colours of the pads of paper are compared to a chart to determine the results. Dipstick assays can occasionally be used to estimate an approximate or semi-quantitative concentration based on the intensity or shade of colour that is produced. As seen in figure 12.2, based on the intensity or shade of colour that is produced, dipstick assays sometimes allow a user to determine an

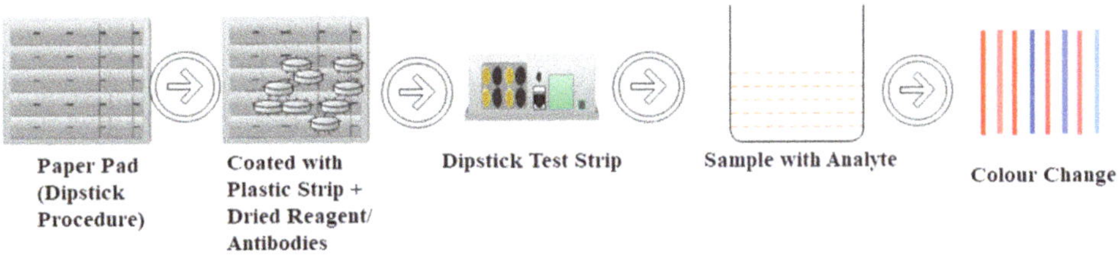

Figure 12.2. Mechanism of paper-based POC assay.

approximate or semi-quantitative concentration of the analyte. The main advantages of dipstick assays are their simplicity, low cost, and ability to test for multiple analytes simultaneously. The main disadvantages of dipstick assays are that they typically have poor limits of detection and poor specificity (Mambatta *et al* 2015, Dadzie *et al* 2019).

12.5.2.2 Lateral flow assays

In comparison to dipsticks, LFAs are more complicated devices that rely on antibodies to provide high specificity, such as the home pregnancy test. LFA devices contain a sample pad, test line, conjugate pad, control line, and absorbent, which are made up of overlapping porous membranes. The user places the sample on the sample pad, and it wicks across the device, interacting with a labelled conjugate antibody and an immobilized capture antibody. When the antigen (analyte) is present in the sample, the capture antibody holds the tagged antibody in place by their unique interactions with the antigen, generating a coloured band across the strip. To improve the detection capabilities of these assays, more advanced forms of LFAs integrate nanoparticles, enzymes, or oligonucleotides (De Puig *et al* 2017, Syedmoradi *et al* 2017). Figure 12.3 shows how LFAs are currently being utilised to detect illnesses, infections, poisons, and pollutants in a variety of applications (K. M., and Gallotta, A. 2016). LFAs are currently being utilized to detect illnesses, infections, poisons, and pollutants in a variety of applications (Koczula and Gallotta 2016). LFAs were recently developed for the detection of COVID-19 (Broughton *et al* 2020, Choi 2020, Hussein *et al* 2020, Li *et al* 2020) (figure 12.3).

The key benefits of LFAs are that they are easy to use, precise, affordable, and do not require any additional equipment. The main limitations of LFAs are that they

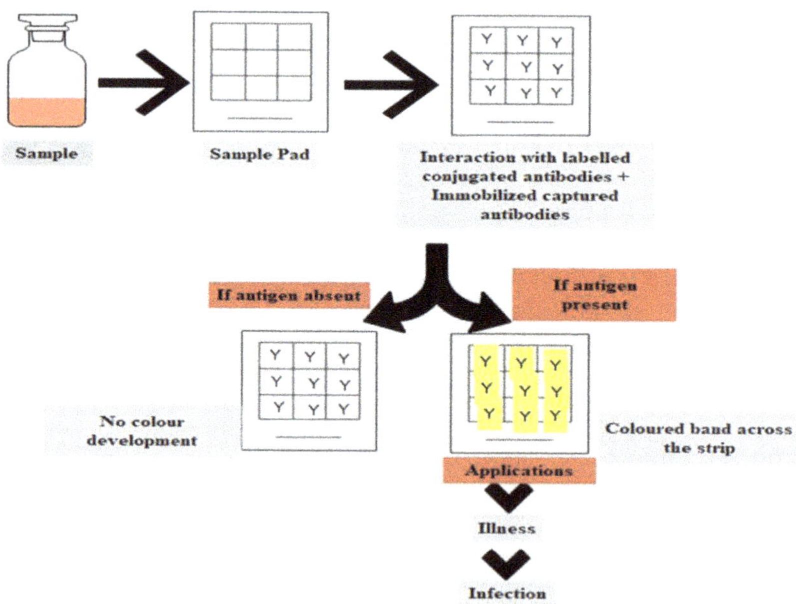

Figure 12.3. Mechanism of lateral flow assays (LFA).

often only provide qualitative (yes/no) answers, that each device can only detect a single analyte, and that they have lower detection limits than laboratory-based assays such as ELISA. MicroPADs are based on dipstick and LFA technologies and attempt to overcome the limits of these two diagnostic platforms (Martinez *et al* 2017).

12.6 Conclusion

The creation of POC diagnostic devices, which potentially reduce the need for expensive and time-consuming laboratory-based analytical processes, is the most prevalent use of paper-based microfluidic devices. This chapter gives a summary of existing methods for producing paper-based microfluidic devices, as well as examples of their uses, a discussion of their current limits, and a forecast for their future. PADs are now a vibrant field of study with a diverse set of applications. The most prevalent PAD manufacturing process is wax-printing and heating, which is utilized to produce huge numbers of devices in a short length of time. However, because of the intrinsic lack of control over the fabrication process in this technology, repeatable PAD characteristics and, as a result, fluidic flow control are not attainable, which are the primary barriers to mass production and commercialization. As a result, generating homogeneous microfluidic channels that are repeatable from device to device remains an unresolved problem.

References

Abe K, Suzuki K and Citterio D 2008 Inkjet-printed microfluidic multianalyte chemical sensing paper *Anal . Chem.* **80** 6928–34

Akyazi T, Basabe-Desmonts L and Benito-Lopez F 2018 Review on microfluidic paper-based analytical devices towards commercialisation *Anal. Chim. Acta* **1001** 1–17

Azimi-Boulali J, Madadelahi M, Madou M J and Martinez-Chapa S O 2020 Droplet and particle generation on centrifugal microfluidic platforms: a review *Micromachines* **11** 603

Broughton J P, Deng X, Yu G, Fasching C L, Servellita V, Singh J and Chiu C Y 2020 CRISPR–Cas12-based detection of SARS-CoV-2 *Nat. Biotechnol.* **38** 870–4

Busek M, Nøvik S, Aizenshtadt A, Amirola-Martinez M, Combriat T, Grünzner S and Krauss S 2021 Thermoplastic elastomer (TPE)–poly (methyl methacrylate)(PMMA) hybrid devices for active pumping pdms-free organ-on-a-chip systems *Biosensors* **11** 162

Caizán-Juanarena L, Borsje C, Sleutels T, Yntema D, Santoro C, Ieropoulos I and Ter Heijne A 2020 Combination of bioelectrochemical systems and electrochemical capacitors: principles, analysis and opportunities *Biotechnol. Adv.* **39** 107456

Camplisson C K, Schilling K M, Pedrotti W L, Stone H A and Martinez A W 2015 Two-ply channels for faster wicking in paper-based microfluidic devices *Lab Chip* **15** 4461–6

Charbaji A, Heidari-Bafroui H, Anagnostopoulos C and Faghri M 2021 A new paper-based microfluidic device for improved detection of nitrate in water *Sensors* **21** 102

Choi J R 2020 Development of point-of-care biosensors for COVID-19 *Front. Chem.* **8** 517

Choi J R, Yong K W, Tang R, Gong Y, Wen T, Yang H and Xu F 2017 Lateral flow assay based on paper–hydrogel hybrid material for sensitive point-of-care detection of dengue virus *Adv. Healthcare Mater.* **6** 1600920

Chowdury M A and Khalid F 2021 Application of microfluidic paper-based analytical device (μPAD) to detect COVID-19 in energy deprived countries *Int. J. Energy Res.* **45** 18275–80

Colozza N, Caratelli V, Moscone D and Arduini F 2021 Origami paper-based electrochemical (bio) sensors: state of the art and perspective *Biosensors* **11** 328

Costa M N, Veigas B, Jacob J M, Santos D S, Gomes J, Baptista P V and Fortunato E 2014 A low cost, safe, disposable, rapid and self-sustainable paper-based platform for diagnostic testing: lab-on-paper *Nanotechnology* **25** 094006

Dadzie I, Quansah E, Puopelle Dakorah M, Abiade V, Takyi-Amuah E and Adusei R 2019 The effectiveness of dipstick for the detection of urinary tract infection *Can. J. Infect. Dis. Med. Microbiol.* **2019** 8642628

De Puig H, Bosch I, Gehrke L and Hamad-Schifferli K 2017 Challenges of the nano–bio interface in lateral flow and dipstick immunoassays *Trends Biotechnol.* **35** 1169–80

Delaney J L, Hogan C F, Tian J and Shen W 2011 Electrogenerated chemiluminescence detection in paper-based microfluidic sensors *Anal. Chem.* **83** 1300–6

Escobar A, Chiu P, Qu J, Zhang Y and Xu C Q 2021 Integrated microfluidic-based platforms for on-site detection and quantification of infectious pathogens: towards on-site medical translation of SARS-CoV-2 diagnostic platforms *Micromachines* **12** 1079

Gerbers R, Foellscher W, Chen H, Anagnostopoulos C and Faghri M 2014 A new paper-based platform technology for point-of-care diagnostics *Lab Chip* **14** 4042–9

Gong M M and Sinton D 2017 Turning the page: advancing paper-based microfluidics for broad diagnostic application *Chem. Rev.* **117** 8447–80

Gonzalez A, Estala L, Gaines M and Gomez F A 2016 Mixed thread/paper-based microfluidic chips as a platform for glucose assays *Electrophoresis* **37** 1685–90

Han K N, Choi J S and Kwon J 2016 Three-dimensional paper-based slip device for one-step point-of-care testing *Sci. Rep.* **6** 1–7

He Y, Huang Q, He Y, Ji H, Zhang T, Wang B and Huang Z 2021 A Low excitation working frequency capacitively coupled contactless conductivity detection (C4D) sensor for microfluidic devices *Sensors* **21** 6381 https://sciencedirect.com/science/article/pii/S0925400521002495

Hu J, Wang S, Wang L, Li F, Pingguan-Murphy B, Lu T J and Xu F 2014 Advances in paper-based point-of-care diagnostics *Biosens. Bioelectron.* **54** 585–97

Hussein H A, Hassan R Y, Chino M and Febbraio F 2020 Point-of-care diagnostics of COVID-19: from current work to future perspectives *Sensors* **20** 4289

Kiss S Z, MacKinnon N and Korvink J G 2021 Microfluidic overhauser DNP chip for signal-enhanced compact NMR *Sci. Rep.* **11** 1–11

Koczula K M and Gallotta A 2016 Lateral flow assays *Essays Biochem.* **60** 111–20

Li Z, Yi Y, Luo X, Xiong N, Liu Y, Li S and Ye F 2020 Development and clinical application of a rapid IgM–IgG combined antibody test for SARS-CoV-2 infection diagnosis *J. Med. Virol.* **92** 1518–24

Lin F, Liu Y, Yu X, Cheng L, Singer A, Shpyrko O G and Doeff M M 2017 Synchrotron X-ray analytical techniques for studying materials electrochemistry in rechargeable batteries *Chem. Rev.* **117** 13123–86

Lin S C, Tseng C Y, Lai P L, Hsu M Y, Chu S Y, Tseng F G and Cheng C M 2016 Based CRP monitoring devices *Sci. Rep.* **6** 1–7

Lu J, Ge S, Ge L, Yan M and Yu J 2012 Electrochemical DNA sensor based on three-dimensional folding paper device for specific and sensitive point-of-care testing *Electrochim. Acta* **80** 334–41

Maccarrone G, Nischwitz S, Deininger S O, Hornung J, König F B, Stadelmann C and Weber F 2017 MALDI imaging mass spectrometry analysis—a new approach for protein mapping in multiple sclerosis brain lesions *J. Chromatogr.* B **1047** 131–40

Mambatta A K, Jayarajan J, Rashme V L, Harini S, Menon S and Kuppusamy J 2015 Reliability of dipstick assay in predicting urinary tract infection *J. Fam. Med. Prim. Care* **4** 265

Männel M J, Baysak E and Thiele J 2021 Fabrication of microfluidic devices for emulsion formation by microstereolithography *Molecules* **26** 2817

Martinez A W, Phillips S T and Whitesides G M 2008 Three-dimensional microfluidic devices fabricated in layered paper and tape *Proc. Natl. Acad. Sci.* **105** 19606–11

Martinez A W, Phillips S T, Butte M J and Whitesides G M 2007 Patterned paper as a platform for inexpensive, low-volume, portable bioassays *Angew. Chem.* **46** 1318–20

Martinez A W, Phillips S T, Whitesides G M and Carrilho E 2010 Diagnostics for the developing world: microfluidic paper-based analytical devices *Anal. Chem.* **82** 3–10

Meredith N A, Quinn C, Cate D M, Reilly T H, Volckens J and Henry C S 2016 based analytical devices for environmental analysis *Analyst* **141** 1874–87

Müller R H and Clegg D L 1949 Automatic paper chromatography *Anal. Chem.* **21** 1123–5

Muniyappan S, Lin Y, Lee Y H and Kim J H 2021 17O NMR spectroscopy: a novel probe for characterizing protein structure and folding *Biology* **10** 453

Nassar O, Jouda M, Rapp M, Mager D, Korvink J G and MacKinnon N 2021 Integrated impedance sensing of liquid sample plug flow enables automated high throughput NMR spectroscopy *Microsyst. Nanoeng.* **7** 1–17

Niculescu Ochoa M., Algorri J. F., Roldán-Varona P., Rodríguez-Cobo L. and López-Higuera J. M. 2021 Recent Advances in Biomedical Photonic Sensors: A Focus on Optical-Fibre-Based Sensing. *Sensors* **21** 6469

Ochoa M, Algorri J F, Roldán-Varona P, Rodríguez-Cobo L and López-Higuera J M 2021 Recent advances in biomedical photonic sensors: a focus on optical-fibre-based sensing *Sensors* **21** 6469

Paut A, Prkić A, Mitar I, Bošković P, Jozić D, Jakić M and Vukušić T 2021 Potentiometric response of solid-state sensors based on ferric phosphate for iron (III) determination *Sensors* **21** 1612

Plata M, Hale W, Sharma M, Werner J M and Utz M 2021 Microfluidic platform for serial mixing experiments with in operando nuclear magnetic resonance spectroscopy *Lab Chip* **21** 1598–603

Przybylska A, Gackowski M and Koba M 2021 Application of capillary electrophoresis to the analysis of bioactive compounds in herbal raw materials *Molecules* **26** 2135

Scott S M and Ali Z 2021 Fabrication methods for microfluidic devices: an overview *Micromachines* **12** 319

Sher M, Zhuang R, Demirci U and Asghar W 2017 based analytical devices for clinical diagnosis: recent advances in the fabrication techniques and sensing mechanisms *Expert Rev. Mol. Diagn.* **17** 351–66

Su M, Ge L, Ge S, Li N, Yu J, Yan M and Huang J 2014 Based electrochemical cyto-device for sensitive detection of cancer cells and *in situ* anticancer drug screening *Anal. Chim. Acta* **847** 1–9

Świontek S, Środa M and Gieszczyk W 2021 Ceramics, glass and glass-ceramics for personal radiation detectors *Materials* **14** 5987

Syedmoradi L, Daneshpour M, Alvandipour M, Gomez F A, Hajghassem H and Omidfar K 2017 Point of care testing: the impact of nanotechnology *Biosens. Bioelectron.* **87** 373–87

Tang C K, Vaze A and Rusling J F 2014 Based electrochemical immunoassay for rapid, inexpensive cancer biomarker protein detection *Anal. Methods* **6** 8878–81

Vella S J, Beattie P, Cademartiri R, Laromaine A, Martinez A W, Phillips S T and Whitesides G M 2012 Measuring markers of liver function using a micropatterned paper device designed for blood from a fingerstick *Anal. Chem.* **84** 2883–91

Wang S, Ge L, Song X, Yu J, Ge S and Huang J *et al* 2012 Paper-based chemiluminescence ELISA: lab-on-paper based on chitosan modified paper device and wax-screen-printing *Biosens. Bioelectron.* **31** 212–8

Wang X, Hagen J A and Papautsky I 2013 Paper pump for passive and programmable transport *Biomicrofluidics* **7** 014107

Yetisen A K, Akram M S and Lowe C R 2013 Paper-based microfluidic point-of-care diagnostic devices *Lab Chip* **13** 2210–51

Yue T, Zhao D, Phan D T, Wang X, Park J J, Biviji Z and Lee A P 2021 A modular microfluidic system based on a multilayered configuration to generate large-scale perfusable microvascular networks *Microsyst. Nanoeng.* **7** 1–13

Zaky Z A, Moustafa B and Aly A H 2021 Plasma cell sensor using photonic crystal cavity *Opt. Quantum Electron.* **53** 1–13

Zhang Y, Cole T, Yun G, Li Y, Zhao Q, Lu H and Tang S Y 2021 Modular and self-contained microfluidic analytical platforms enabled by magnetorheological elastomer microactuators *Micromachines* **12** 604

Zhou J, Zheng Y, Liu J, Bing X, Hua J and Zhang H 2016 A paper-based detection method of cancer cells using the photo-thermal effect of nanocomposite *J. Pharm. Biomed. Anal.* **117** 333–7

IOP Publishing

Paper-Based Diagnostic Devices for Infectious Diseases

Nidhi Puranik, Arpana Parihar and Raju Khan

Chapter 13

Integration of paper-based analytical tools with smartphones and IOMT

Pragati Raghuwanshi, Rachna Parashar, Tanusha Pathak and Aushtosh Singh Raghubanshi

For point-of-care testing (POCT) of numerous infections affecting human health, paper analytic devices combined with the Internet of Medical Things (IoMT) have gained recognition in recent years. The sensors based on these phenomena are intended to be low cost, portable, environmentally friendly, and provide an accurate, simple, and quick response. This chapter is based on the basic idea of detecting elements of paper-based analytical devices with smartphones and the IoMT, taking into account the growing relevance of paper-based analytical devices in the healthcare arena. The most current studies on paper-based analytical tools are summarized in this chapter, along with the issues and solutions that have been solved.

13.1 Introduction

A person's health is critical for leading a confortable and prosperous life. The World Health Organization (WHO) defines health as "a state of complete physical, mental and social well-being and not merely the absence of disease or infirmity". Healthcare is maintaining or increasing one's health using prevention, diagnosis, and treatment to prevent disease and assist with injury. Manual management is used in most traditional healthcare situations, and the upkeep of patient demographic information, case histories, diagnostics, medication, billing, and drug inventory management can result in human errors and will impacts patients [1].

With recent improvements in quality of life and medicine extending people's lives, it is more necessary to keep track of the health of patients and healthy people. Because the current healthcare system in North America makes this impossible, wireless gadgets that can be utilized from home are required. Biomedical wearables have gained popularity in the recent decades. There are various reasons for this, the most important are the high cost of healthcare, longer wait times, and increased public awareness of

doi:10.1088/978-0-7503-5820-0ch13 © IOP Publishing Ltd 2023

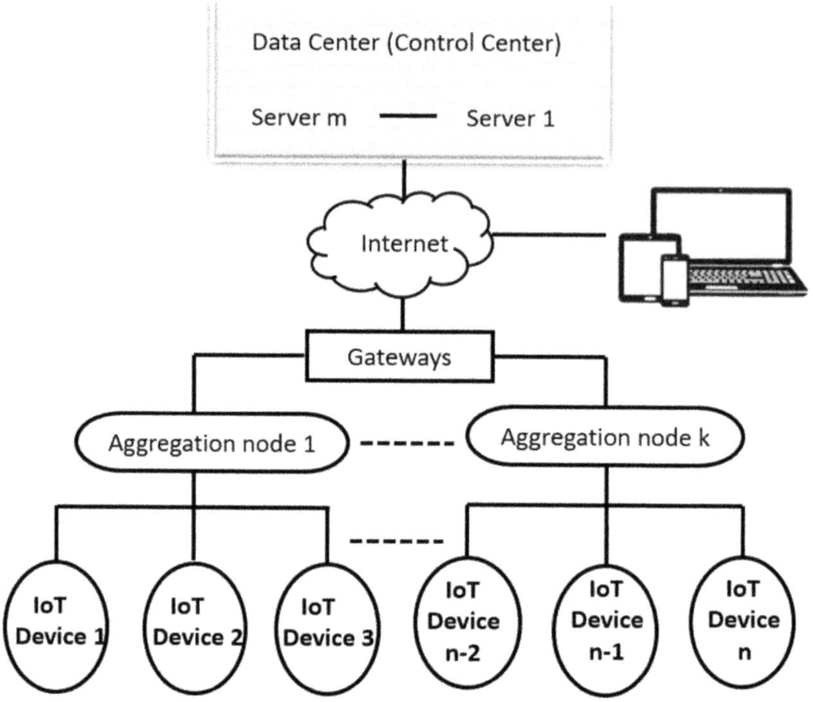

Figure 13.1. Example of Internet of Things System, where *n*—IoT devices, *k*—aggregation nodes, *m*—servers.

how to enhance the quality of life [2]. Medical devices that exchange data across a network without requiring human-to-computer or human-to-human contact are called 'Internet of Medical Things' (IoMT) devices. In the healthcare and medical domains, the Internet of Things (IoT) plays a critical role. The development of intelligent sensors, intelligent devices, and sophisticated lightweight communication protocols enabled the interconnection of medical things to monitor biological signals and diagnose patient ailments without the need for human involvement, dubbed the IoMT [3]. In simpler terms, IoMT is generally perceived to be the application of the basics, ideas, tools, techniques, and concepts of the well-known internet approach to the medical and healthcare sectors and domains. In order to connect the available healthcare resources and other medical services utilizing the most advanced internet-based technology, we needed all of our efforts to build a functional network of services. The proposed IoMT principles are crucial when providing medical care in remote locations. Healthcare, medical operations, and services have changed due to implementing IoMT principles and methodologies [4] (figure 13.1).

13.2 IoMT communications and devices

Medical equipment uses four communication networks to connect in real-time. These categories include body area networks (BAN), home area networks (HAN), neighbourhood area networks (NAN), and wide area networks.

A BAN is a medium for transmitting patients' vital signals, measured by a wearable or portable sensor. According to Kocabas *et al* in [5], biomedical signals can encrypt communications between medical equipment. Later, Poon *et al* provided a low-power bio-identification approach [6] by securing the communication between BAN sensors using an inter-pulse interval (IPI). Venkatasubramanian *et al* [7] used a physiological signal for BAN sensor communications that agrees over a secret key of the symmetric key cryptosystem. As a result, the medical data obtained is transferred to the controller in two ways:

Smartphone: sends collected data to a base station (BS), which directs it until it reaches the medical data centre via a mobile network.

Wireless medical device: sends data using one of several wireless communication protocols, including Zigbee [8], Bluetooth [9], and Wi-Fi [10].

A HAN employs a controller to communicate and transfer the obtained data to an accessible access point (AP) in the patient's home. Transmissions can be made via Wi-Fi or, in the case of a Femtocell AP [11], LTE/LTE-A [12].

A NAN is a network that allows users to connect to the internet rapidly. It has been used to set up wireless communication between nearby regions, residences and their surroundings. It might be built around an omnidirectional antenna that allows a single AP to cover at least a half-mile radius [13].

Wide area network: the communication between a mobile BS or an access point to the mobile/internet (remote) medical infrastructure is referred to as a wide area network (WAN). A WAN ensures real-time data transfer to emergency response teams in the event of an emergency. Once received, the AP can also deliver the data to cloud services for storage at the designated server (table 13.1).

Table 13.1. A collection of IoMT connectivity protocols.

Protocol	Range	Classification	Description
LTE or 4G	Medium range	Wireless	Cellular technologies that link accessible and personal medical equipment long-distance, high-power, dependable medical interconnections.
Wi-Fi,1x, 802	Medium range	Wireless	Real-time, reliable, long-range, and high-power medical connections.
Z-wave	Medium range	Wireless	It is used in low data rate medical interconnections, which include tele-home healthcare and sending alerts.
6LoWPan	Medium range	Wireless	Used for low-power wireless LANs in healthcare
(IP) Internet protocol	Long range	Wireless	Communications for IoMT and e-healthcare were handled by the software.
Zigbee	Medium range	Wireless	Used for low data rate medical connections with minimum latency and energy consumption.
(M2M) Machine-to-machine	Long range	Wireless	Real-time remote patient monitoring and error detection enhanced patient care and attention.

13.3 Applications of IoMT

IoMT technology has several advantages in terms of healthcare applications. Some of the standard applications are listed below.

13.3.1 Real-time health monitoring

A patient's vital signs might be monitored in real-time, allowing patients and medical personnel to interact quickly. Minimizing the number of doctor visits reduces the cost of medical treatment. Another advantage of IoMT is that it improves the health and lifestyle of patients. Quick access to a patient's vital signs makes an early diagnosis, prescription, and medication through a wearable device conceivable. Innovative medical technology: it involves innovative medical tools and kits that paramedics use to offer quick aid to patients who require emergency medical attention and support. One example is the employment of medical drones to carry out such a duty [14]. Since medical drones can reach the emergency scene most quickly, they were initially developed to respond to situations involving patients experiencing cardiac arrests. Since paramedics can become delayed in traffic and be unable to arrive as quickly as required, the drones would be instructed to fly to specific locations, saving time and, in turn, saving lives. This promotes the use of sophisticated medical robots [15] to perform surgical procedures in a hospital environment. Medical technologies based on artificial intelligence (AI) and virtual/augmented reality have also been used for various medical applications. This involves using virtual reality to carry out numerous realistic tasks, including training simulations [16], emergency training [17], and CPR instruction [18]. For a greater accuracy rate, AI-based medical technologies are also being deployed. In order to find the most effective cancer treatment, IBM Watson and Gene Network Sciences (GNS) Healthcare AI systems explore molecular connections [19].

13.3.2 Personal emergency response systems

Personal emergency response systems (PERS) are being used more often to remotely convey crucial signals to the hospital [20] based on a predictive risk assessment approach to inform patients and physicians in real-time of any unexpected medical occurrence (examples: stroke, cardiac arrest, seizure, etc). Location-based PERS are now being updated [21] for greater accuracy and quicker reaction times. A classic example is an intelligent belt from Active-Protective, worn around a patient's waist which transmits real-time data using Bluetooth and AI [22].

Ingestible cameras: these innovative and reasonably priced capsules that can be ingested by a patient (*in vivo*/*in vitro*) to give real-time visual monitoring of internal organs for the early diagnosis of chronic illnesses and cancer [23]. Ingestible devices rely on a tracking/recording system, a camera or x-ray capsule, and the diagnostics toolkit for analysis. The swallowable data recorder capsule medical device [24], the ingestible endoscopic optical scanning device [25], and the ingestible hydrogel device [26] are just a few examples of the numerous ingestible devices that have been introduced.

Real-time patient monitoring (RTPM): the millennial generation's high reliance on smart gadgets as an integral part of their everyday life is a new trend which is currently evolving [27]. According to the sensors connected to the patient's body, RTPM is utilized to assure real-time, economic remote consistent monitoring, either through homecare telehealth or telecare monitoring systems [28]. This might involve monitoring heart rate, blood sugar, breathing, and glucose levels. There are a lot of new RTPM developments out there right now, such as linked inhaler delivery systems, an app for the Apple Watch that tracks depression, Apple's Research Kit for Parkinson's Disease, and ADAMM intelligent asthma monitoring, to name a few [29] for heart diseases.

The most crucial monitoring is that of the heart because the measured vital signs indicate numerous ailments concealed in essence, such as arrhythmia. In most instances, ECG electrodes will be attached to the patients' chests to measure their physiological data. After signal conditioning, digitization, and packetizing, the vitals will be broadcast to a central server. The server could be remote in a care facility or a cloud-based server. The graphical user interface (GUI) between the physicians and the server will be developed as a smartphone app or a web page. The doctor may be able to see the patient's condition in real-time and take necessary measures. Several pieces of research demonstrate the creation of important signal detecting nodes with internet connectivity that can offer real-time signal status showing an android-based remote monitoring system with sensors such as a pedometer and a pulse oximeter. Some other senses also include an ECG monitoring system for heart patients. The use of an Arduino sensor and multi-parameter monitoring system with a defibrillator device is also presented in various studies [30].

- *Brain and neurological diseases*

  Patients suffering from disorders such as epilepsy, Alzheimer's, dementia, stroke, and Parkinson's, among others, obtained significant comfort in using IoMT to monitor brain and neurological signals. Besides that, IoT-based systems are now being developed to monitor the activity of psychiatric patients in terms of improving research and providing unique approaches to the patients [35]. The acquiring sensors are either contact-based or contact-less. In the signal acquisition node, Galvanic skin response sensors, EEG sensors, wristwatches with integrated multi-sensors, Kinect with gesture recognition, salivary alpha-amylase biosensors, cameras, and other sensors are commonly employed. A camera-based system using an HC-V720 high-definition camera to capture the patient's movement has been created to monitor patients with neurodegenerative illnesses. Other methods for stress level tracking include blood pressure monitoring, based on the textile-based autonomic nervous system, which includes a t-shirt with embedded sensors and wireless sensor tag-based wristwatches that are also used in monitoring neurological activities of patients [31].
- *Diabetic patients*

  Patients with diabetic difficulties should have their glucose levels evaluated on a regular basis to ensure that their diet is suitable and that their glucose levels are under control. Many gadgets are commercially available that enable users to track their blood sugar levels from the comfort of their

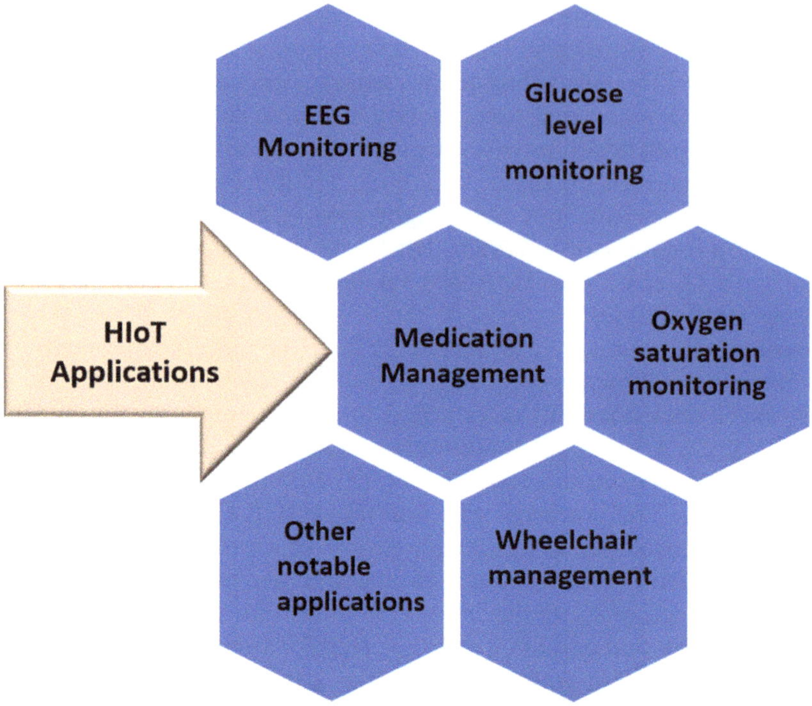

Figure 13.2. Applications of IoMT in healthcare.

homes. Although, these do not provide real-time surveillance with a doctor or clinician. IoMT allows this to happen by constructing clever and low-power nodes that measure a patient's glucose level and make it available to clinicians in real-time via mobile or online applications. In the following section, we will go through some of the remote monitoring solutions for diabetes patients [31].

The sensor node is coupled with a smartphone through Bluetooth in a Bluetooth-based glucose monitoring system. The monitoring app on the smartphone can display the measured numbers in a visual format.

A long-term monitoring solution for diabetes patients with an implanted sensor for glucose monitoring. The individuals' glucose levels are evaluated after every 2 min; the remote server is updated.

A near-infrared (NIR) based non-invasive glucose monitoring system, depending upon the variations of the received signal intensity from the NIR sensor, predicts the blood glucose level of diabetic patients (figure 13.2).

13.4 Paper-based devices with smartphones and IoMT

Paper-based diagnostic devices must fulfil the following requirements in order to be used in place of complicated equipment: high sensitivity and selectivity, low limit of detection (LOD), low sample volume, rapid response, affordable cost, and user-friendly format. Paper meets some of these criteria: it is affordable, biocompatible, and plentiful; it does not require external pumping and works by capillary action, and it is readily manipulated, disposed of, and scaled [32]. POC devices have largely been built thus far using cellulose- and nitrocellulose-based materials. Cellulose is a linear chain molecule composed of glucose subunits that is fibrous, porous, hydrophilic, biodegradable, and insoluble in water. The majority of the materials used to construct dipsticks and microfluidic paper-based analytical devices (PADs) are cellulose-based. Nitrocellulose is made by partially nitrating cellulose, which makes it more porous and changes its hydrophilic to hydrophobic characteristics [33]. Because of its propensity to bind irreversibly and hydrophobically to proteins through absorption, nitrocellulose membranes are used in lateral flow assays (LFAs) and commercial diagnostics. For the preparation of paper-based diagnostic devices, the porosity and surface chemistry of these materials is critical. Several organizations have examined the most recent work on paper-based sensing systems [34]. Initially, paper-based diagnostic devices were solely intended to provide qualitative, positive/negative findings (e.g., pregnancy tests); nevertheless, they have since been shown to be capable of quantitative analysis. Materials with at least one dimension in the 1100 nm range are classified as nanoparticles. Semiconductors, metals, carbon-based materials and polymers, are examples of possible forms and materials [35]. The current decade has seen the development of paper-based devices in healthcare that are integrated with smartphones and IoMT platforms and are frequently used for point-of-care testing for human health [36–40]. The data acquired by this can be used using a normal analytical-chemical instrument, such as IT communication equipment, diffuse reflectance spectroscopy, or electronic devices like scanners and mobile phones. Smartphones are increasingly ubiquitous, and they are said to play a vital part in performing POCT in a sustainable and cost-effective manner. They retain analytical reading capabilities through the screen, which may serve as both a display and a controller, as well as a possible source of signal capture via an integrated camera, audio connection, power connector, and ambient light sensors. They are a well-known medium for large storage (device and cloud storage) for data collecting and analysis via different applications, as well as data transfer by wire or wireless (Bluetooth, NFC, Wi-Fi, and so on) systems. These gadgets are connected to the internet of things (IoT). Colorimetric images/electrical signals may be compared to data samples in a database using internet connections, and a correct data interpretation can be provided in no time [41].

Machine learning (ML) and AI have been shown to be more effective methods for predicting patterns by comparing previously stored data. This is extremely useful for human health, water, food/beverage analysis, and environmental situations. Fifth-generation (5G) smartphones offer extremely high capabilities in terms of signal monitoring, data transport, and data analysis. It can detect visual stimulation with high sensitivity and picture resolution using a high-definition (HD) camera, as well as quickly evaluating data using high-speed internet and CPU [42].

Paper-based sensing devices meet all of the ASSURED law's requirements and provide long-term solutions. It is cost-effective, environmentally beneficial, and simple to use for customers. By combining electrical and optical sensing modalities, it is conveniently applicable to all diagnostic tests. It has been shown to identify and isolate a wide range of bio-targets and pathogens in a variety of matrices, including plasma, whole blood, and peritoneal dialysis fluid. The information generated during blood type testing in a paper-based sensor is read using an Android app [43].

The barcode-like design was created to make it easier to analyse length-based information using a smartphone, and it is said to have fewer environmental effects than electrical and colorimetric signals. The generated findings were preserved as electronic data and sent to the patient/professionals through text message [44]. Moazeni *et al* [45] have produced peptide-modified plastic-paper printed active devices (PADs) for the detection of alpha-fetoprotein (AFP) in human blood. To improve the sensitivity and stability of the immobilized antibody, the upper surface of the chromatography paper was modified with a silver graphene electrode (20% Ag) and diphenylalanine in the detection zone. Phosphate buffer saline (PBS) and plasma, it has detection limits of 1 and 10 ng ml^{-1}, respectively. Adkins *et al* [46] developed an electrochemical and colorimetric approach for detecting faecal indicator bacteria (FIB), and two different methods were used to solve the disadvantages of each method. As a result, the colorimetric method's detection limit is higher than the electrochemical methods, yet the detection time is the same. Overall, the advancement of POC testing technology necessitates not only the automation of manual tasks, but also systematic data collecting, monitoring, and planning in order to maintain the existing infrastructure. Several studies examine smartphone and IoMT-based sensing platforms [47, 48] paper-based devices in healthcare [49, 50], and IoMT in biosensing systems [51, 52] independently. However, a supplementary study is required in order to explore them in an integrated manner.

13.5 Various sensing mechanisms explored in IoMT and smartphone analysis assisted paper devices

The following different biosensor techniques are used to characterize the sensing mechanism for paper-based analytical devices: electrochemistry, colorimetry, photo electrochemistry, fluorescent chemiluminescence (CL), nanoparticle-based sensing, electrochemiluminescence (ECL), and spectrometry sensing, etc.

13.5.1 Colorimetric sensing

Colorimetric biosensors have gained popularity in recent years as POC diagnostics have become more crucial. To find variations in the absorbance or reflectance of conjugates, colorimetric tests are utilized [53]. This detection approach enables equipment-free measurements on the field, resulting in low costs and portability [54]. Modern smartphone technologies employ inexpensive complementary metal oxide semiconductor (CMOS) arrays to capture and convert the amount of light hitting a pixel into electrical data [55]. Each pixel in these devices has multiple transistors that amplify and transfer the charge. The colour of incident light is not detectable by a CMOS sensor. A colour filter is added to the sensor for this reason, allowing each pixel to detect only one colour, either red, green, or blue. To mimic the sensitivity of the human eye, the array comprises half green light sensors and a quarter of each red and blue light sensor. This filter is called a Bayer pattern [56]. Because of this, colorimetric sensors can detect colour changes brought on by structural changes with the help of basic illumination and an algorithmically sound smartphone app. For practical analysis, a variety of software has been created, including ImageJ, Fiji, The Image Studio, and Image Lab [57, 58]. However, controlling the ambient light conditions for repeatability and sensitivity of the study is difficult, extra units for smartphones have recently been recommended for interference-free, reliable analysis [59].

13.5.2 Electrochemical sensing

A molecular sensing device known as an electrochemical biosensor consists of a biological detecting element and an electrode transducer that converts the biological recognition into an electrical signal [60]. For electrochemical sensing, three electrodes are often needed: a working electrode, also known as the sensing or redox electrode, a counter electrode, and a reference electrode, which is frequently manufactured from Ag/AgCl. Amperometric and potentiometric measures are the most used measuring methods. When a constant potential is given to a system, amperometry is used to measure changes in current that are related to the reduction or oxidation of electroactive species during a biological reaction. Potentiometric instruments detect the build-up of a charge potential at the working electrode in relation to the reference electrode in an electrochemical cell [61].

Since the 1970s, electrochemical biosensors have been studied to detect proteins, glucose, and DNA employing aptamers, functional polymer surface, and antibodies as capture molecules. Several groups have studied this vast area of study, highlighting its relevance. For their great sensitivity, mobility, low cost, and simplicity, electrochemical biosensors have become popular POC diagnostic platforms in the last decennium [62].

Various portable electrochemical sensor units for smartphones have been developed over the last decade. Screen-printed electrodes (SPEs) for the measurement of various analytes have been developed, including antibodies, proteins, and nucleic acids [63, 64]. Aymerich *et al* designed another potentiostat based on a smartphone that uses cutting-edge circuit readout digitalization methods and a lab-on-a-chip idea [65]. This USB-powered gadget measured the blood's ethanol content and provided sensitive readings for prohibited ethanol levels. For simultaneous CV and DPV measurements of electroactive biomolecules, another USB-powered apparatus was created [66]. Ascorbic acid, uric acid, and dopamine were tested in simulated urine using SPEs, a coin-sized detector, and a smartphone. Wireless designs that transport data via Bluetooth, a phone, or a modified electrode have also been created [67]. The hand-held detector was used to measure CV and EIS for glucose and volatile organic chemicals, respectively. In these the system was managed by a smartphone app, which also analysed data and displayed findings instantly. Finally, a smartphone cover with a potentiostat, Bluetooth data transfer, and a permanent bare three-electrode system was created [68]. A specialized application locates a magnetic enzyme pellet on a magnetic sensor surface. The built-in potentiostat in the case monitors the blood's glucose levels once a blood sample is dropped over the enzyme pellet and shows the findings on the smartphone screen. All of these gadgets have a cheap potentiostat, and a phone app may be used to perform the analysis. Electrochemical sensing platforms include a single electrode on a three-electrode system, a microelectrode array (MEA), and a PAD [69]. Among them, PADs are the next generation POC design because they enable multiplexed analysis on paper at low cost [70].

13.5.3 Fluorescence sensing

In fluorescence-based tests, smartphones embrace the light produced following radiative transfer from the target sample. These include quantum dots, small molecule fluorophores and fluorescent nanoparticles [71]. Low molecular weight, water-soluble small molecule fluorophores have responsive groupings that allows the capturing of agents like peptides, antibodies or nucleic acids. Because they have tiny molecular weights, they tend to behave like the attached biomolecules, rather than the fluorophore itself [72, 73]. QDs are semiconductor nanoparticles that glow when excited. A functional polymer encapsulates QDs to give them water solubility and biocompatibility without affecting their optical characteristics [74]. The majority of nanoparticles are efficient FRET or electron transfer fluorescence quenchers [71, 75, 76].

Fluorescence-based sensing has several benefits over colorimetric systems, including selectivity, sensitivity, and speed [77]. Because emission wavelengths are limited, smaller concentrations may be measured. Also, because the excitation source strength may be modified, lower detection limits can be reached [78]. However, background excitation light interferes with fluorescence-based POC sensing devices, causing results to be inaccurate. Using cost-effective, effective filters to increase the signal-to-noise ratio leads to minimum sensitivity [79, 80]. For the purpose of enabling and enhancing fluorescence-based measurements on paper, a smart surface or a device linked to or wirelessly connected to smartphones has been designed to filter out such signals.

When upconversion phosphors are activated by near-infrared (NIR) light, they exhibit an anti-Stokes luminescence known as upconversion fluorescence. Upconversion phosphors were used to avoid background fluorescence and scattering light since they were stimulated in the NIR range. Upconversion nanoparticles (UCNPs) have been described as solid compact laser systems, infrared quantum counter detectors, fluorescent labels for biomolecule detection, and optical data storage in the literature. Because of their remarkable biomimetic qualities, they have been employed as smart surfaces for fluorescence and luminescence-based sensor systems. He *et al* reported the first UCNPs and paper-based biosensor to identify matrix metalloproteinase-2, a significant blood biomarker (MMP-2) [81]. Over the last decade, researchers have looked into smartphone-based biosensors that use UCNPs.

Currently, smart platforms are employed to detect brain natriuretic peptide (BNP) and tumorigenicity suppression 2 using paper-based platforms with fluorescent materials or nanoparticles, primarily UCNPs (ST2), dipicolinic acid (DPA), cocaine, *E. coli* O, *Salmonella* spp, and influenza A.

Over the last decade, several researchers have focused on improving smartphone imaging technologies for POC diagnostics. A USB-powered excitation module was presented by Shah *et al* to enable radiometric smartphone fluorescence measurements without the need for optical filters or other accessories. It links UV light-emitting diodes (LED) with long Stokes shift quantum dots. When the device was used to detect influenza A nucleoprotein using the LF assay, the LOD was found to be 2.0 fmol, which is more than two orders of magnitude superior to tests created for smartphones using gold nanoparticles.

For early detection and real-time prognosis of HF at the bedside, a straightforward, hand-held multiplexed home prognosis platform was created employing UCNP-based LF immunoassays and a smartphone-based reader. The capacity to translate a clinical sample into a result on a smartphone allowed for the very sensitive and precise identification of heart failure biomarkers, brain natriuretic peptide (BNP), and suppression of tumorigenicity 2 (ST2). The stated LODs for BNP and ST2 are just one order higher than the clinical cut-off values, at 5.0 pg mL^{-1} and 1.0 ng mL^{-1}, respectively.

13.6 Challenges, limitations, and future scope

The healthcare business has seen significant technological advancements and applications in tackling healthcare-related concerns in recent years. These have substantially ameliorated healthcare services that may be accessed instantly. IoT has effectively altered the healthcare industry through the use of connectivity, cloud-based services, and sensing systems. IoT, like other technologies, has obstacles and issues that might be explored further in the future. Some of the difficulties have been examined in more detail in the following section.

13.6.1 Cost of servicing and maintenance

Rapid technical breakthroughs have recently occurred, necessitating periodic upgrades of IoT-based devices. A vast number of connected medical devices and sensors are used in every IoT-based system. Substantial maintenance, service, and upgrade expenses are involved which may have an influence on the company's as well as end-users' financials. As a result, sensors that can be operated with fewer maintenance costs must be included.

13.6.2 Power consumption

The majority of IoT devices are powered by batteries. It is difficult to change a sensor's battery once it has been installed. Consequently, the system was powered by a large battery. Presently, scientists around the world are attempting to create medical equipment that can produce their own power. These systems may be able to assist in alleviating the global energy issue to some extent.

13.6.3 Standardization

In the healthcare industry, a large number of distributors provide a wide range of products. The bulk of these goods claim that they adhere to recognized design principles and procedures. A lack of legitimacy exists, though. In standardizing various IoT devices using communication protocols, aggregation of data, and gateway connections, a specialist organization must be established. It's also important to consider the standardization and validation of the electronic health records that HIoT devices record. Various organizations and standardization bodies, including the Internet Protocol for Smart Objects (IPSO), the European Telecommunications Standards Institute (ETSI), and the Information Technology and Innovation Foundation (IETF), work with researchers to create working groups for device standardization.

13.6.4 Data security and privacy

Real-time monitoring has evolved as a result of cloud computing. Cyberattacks have increased as a result. This may lead to mismanagement of patient data and impair the therapy process. Several precautions must be taken while developing an IoMT system to avoid this malicious assault. If an IoMT network contains medical or sensor equipment, it must analyze and implement authorization monitoring, protection booting, high availability, and authentication mechanisms methods. Similarly, network protocols like Wi-Fi, Bluetooth, and Zigbee must provide safe routing and message integrity checking. Since the IoT is a system in which each user is linked to a server, any weakness in IoT safety may violate patient privacy. This could be addressed by integrating sophisticated algorithms and cryptographies into a more secure environment.

13.6.5 Scalability

This refers to a device's capacity to acclimate itself to environmental changes. The system that is more scalable operates faster and more efficiently with the resources available. Thus, scalability is critical in device design. System efficiency is increased both today and in the future as a result. The IoMT technology connects medical equipment, sensors, and actuators to communicate data over the internet. The lack of homogeneity across linked devices reduces scalability and must be managed efficiently.

13.6.6 Identification

Professionals in healthcare manage several patients and caregivers. When a patient has several health conditions, he sees many doctors. To minimize confusion and ensure the seamless running of the healthcare system, it is critical to interchange patient, caregiver, and doctor identities throughout a single treatment session.

Self-configuration IoT devices must empower consumers by allowing manual setup. This will allow users to adjust system settings to meet application and environmental demands.

13.6.7 Discovering new diseases

New healthcare apps are constantly being added to mobile technologies. Despite the enormous number of healthcare mobile apps accessible, the ailments for which these apps were built are still restricted. Thus, additional illnesses that were previously ignored or under-researched must be included. This will broaden the range of IoT applications.

13.6.8 Environmental impact

Combining biological sensors with semiconductor-rich devices is necessary to build an IoT system. The fabrication uses a lot of harmful chemicals and metals. This may harm the environment. Thus, an appropriate regulating agency must be established to oversee sensor fabrication. More study is needed on biodegradable sensor materials.

13.7 Conclusion

With an increased risk of health hazards, advancement in medical care has become a necessity. IoMT and the integration of medical devices using paper and smartphones have made healthcare easy and convenient. IoMT has made patient care convenient, and medical records have become easily accessible to physicians and caregivers. However, more research is needed for the advancement of these devices as stated above.

References

[1] Vishnu S, Ramson S J and Jegan R 2020 Internet of medical things (IoMT)—an overview *2020 5th Int. Conf. on Devices, Circuits and Systems (ICDCS)* (Piscataway, NJ: IEEE) pp 101–4

[2] Qureshi F and Krishnan S 2018 Wearable hardware design for the internet of medical things (IoMT) *Sensors* **18** 3812

[3] Joyia G J, Liaqat R M, Farooq A and Rehman S 2017 Internet of medical things (IoMT): Applications, benefits and future challenges in healthcare domain *J. Commun.* **12** 240–7

[4] Singh R P, Javaid M, Haleem A, Vaishya R and Ali S 2020 Internet of Medical Things (IoMT) for orthopaedic in COVID-19 pandemic: roles, challenges, and applications *J. Clin. Orthop. Trauma* **11** 713–7

[5] Yaacoub J P A, Noura M, Noura H N, Salman O, Yaacoub E, Couturier R and Chehab A 2020 Securing internet of medical things systems: limitations, issues and recommendations *Future Gener. Comput. Syst.* **105** 581–606

[6] Poon C C Y, Zhang Y-T and Bao S-D 2006 A novel biometrics method to secure wireless body area sensor networks for telemedicine and m-health *IEEE Commun. Mag.* **44** 73–81

[7] Venkatasubramanian K K, Banerjee A and Gupta S K S 2010 PSKA: usable and secure key agreement scheme for body area networks *IEEE Trans. Inf. Technol. Biomed.* **14** 60–8

[8] Alliance ZigBee 2006 Zigbee-2006 specification (http://zigbee.org/)

[9] Bhagwat P 2001 Bluetooth: technology for short-range wireless apps *IEEE Internet Comput.* **5** 96–103

[10] Wi-Fi Alliance 2010 Wi-fi certified wi-fi direct. White paper.

[11] Doppler K, Rinne M, Wijting C, Ribeiro C B and Hugl K 2009 Device-to-device communication as an underlay to LTE-advanced networks *IEEE Commun. Mag.* **47** 42–9

[12] Chandrasekhar V, Andrews J G and Gatherer A 2008 Femtocell networks: a survey *IEEE Commun. Mag.* **46** 59–67

[13] Ye F, Qian Y and Hu R Q 2015 Energy efficient self-sustaining wireless neighborhood area network design for smart grid *IEEE Trans. Smart Grid* **6** 220–9

[14] Haidari L A, Brown S T and Ferguson M *et al* 2016 The economic and operational value of using drones to transport vaccines *Vaccine* **34** 4062–7

[15] Li M and Taylor R H 2004 Spatial motion constraints in medical robot using virtual fixtures generated by anatomy *2004 Proc. ICRA'04. 2004 IEEE Int. Conf. on Robotics and Automation* vol 2 *(Piscataway, NJ)* (IEEE) pp 1270–5

[16] McCarthy C J and Uppot R N 2019 Advances in virtual and augmented reality—exploring the role in health-care education *J. Radiol. Nurs.* **1** 105–5

[17] Munzer B W, Khan M M, Shipman B and Mahajan P 2019 Augmented reality in emergency medicine: a scoping review *J. Med. Internet Res.* **21** e12368

[18] Balian S, McGovern S K, Abella B S, Blewer A L and Leary M 2019 Feasibility of an augmented reality cardiopulmonary resuscitation training system for health care providers *Heliyon* **5** e02205

[19] Agrawal P 2018 Artificial intelligence in drug discovery and development *J. Pharmacovigil.* **6** 1–2

[20] Tran B Personal emergency response (per) system, September 10 2013. US Patent 8,531,291.

[21] Patel V, Chesmore A, Legner C M and Pandey S 2022 Trends in workplace wearable technologies and connected-worker solutions for next-generation occupational safety, health, and productivity *Adv. Int. Syst.* **4** 2100099

[22] Peabody S R 2012 System containing location-based personal emergency response device, February 14, 2012. US Patent 8,116,724.

[23] Kiourti A, Psathas K A and Nikita K S 2014 Implantable and ingestible medical devices with wireless telemetry functionalities: a review of current status and challenges *Bioelectromagnetics* **35** 1–15

[24] Marshall D R 2003 Swallowable data recorder capsule medical device, October 14, 2003. US Patent 6,632,175.

[25] Bandy W R, Jamieson B G, Powell K J, Salsman K E, Schober R C, Weitzner J and Arneson M R 2013 Ingestible endoscopic optical scanning device, September 10, 2013. US Patent 8,529,441

[26] Liu X, Steiger C, Lin S, Parada G A, Liu J, Chan H F, Yuk H, Phan N V, Collins J and Tamang S *et al* 2019 Ingestible hydrogel device *Nat. Commun.* **10** 493

[27] Toohey S L, Wray A, Wiechmann W, Lin M and Boysen-Osborn M 2016 Ten tips for engaging the millennial learner and moving an emergency medicine residency curriculum into the 21st century *West. J. Emerg. Med.* **17** 337

[28] McFarland S, Coufopolous A and Lycett D 2019 The effect of telehealth versus usual care for home-care patients with long-term conditions: a systematic review, meta-analysis and qualitative synthesis *J. Telemed. Telecare* **27** 69–87

[29] Kang M, Park E, Cho B H and Lee K-S 2018 Recent patient health monitoring platforms incorporating internet of things-enabled smart devices *Int. Neurourol. J.* **22** S76

[30] Serhani M A, T El Kassabi H, Ismail H and Nujum Navaz A 2020 ECG monitoring systems: review, architecture, processes, and key challenges *Sensors (Basel, Switzerland)* **20** 1796

[31] Ahmed Q A and Al-Neami A Q H 2020 A smart biomedical assisted system for Alzheimer patients *IOP Conf. Ser.: Mater. Sci. Eng.* **881** 012110

[32] Quesada-Gonzalez D and Merkoci A 2015 Nanoparticle-based lateral flow biosensors *Biosens. Bioelectron.* **73** 47–63

[33] O'Sullivan A C 1997 Cellulose: the structure slowly unravels *Cellulose* **4** 173–207

[34] Pelton R 2009 Bioactive paper provides a low-cost platform for diagnostics *TrAC Trends Anal. Chem.* **28** 925–42

[35] Zamborini F P, Bao L and Dasari R 2012 Nanoparticles in measurement science *Anal. Chem.* **84** 541–76

[36] Tseng C C, Yang R J, Ju W J and Fu L M 2018 Microfuidic paper-based platform for whole blood creatinine detection *Chem. Eng. J.* **348** 117–24

[37] Kou X *et al* 2020 Smartphone-assisted robust enzymes@MOFs-based paper biosensor for point-of-care detection *Biosens. Bioelectron.* **156** 112095

[38] Puneeth S B and Goel S 2021 Handheld and 'Turnkey' 3D printed paper-microfuidic viscometer with on-board microcontroller for smartphone based biosensing applications *Anal. Chim. Acta* **1153** 338303

[39] Franco M de O K, Suarez W T, dos Santos V B, Resque I S, dos Santos M H and Capitán-Vallvey L F 2021 Microanalysis based on paper device functionalized with cuprizone to determine Cu^{2+} in sugar cane spirits using a smartphone *Spectrochim. Acta* A **253** 119580

[40] Huang L *et al* 2021 Miniaturized paper-based smartphone biosensor for diferential diagnosis of wild-type pseudorabies virus infection versus vaccination immunization *Sensors Actuators* B **327** 128893

[41] Quesada-González D and Merkoçi A 2015 Nanoparticle-based lateral fow biosensors *Biosens. Bioelectron.* **73** 47–63

[42] Jiao Y *et al* 2020 3D vertical-fow paper-based device for simultaneous detection of multiple cancer biomarkers by fuorescent immunoassay *Sensors Actuators* **306** 127239

[43] Shafee H *et al* 2015 Paper and fexible substrates as materials for biosensing platforms to detect multiple biotargets *Sci. Rep.* **5** 1–9

[44] Guan L, Tian J, Cao R, Li M, Cai Z and Shen W 2014 Barcode-like paper sensor for smartphone diagnostics: an application of blood typing *Anal. Chem.* **86** 11362–7

[45] Moazeni M, Karimzadeh F and Kermanpur A 2018 Peptide modifed paper based impedimetric immunoassay with nanocomposite electrodes as a point-of-care testing of Alpha-fetoprotein in human serum *Biosens. Bioelectron.* **117** 748–57

[46] Adkins J A, Boehle K, Friend C, Chamberlain B, Bisha B and Henry C S 2017 Colorimetric and electrochemical bacteria detection using printed paper- and transparency-based analytic devices *Anal. Chem.* **89** 3613–21

[47] Kanchi S, Sabela M I, Mdluli P S, Inamuddin and Bisetty K 2018 Smartphone based bioanalytical and diagnosis applications: A review *Biosens. Bioelectron.* **102** 136–49

[48] Bender L J, Yue K R Y, To J M, Deacken L and Jadad R A 2013 A lot of action, but not in the right direction: systematic review and content analysis of smartphone applications for the prevention, detection, and management of cancer *J. Med. Internet Res* **15** e287

[49] Darwish N T, Sekaran S D and Khor S M 2018 Point-of-care tests: a review of advances in the emerging diagnostic tools for dengue virus infection *Sensors Actuators* B **255** 3316–31

[50] Sher M, Zhuang R, Demirci U and Asghar W 2017 Paper-based analytical devices for clinical diagnosis: recent advances in the fabrication techniques and sensing mechanisms *Expert Rev. Mol. Diagn.* **17** 351–66

[51] Quesada-Gonzalez D and Merkoci A 2015 Nanoparticle-based lateral flow biosensors *Biosens.Bioelectron.* **73** 47–63

[52] Holzinger M, Le Goff A and Cosnier S 2014 Nanomaterials for biosensing applications: a review *Front. Chem.* **2** 63

[53] Kishnani V, Park S, Nakate U T, Mondal K and Gupta A 2021 Nano-functionalized paper-based IoT enabled devices for point-of-care testing: a review *Biomed. Microdevices;* **24** 2

[54] Vilela D, Gonzalez M C and Escarpa Á 2012 Sensing colorimetric approaches based on gold and silver nanoparticles aggregation: Chemical creativity behind the assay. A review *Anal. Chim. Acta* **751** 24–43

[55] Bigas M, Cabruja E, Forest J and Salvi J 2006 Review of CMOS image sensors *Microelectron. J.* **37** 433–51

[56] Menon D and Calvagno G 2011 Color image demosaicking: An overview *Signal Process. Image* **26** 518–33

[57] Schindelin J *et al* 2012 Fiji: an open-source platform for biological-image analysis *Nat. Methods* **9** 676–82

[58] Schneider C A, Rasband W S and Eliceiri K W 2012 NIH Image to ImageJ: 25 years of image analysis *Nat. Methods* **9** 671–5

[59] Roda A, Michelini E, Zangheri M, Di Fusco M, Calabria D and Simoni P 2016 Smartphone-based biosensors: A critical review and perspectives *TrAC Trends Anal. Chem.* **79** 317–25

[60] Wang J 2006 Electrochemical biosensors: towards point-of-care cancer diagnostics *Biosens. Bioelectron.* **21** 1887–92

[61] Grieshaber D, MacKenzie R, Vörös J and Reimhult E 2008 Electrochemical biosensors—sensor principles and architectures *Sensors (Basel)* **8** 1400–58

[62] da Silva E T S G, Souto D E P, Barragan J T C, Giarola J de F, de Moraes A C M and Kubota L T 2017 Electrochemical biosensors in point-of-care devices: recent advances and future trends *Chem. Electro. Chem.* **4** 778–94

[63] Sun A C, Yao C, Venkatesh A G and Hall D A 2016 An efficient power harvesting mobile phone-based electrochemical biosensor for point-of-care health monitoring *Sensors Actuators* B **235** 126–35

[64] Sun A, Wambach T, Venkatesh A G and Hall D A 2014 A low-cost smartphone-based electrochemical biosensor for point-of-care diagnostics *2014 IEEE Biomedical Circuits and Systems Conf.* pp 312–5

[65] Aronoff-Spencer E, Venkatesh A G, Sun A, Brickner H, Looney D and Hall D A 2016 Detection of Hepatitis C core antibody by dual-affinity yeast chimera and smartphone-based electrochemical sensing *Biosens. Bioelectron.* **86** 690–6

[66] Aymerich J, Marquez A, Terés L, Muñoz-Berbel X, Jimenez C, Domínguez C, Serra-Graells F and Dei Ḿ 2018 *Biosens. Bioelectron.* **117** 736–42

[67] Ji D, Liu Z, Liu L, Low S S, Lu Y, Yu X, Zhu L, Li C and Liu Q 2018 Simultaneous electrochemical detection of ascorbic acid, dopamine and uric acid based on graphene anchored with Pd-Pt nanoparticles *Biosens. Bioelectron.* **119** 55–62

[68] Ji D, Liu L and Li S *et al* 2017 Smartphone-based cyclic voltammetry system with graphene modified screen printed electrodes for glucose detection *Biosens. Bioelectron.* **98** 449–56

[69] Liu L, Zhang D and Zhang Q *et al* 2017 Smartphone-based sensing system using ZnO and graphene modified electrodes for VOCs detection *Biosens. Bioelectron.* **93** 94–101

[70] Catarino R, Vassilakos P and Scaringella S *et al* 2015 Smartphone use for cervical cancer screening in low-resource countries: a pilot study conducted in Madagascar *PLoS One* **10** e0134309

[71] Zhang H, Uselman R R and Yee D 2011 Exogenous near-infrared fluorophores and their applications in cancer diagnosis: biological and clinical perspectives *Expert Opin. Med. Diagn.* **5** 241–51
[72] Luby B M, Charron D M, MacLaughlin C M and Zheng G 2017 Activatable fluorescence: From small molecule to nanoparticle *Adv. Drug. Deliv. Rev.* **113** 97–121
[73] Achilefu S, Dorshow R B, Bugaj J E and Rajagopalan R 2000 Novel receptor-targeted fluorescent contrast agents for *in vivo* tumor imaging *Invest. Radiol* **35** 479–85
[74] Ke S, Wen X and Gurfinkel M *et al* 2003 Near-infrared optical imaging of epidermal growth factor receptor in breast cancer xenografts *Cancer Res.* **63** 7870–5
[75] Bunz U H and Rotello V M 2010 Gold nanoparticle-fluorophore complexes: sensitive and discerning 'noses' for biosystems sensing *Angew. Chem. Int. Ed. Engl.* **49** 3268–79
[76] Wolfbeis O S 2015 An overview of nanoparticles commonly used in fluorescent bioimaging *Chem. Soc. Rev.* **44** 4743–68
[77] Wang Q X, Xue S F and Chen Z H *et al* 2017 Dual lanthanide-doped complexes: the development of a time-resolved ratiometric fluorescent probe for anthrax biomarker and a paper-based visual sensor *Biosens. Bioelectron.* **94** 388–93
[78] Jung H S, Chen X, Kim J S and Yoon J 2013 Recent progress in luminescent and colorimetric chemosensors for detection of thiols *Chem. Soc. Rev.* **42** 6019–31
[79] Lee L G, Nordman E S, Johnson M D and Oldham M F 2013 A low-cost, high-performance system for fluorescence lateral flow assays *Biosensors (Basel)* **3** 360–73
[80] Williams G, Backhouse C and Aziz H 2014 Integration of organic light emitting diodes and organic photodetectors for lab-on-a-chip bio-detection systems *Electronics* **3** 43–75
[81] Zhang H, Wu M, Ta H T, Xu Z P and Zhang R Recent development and applications of sensors for the detection of matrix *Adv. Mater. Technol.* **25** 2201786

Chapter 14

The futuristic paradigm shift in the field of biosensing applications

Arpana Parihar, Ayushi Singhal, Vedika Khare and Raju Khan

A widespread diagnostic initiative to detect diseases early could save countless lives and money every year. Early diagnosis of infectious diseases and oncological disorders has certain limitations, and existing methods rely on expensive technology and expert staff, which makes it difficult to implement in resource settings. The revolutionary changes in the field of disease biomarker biosensing hold promise in this context. The challenges and technological constraints that must be solved in order to obtain precise disease diagnoses, as well as how these roadblocks have hampered the progress of point-of-care sensors are discussed in this chapter. Further, advances in the field of disease biosensing and their widespread usage as disease detection platforms are highlighted.

14.1 Introduction

The use of biosensors and devices as medical equipment for health, diagnosis, and preventive medicine has received great attention in recent years. Medical devices that can be employed in daily life are needed around the world as a method to manage an aging society (particularly for testing, diagnosis, and sensing) to limit the rise in lifestyle-related illnesses and their severity [1, 2]. Wearable biological and chemical devices are significant personal gadgets that will be key players in this endeavor. Currently, health management and illness prevention are the main medical uses of diagnostic technologies. They should also keep the rising cost of medical and nursing care under control. The paper-based biosensors and diagnostic tools are used in the sectors of medicine, welfare, and healthcare worldwide as tools for health and preventative medicine [2, 3]. A biosensor is a device or system that combines a biological and an electrical component to produce a quantifiable signal. The electronic component detects, records, and communicates information on physiological changes in the environment as well as detecting the presence of

doi:10.1088/978-0-7503-5820-0ch14

© IOP Publishing Ltd 2023

various chemical or biological compounds [4]. Biosensors are available in a variety of sizes and forms, and they can detect and measure even minute amounts of illnesses, hazardous substances, and pH levels. An analyte, bioreceptor, transducer, electronics, and display comprise a typical biosensor. An analyte is a material whose constituents are being identified or detected (e.g., glucose, alcohol, ammonia, and lactose). Biomolecules (molecules) or biological elements that may detect the specific target (i.e., analyte) are referred to as bioreceptors [5]. Enzymes, cells, aptamers, deoxyribonucleic acid (DNA or RNA), and antibodies are examples. A transducer is an electronic device that converts energy from one form to another. A biosensor would not be complete without a transducer. It translates a bio-recognition signal into an electrical signal indicating the quantity or presence of a chemical or biological target [6]. The signal may be transformed and processed before being shown. The transducer's electrical impulses are amplified and transformed to digital form. The display unit quantifies the processed signals. The display unit is made up of a user interpretation system, such as a computer or printer, that outputs the associated response for the user to read and understand. The output might be a numerical, graphical, or tabular value, or a figure, depending on the end-users requirement. Leland Charles Clark Jr., the inventor of biosensors, explained the components of a biosensor in his study. A study [7] concentrated on an electrode capable of monitoring blood oxygen levels. Clark demonstrated the use of an amperometric enzyme electrode for glucose detection in an experiment [8, 9]. In 1967, Updike and Hicks refined Clark's work by developing the first working enzyme electrode, which consisted of glucose oxidase placed on top of an oxygen sensor [10]. Figure 14.1 depicts the evolution of biosensors from the past to the present day.

Paper-based biosensors have been used to replace expensive and complicated analytical instruments used in healthcare with compact and widely-used sensors suited for medical applications [1–5]. It is crucial for the advancement of healthcare and medical monitoring to include biosensors in the Internet of Things (IoT) in order to improve quality of life (QoL). Devices that use optical, piezoelectric, and electrochemical transducers to detect analytes have advanced markedly over the past 50 years [4–6]. Due to their good performance, portability, ease of use, and low cost, paper-based sensors are starting to be employed in a range of analytical, medical

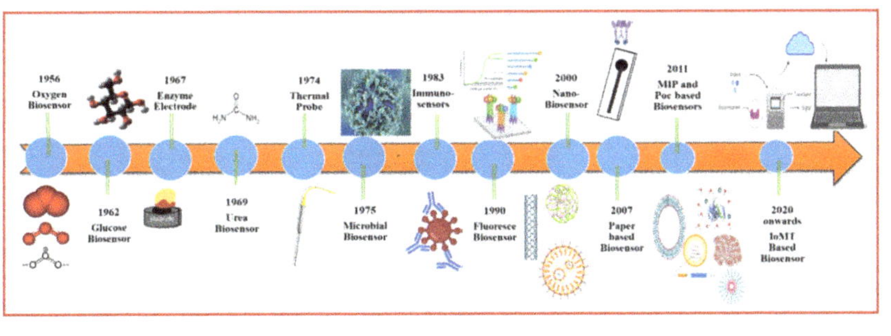

Figure 14.1. Evolution in biosensors technology.

diagnostic, and screening applications. Portable analyzers have been created to detect metabolites and electrolytes in addition to the advancements in biosensors [7–10]. The types of biosensors and various paper-based integrated biosensor platforms are discussed in this chapter. Further futuristic paradigm shifts and challenges will be emphasized.

14.2 Types of biosensor

Biosensors are used to detect biomolecules that belong to a diverse group. Bioreceptors are the most significant component in biosensor fabrication. Figure 14.2 shows the various categories of biosensors, including enzyme-based biosensors, immune-sensors (high specificity and sensitivity; especially helpful in prognosis), aptamer or nucleic acid-based biosensors (high specificity for microbial strains and nucleic acid-containing analyte), and microbial or whole-cell biosensors [10, 11]. The second group is based on the transducer, with the most common types being electrochemical (amperometric, impedance, conductometric, and potentiometric) biosensors, followed by electronic biosensors, thermal biosensors, optical sensors, and mass-based or gravimetric sensors [12–15]. The pairings of bioreceptors and analytes constitute another categorization, however this one is more restricted. Both the detection systems (optical, electrical, electronic, thermal, mechanical, and magnetic) and the technologies (nano, surface plasmon resonance (SPR), biosensors-on-chip (lab-on-chip), are subdivided into distinct categories [16, 17].

14.2.1 Electrochemical biosensors

Electrochemical biosensors are the most researched and widely employed biosensors, with their working principles based on the analyte's and transducer's electrochemical properties. The sensitivity, selectivity, and detection capabilities of electrochemical biosensors are all high. On the transducer surface, an electrochemical reaction occurs between the bioreceptor and the analyte, resulting in visible electrical signals in the form of current, voltage, impedance, and capacitance [12, 18]. Electrochemical biosensors are subdivided as amperometric, conductometric, impedimetric, potentiometric, and voltammetric based on the transduction principle [19]. Two or three

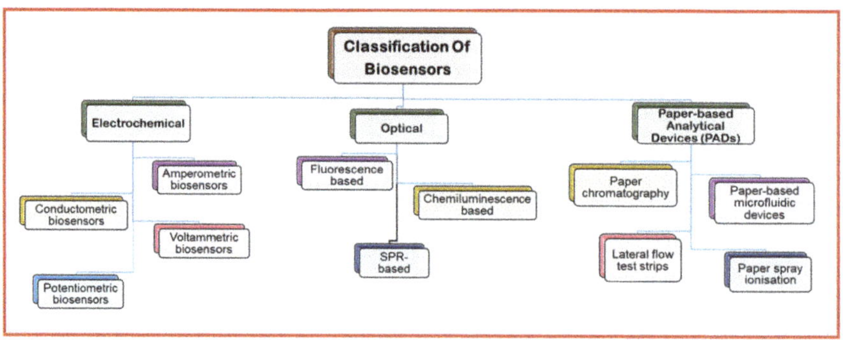

Figure 14.2. Types of biosensor.

electrodes make up amperometric biosensors. When a constant voltage is given to the working electrode with respect to the reference electrode, the sensors detect the current that is generated at the working electrode as a result of electrochemical oxidation or reduction of electroactive species. There is a direct correlation between the amount of analyte present in a solution and the amount of current that is produced on the working electrode's surface [20, 21]. Conductometric biosensors are able to detect an electrochemical process by measuring the difference in conductance that exists between two electrodes (change in conductivity properties of the analyte). For the purpose of frequently monitoring the metabolic activity of living biological systems, biosensors that measure conductivity and impedance are typically utilized [22, 23]. Because of the interaction between the analyte and the bioreceptor, potentiometric biosensors are able to quantify the charge that has accumulated at the working electrode in comparison to the reference electrode when there is no current flowing. Utilizing ion-selective electrodes in conjunction with ion-sensitive field-effect transistors allows for the conversion of a biological process into a potential signal [17, 24].

Voltammetric biosensors work by measuring the current that flows through the sensor during a carefully modulated shift in the voltage that is being applied. These sensors offer two benefits: very sensitive readings and the ability to detect a large number of analytes at the same time [25, 26]. Figure 14.3 contains the schematics that display the device's components, manufacturing process, and operation. Functions and components are illustrated in figure 14.3(A) in a stepwise way. Figure 14.3 also contains

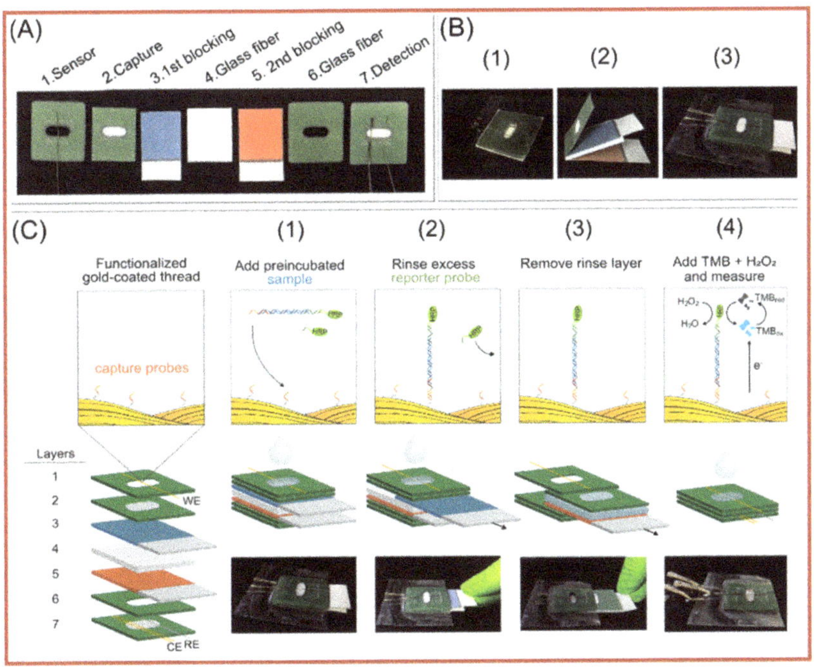

Figure 14.3. Schematics depicting the device's components, manufacturing, and operation. (A) Functions and components, (B) fabrication steps, and (C) working principle of the sensor [27]. Reprinted from [27] with permission of ACS.

the schematics that depict the device's manufacturing process. The first phase demonstrates the sensor, which is a wax layer that contains a hollow channel and a space for a capture probe-modified gold thread working electrode (WE). In the second stage, there is a presentation of a capture compartment that has a wax layer and a paper channel that is hydrophilic. In the third chamber, there is a layer of blocking, and in the fourth chamber, there is a layer of glass fibre absorbent pad. The fifth compartment includes a second blocking phase that consists of a moveable wax layer that has an aflange, which is then followed by the spacer. In figure 14.3(B), the fabrication of the sensor includes alignment and lamination, as well as the preparation of the movable layers. These layers are prepared by taping the capture, glass fibre, and second blocking layers together, and then inserting the first blocking layer between the capture and glass fibre layers. In the last step, the moveable layers are positioned within the laminated layers (between the detection layer and the spacer layer), and the functionalized working electrode is positioned on top of the detection layer. Figure 14.3 is an illustration of the sensor's operational methodology (C). Here, the sample of RPA product-HRP conjugates is added to the top of the device, and then it is hybridized with the capture probe on the gold thread, which is followed by blocking, and then the capture, glassfiber, and second blocking layers are simultaneously applied. Following the transfer of this sample to the three-electrode sensor layer, where it would interact with the TMB + H_2O_2 enzymatic substrate, chronoamperometric measurements were carried out [27].

14.2.2 Optical biosensors

Optical biosensors are analytical devices that combine a bioreceptor component with an optical transducer design to create a biosensor. This sort of biosensor is capable of detecting a wide range of chemicals. The operating principle of an optical biosensor, which generates signals based on sample concentration and allows for real-time parallel analysis, enables label-free, real-time parallel analysis. Enzymes, antibodies, aptamers, whole cells, and tissues are all involved in the biorecognition process performed by optical biosensors. In optical biosensors, the transduction process alters the absorbance, transmission, reflection, refraction, phase, intensity, frequency, and/or polarization of light in response to physical or chemical changes caused by biological recognition components. This shift might also be induced by a shift in light polarization. Depending on the state of this premise, optical biosensors are classified as label-free or label-based. The contact of the analytes with the transducer generates the signal that is detected in label-free sensing. In contrast, calorimetric, fluorescence, or luminescent methods can be used to generate the optical signal in label-based sensing. SPR, optical waveguide interferometry, evanescent wave (EW) fluorescence, chemiluminescence, fluorescence, and refractive index are all names for surfaced-enhanced fluorescence. Cheiluminescence is another term for surface-enhanced fluorescence. Raman scattering is an example of an optical idea that might be employed in the development of optical biosensors [13, 28–30].

14.2.2.1 Optical biosensors based on fluorescence

Fluorescence is an optical phenomena that includes the labelling of the analyte or molecules being detected. As a result of this incident, there has been a lot of interest in the development of fluorescence-based optical biosensors. Because of its high selectivity, sensitivity, and fast reaction time, this type of biosensor is the most intensively studied for medical diagnostic, environmental, and food quality monitoring applications [31]. This biosensor employs a variety of fluorescent dyes, including QDs, dyes, and fluorescent proteins. There are three types of fluorescence-based biosensors: fluorescent quenching (turn-off), fluorescent amplification (turn-on), and fluorescence resonance energy transfer (FRET) [17, 32]. Because of their increased sensitivity, optical biosensors based on fluorescence resonance energy transfer (FRET) have recently controlled the research of the intercellular process. Long-range multipole interactions in the FRET process transmit non-radiative energy from an excited donor molecule (D) to the lowest-energy acceptor molecule (A). FRET-based optical sensors are widely used in medical applications such as cancer treatment and aptamer testing because they can respond to changes in angstroms to nanometers [17, 29]. To detect lead ions, Liu *et al* created a carbon dots (CDs)/Au NR assembly-based FRET sensor. With a detection limit of 0.05 M, the linear range was achieved from 0 to 155 M [33].

14.2.2.2 Optical biosensors based on chemiluminescence

When light energy is released as a result of a chemical reaction, it is referred to as chemiluminescence. Chemiluminescence-based biosensors have received a great deal of interest due to their simplicity, low detection limit, wide calibration range, and inexpensive equipment cost [34]. Martina *et al* present a smartphone-based biosensor that detects and quantifies Ochratoxin A (OTA) in wine and instant coffee using a combination of the LFIA method and chemiluminescence (CL) detection. The biosensor can detect OTA quantitatively in wine and coffee samples up to 25 g l^{-1} with detection limits of 0.3 and 0.1 g l^{-1}, which are lower than European law limits [35].

14.2.2.3 SPR-based optical biosensor

Surface plasmon waves are utilized in SPR-based biosensors to detect changes in refractive index produced by molecule interaction with a metal surface. This biosensor is label-free and relies on the SPR principle [36]. When polarized light collides with a metal surface at the interface of two mediums with differing refractive indices, electron charge density waves known as plasmons form at a certain angle, according to the SPR phenomenon. The SPR phenomenon causes the intensity of reflected light to decrease in contrast to incoming light at a particular angle known as the resonance angle [37], depending on the thickness of the layer at the metal surface. The intensity decreases in proportion to the bulk on the surface. Belal *et al* suggested a new optical biosensor based on surface plasmon resonance that uses SnSe allotropes and a BlueP/MoS_2 heterostructure. According to the findings, the developed sensor has sensitivity of 168 deg/RIU, 179 deg/RIU, 184 deg/RIU, 187 deg/RIU, 187 deg/RIU, and 185 deg/RIU with a maximum quality factor of 24.83 RIU1 and detection accuracy of 0.54 deg/RIU [38].

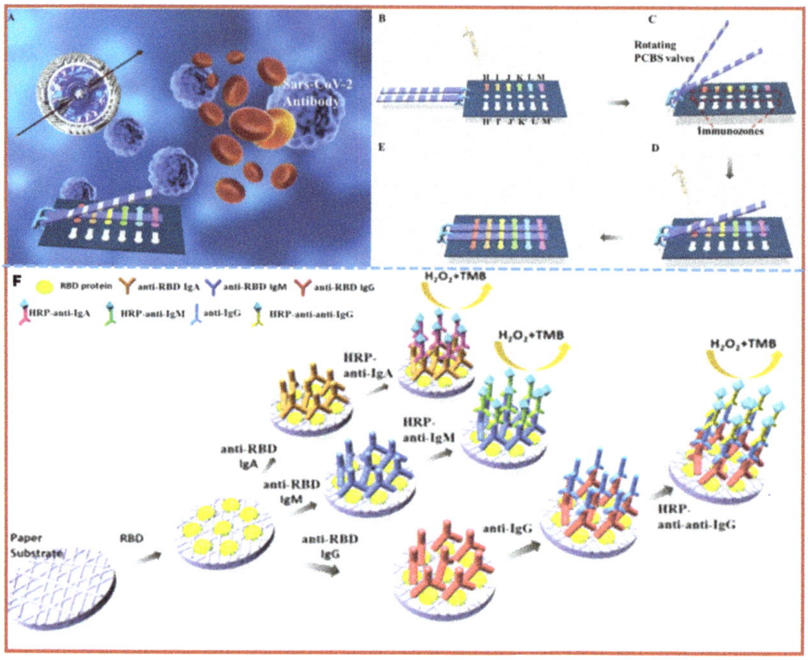

Figure 14.4. The PFST-PADs serological test. (A) PFST-PADs diagram for SARS-CoV-2 analysis. (B) A paper-based valve device with two long-arm channels and six circular reaction zones. (C) Rotate the paper-based device's long-arm PCBS valves. (D) The six circular reaction zones are connected to the reservoirs. (E) A paper-based valve device was used to shut the long-arm channels ('ON' state), allowing dyes to pass through. On the PFST-PADs. (F) A schematic diagram of the anti-RBD IgA/IgM/IgG immunoassay method is shown. Reprinted from [39] with permission of ACS

Figure 14.4 depicts the PFST-PADs serological test. In this study, PFST-PADs with two long-arm channels (H, I, J, K, L, M, and H′, I′, J′, K′, L′, M′) and six circular reaction zones (H, I, J, K, L, M, and H′, I′, J′, K′, L′, M′) ('OFF' state) were employed for SARS-CoV-2 investigation. The long-arm PCBS valves of the paper-based device revolved. The reservoirs H, I, J, K, L, and M are linked to the six circular reaction zones. To close the long-arm channels ('ON' state), a paper-based valve mechanism was utilized, enabling dyes to pass through. Figure 14.4 depicts the working principle of the anti-RBD IgA/IgM/IgG immunoassay technique [39].

14.3 Paper-based biosensors

In recent decades, paper, a ubiquitous and multifunctional material, has attracted a lot of interest, particularly when Whiteside's group announced paper-based microfluidics in 2007 [40]. This ubiquitous substance is transparent, lightweight, easily accessible, and adaptable [41]. Traditional (bio) chemical studies can benefit from paper-based analytical devices (PADs), which require less sample, are easier to use, and are less expensive [42]. PADs may also create a wide range of detecting capabilities by including signal transduction devices (colorimetry, fluorescence, chemiluminescence, current, and so on). This feature permits the construction of various PADs based on the inherent qualities of the target analyte as well as practical considerations. PADs are used in a variety of applications, including paper chromatography, lateral flow test strips, and paper-based microfluidic devices [43–49]. Lui *et al* developed a simple and cost-effective electrochemical biosensor for portable, ultrasensitive, and quantitative cancer detection by integrating a metal–organic framework (MOF)-functionalized paper with a screen-printed electrode (SPE). This label-free paper-based biosensor's detection limit for an ultrasensitive exosome test is 5 ×103 particles per ml, which is higher than most previously described approaches [50].

Liu *et al* discuss the fabrication of a colorimetric paper-based immunochip that detects cyanotoxins in water swiftly using nanozyme catalysis and a smartphone readout device. It can detect 13 MCs/NODs variations in the sub-microgram per litre range with a detection limit of less than 0.7 g l^{-1} and significant recovery percentages ranging from 88% to 120% in varied water matrices [51]. Huang *et al* created a paper-based smartphone biosensor detecting device (paper-biosensor) based on a blocking immunoassay to distinguish between wild-type pseudorabies virus infection and vaccine immunization. PRV was labelled with latex beads (LBs), and the test line was coated with PRV gE-mAb (T-line). The agreement between their approach and the most extensively used commercial gE-ELISA kit in testing of swine clinical samples ($n = 101$) was 98% [52]. Boonkaew *et al* presented a sequential ePAD for sequential immunosensing fluid administration on a single paper platform with dual flow characteristics (fast/delayed) for simultaneous detection of hepatitis B surface antigen (HBsAg) and hepatitis C core antigen (HCCAg) (HCVcAg). The suggested ePAD has a detection limit of 18.2 pg ml^{-1} for HBsAg and a detection limit of 1.19 pg ml^{-1} for HCVcAg [53]. Davidson *et al* discuss the invention of a paper-based device that detects nucleic acids of pathogens of interest in complicated samples by creating a colorimetric response visible to the naked eye using loop-mediated isothermal amplification (LAMP). Using image analysis and a detection limit of 200 genomic copies per L of patient saliva, the resultant device could identify the virus in 60 min and had 97% analytical sensitivity and 100% specificity [54]. One of the researchers developed a chikungunya virus DNA detection platform by skillfully combining the ultra-high charge transfer efficiency of gold nanoparticles (Au) with the biocompatibility of magnetic nanoparticles (Fe_3O_4) (CHIKV). The inclusion of electrochemical paper analytical devices (ePADs) adds to the sensor's appealing properties, as paper is a low-cost substrate that may facilitate platform mass manufacturing [55]. The setup of paper analytical devices (ePADs) is shown in figure 14.5. For quick multiple detections of food borne pathogens, a novel designed paper-embedded microchip based on LAMP has been created [56].

Because it can give speedy analysis and data without the need for laboratory testing, the paper-based biosensor has potential for future *in situ* applications. Electrochemical and optical detection play a vital role in interpreting data from qualitative to quantitative determination. Because of its unique characteristics, such as mobility, specificity, sensitivity, simplicity, and affordability, researchers are interested in developing electrochemical and optical paper-based biosensors. It also

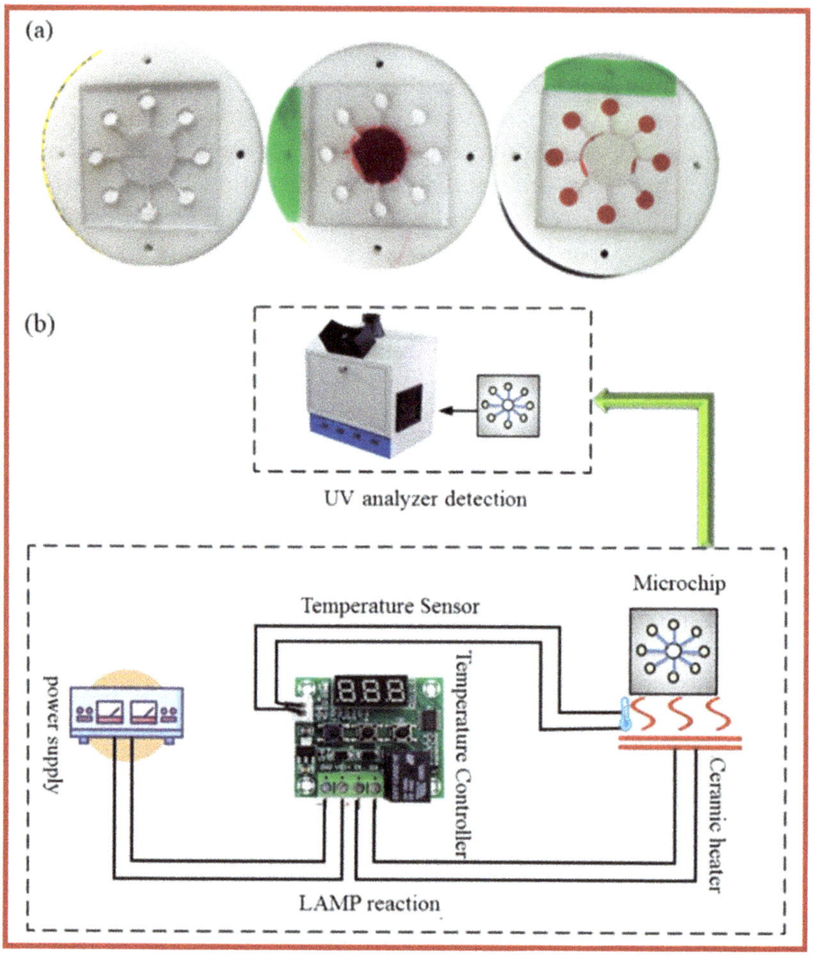

Figure 14.5. Experiment setup. (a) The red ink solution is injected into the reaction chamber. (b) Diagram of the overall structure of the micro-device. Reprinted from [56] with permission of Springer.

allows for rapid data and analysis without the need for a laboratory. As a result, the development of electrochemical and optical paper-based biosensors is crucial, especially in developing countries with limited resources and healthcare facilities. Apart from that, the use of these biosensors is not limited to the detection of microorganisms; they have been used in a variety of disciplines, including environmental and food testing [57–62].

14.3.1 Paper-based microfluidic devices

The use of microfluidics-based innovations has revealed hidden capabilities of paper-based devices that can be used to overcome a number of LFA-related restrictions. In addition to a number of flow improvements, μ-PAD also made multiplexing and quantitative analysis possible [63, 64]. There have been reports of

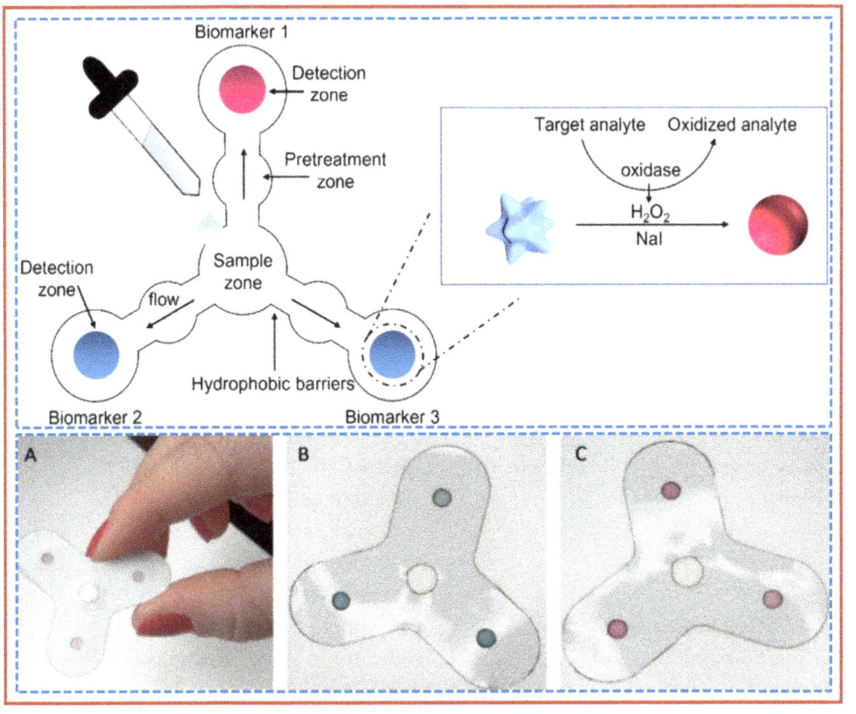

Figure 14.6. A monolithic paper-based device is used to detect three salivary indicators at the same time. (A) The final device picture is inserted in the PVC mask. (B, C) Images of the suggested prototype with the specified mask after the assay on the three analytes injected saliva at the start of the test (B) and after 10 min of response (C). Reprinted from [61] with permission of MDPI.

numerous different types of paper-based microfluidic systems where analysis may be carried out utilizing chemiluminescence, electrochemistry, spectroscopy, and peizo-resistive micro-electro mechanical system (MEMS) based sensing [65]. A variety of paper-based biosensors have also been employed to allow colorimetric biosensing methods. These biosensors basically provide two methods: enzyme-mimetic systems and enzyme-assisted systems. While enzyme-mimetic systems have excellent specificity and sensitivity over a wide temperature range, enzyme-aided systems are well known for their high specificity and sensitivity [66]. Figure 14.6 depicts the simultaneous detection of three salivary biomarkers using a monolithic paper-based device. The device was made with a CO_2 laser cutter. A drop of saliva is put in the middle (sample zone). Saliva travels through the pretreatment zones, which have been marked with a blue colloidal solution of MGNPs and functionalized with a layer of oxidase enzymes, one for each sensing region, before reaching the detecting zones. The inset depicts a colorimetric detection technique based on target-induced reshaping of plasmonic MGNPs mediated by H_2O_2 (a byproduct of biomarker oxidation by the particular oxidase enzyme) in the presence of NaI. For non-physiological amounts of the target analyte, this reaction causes a noticeable colour shift from blue to pink [67]. Table 14.1 includes all the recent development in the field of biosensing devices for analyte detection.

Table 14.1. Recent development in biosensors with their type, analyte, and limit of detection.

Sr. no	Biosensor	Type	Analyte	Limit of detection	References
1.	Amperometric glucose biosensor	Electrochemical	Glucose	0.089 mM	[21]
2.	Enzyme conductometric biosensor	Electrochemical	Dopamine	7.8 μM	[23]
3.	Potentiometric urea biosensor	Electrochemical	Urea	0.77 μM	[76]
4.	Layer-by-layer assembled voltammetric biosensor	Electrochemical	Serotonin (5-hydroxytryptamine, 5-HT)	2 nM	[26]
5.	Aptamer-based biosensor	Electrochemical	SARS-CoV-2 (severe acute respiratory syndrome coronavirus 2)	1.30 pM	[77]
6.	Off-on FRET biosensor	Optical	Pb^{2+} ions	0.05 μM	[33]
7.	Smartphone-based biosensor	Optical	Ochratoxin A (OTA)	0.3 and 0.1 μg l^{-1}	[34]
8.	SPR biosensor	Optical	Cancerous cells		[38]
9.	Porous silicon single layer biosensor	Optical	NGAse substrate	0.51 μM min^{-1}	[78]
10.	Gold nanoparticles based biosensors	Optical	Influenza virus	0.1 $pg.ml^{-1}$	[79]
11.	Metal–organic framework (MOF)-functionalized paper based	Electrochemical	Exosome	5×10^3 particles/ml	[50]
12.	Nanozyme enhanced paper-based biochip	ELISA technology	13 variants of cyanotoxins.	<0.7 g l^{-1}	[51]
13.	Miniaturized paper-based smartphone biosensor	ELISA technology	PRV (pseudorabies virus infection)-gE antibody		[52]
14.	Sequential ePAD	Electrochemical	Hepatitis B surface antigen (HBsAg) Hepatitis C core antigen (HCCAg)	18.2 pg ml^{-1} 1.19 pg ml^{-1}	[53]
15.	Paper-based	Optical (colorimetric response)	SARS-CoV-2	200 genomic copies per μl	[54]

(*Continued*)

Table 14.1. (*Continued*)

Sr. no	Biosensor	Type	Analyte	Limit of detection	References
16.	Paper-based DNA biosensor	Electrochemical	Chikungunya virus DNA (CHIKV)	0.1 nM	[55]
17.	Electrochemical paper-based biosensor	Electrochemical	Cytokine and cancer biomarkers		[57]
18.	Paper-based biosensors	Optical (colorimetric)	Glucose-6-phosphate dehydrogenase (G6PD)		[58]
19.	Flexible paper-based label-free electrochemical biosensor	Electrochemical	miRNA-21	5 pM	[59]
20.	Low-cost paper-based biosensor	Optical (colorimetric)	Phenolic contaminants	0.5 μM	[60]

14.4 Paradigm shift and challenges in the field of fabrication of biosensor-based devices

The future of paper-based sensors seems bright right now. Every month, a number of innovative sensing systems with enhanced analytical performance are launched. Despite this incredible efficiency, the development of bioanalytical devices is still significantly reliant on trial and error throughout the whole manufacturing and optimization process. Although this technique has been successful thus far, it is vital to remember that most changes are either small or very seldom successfully executed in the market. In this case, we believe designers would benefit from a more computerized procedure that would allow for a faster and more efficient analytical performance of their product [68, 69]. This will result in considerable savings in development costs and a higher possibility of the product reaching the market. Similarly, utilizing AI models during data processing may result in a valuable tool for increasing the sensitivity and specificity of the sensor without changing the hardware or biological components [70]. Aside from the obstacles in creating technology and the lack of a consistent model of diagnosis, socio-economic considerations must be considered in order to undertake a substantial cancer diagnostic campaign. Because changes in a patient's biomarkers may be connected to other medical illnesses, even a highly sensitive test capable of detecting many cancer biomarkers would be unable to produce a definitive positive or negative diagnosis. As a result, a skilled oncologist should carefully assess the test results as well as the symptoms of patients. This necessitates the formation and deployment of a large number of healthcare professionals in the context of a mass-diagnosis campaign, as well as possible changes to existing infrastructure (i.e., storage and disposal of samples and tests). Another challenge is managing the implications of such a diagnosis on a patient's life [60]. People may delay getting examined for cancer because the prospect of it gives them so much emotional anguish. Patients who have been diagnosed with cancer may require psychological support, which should begin as soon as the test findings are available. In addition to the psychological strain of the test, the patient must be guaranteed that the results are secret. In actuality, a compromise in data privacy may result in job discrimination as well as a significant rise in the cost of health and life insurance. It follows that it is crucial to provide a strong socio-economic foundation for a major cancer-diagnosis campaign in order for it to be implemented successfully. Many experts agree that it is crucial to mine biological and therapeutic data as early as possible. In addition to traditional data analytics, 'big data' analytics (BDA), is another crucial healthcare component that may be able to aid with some of the difficulties. BDA is characterized as an information management strategy and a collection of tools for extracting more value from health data. Big data offers fresh chances to archive and index previously useless, compartmentalized, or unstructured data for further use by healthcare stakeholders. By converting these once useless data into fresh predicted insights and useful information, BDA provides new insight into the disease. The mass production of point-of-care testing (POCT) devices is another challenge that can be resolved using 3D printing via the additive manufacturing process [71].

Smartphones are ubiquitous and are said to play a significant role in sustainable and low-cost POCT. They include an inbuilt camera, audio jack, power connector, and ambient light sensors, as well as analytical reading capabilities via the screen, which may also operate as a display and controller. They are massive storage media (device and cloud) for data collection, processing, and transmission over wired or wireless (Bluetooth, NFC, Wi-Fi) systems. Devices for the IoT. Colorimetric images/electronic signals can be compared with database data samples via internet connections for rapid, reliable data interpretation. By comparing prior data in a database, ML and AI are better at forecasting patterns. This aids in the analysis of human health, water, food and drink, and environmental elements. 5G devices excel in signal detection, data transfer, and data processing [72]. They can detect visual stimuli with great sensitivity, and have high definition (HD) cameras, fast internet, and a CPU [73].

The integration of nanomaterials improves the sensitivity, specificity, reaction time, and recovery in complex media of microbial sensors, which has several advantages for the detection of microbes [74]. A thorough understanding of the interactions between nanomaterials in these detection techniques, such as charge transfer capabilities, plasmonic resonance, and nanoparticle size-dependent signal amplification, might expedite the creation of highly accurate pathogen detection platforms (figure 14.7). Because nanomaterials work with optical, electrochemical, and piezoelectric detection platforms, detection is flexible and relatively inexpensive. The spread of the COVID-19 pandemic has rekindled interest in the creation of highly contagious pathogenic detection methods other than PCR, ELISA, and flow cytometry. According to the WHO's 'ASSURED' (cheap, specific, sensitive, rapid, user-friendly, equipment-free,

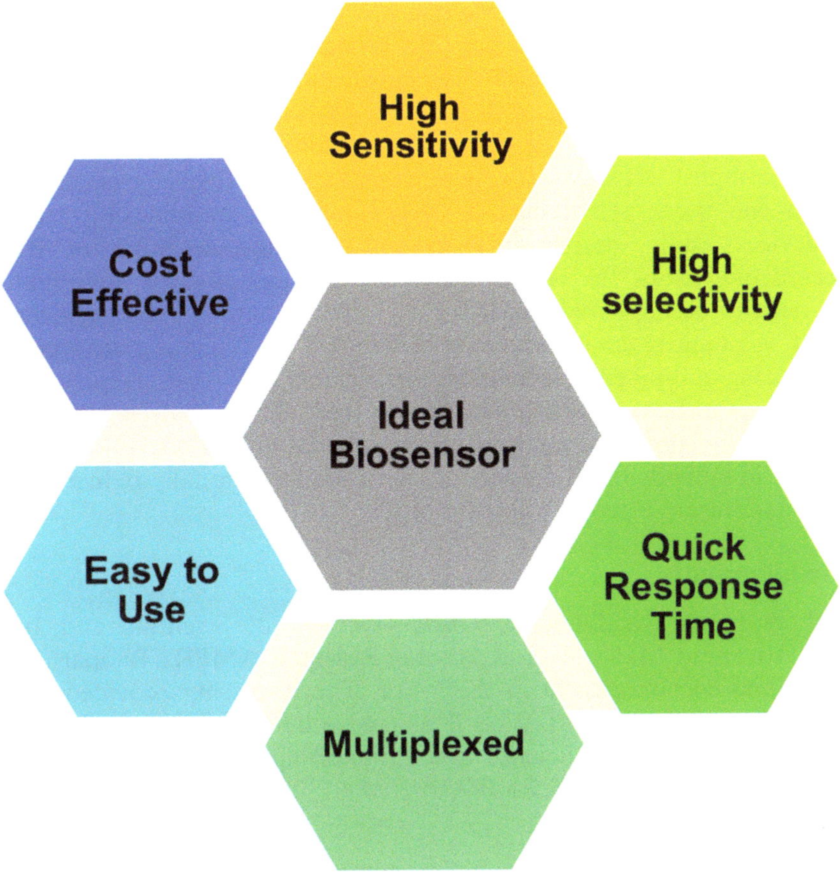

Figure 14.7. Requisite features of ideal biosensor-based devices.

deliverable to end users) standards, the combination of nanosensors into an affordable paper strip or smartphone system broadens the use of nanomaterials for POCT of infectious diseases [4, 70, 75]. These POCT devices have the ability to quickly assess the risk of infection at the clinical bedside, hence lowering the danger to medical workers and assisting in preventing the spread of epidemic diseases.

14.5 Concluding remarks

Our battle against diseases cannot afford to rely on present laboratory-based detection methods; instead, we must strive for the broad use of point-of-care diagnostic devices that meet the REASSURED standards. In this context, paper-based sensors appear to be the most promising option since they combine great analytical performance with cost-effectiveness and environmental friendliness. Recent advances in nanotechnology have enabled the development of multiplexed and ultrasensitive paper-based sensors capable of detecting a wide spectrum of signals. Although the idea for POCT devices was first developed to help with various illness diagnoses, over time the paradigm has changed to emphasize the devices' value in creating a state of wellbeing. To make the POCT tool accessible to all societal groups, extensive research has been done. The ability of paper-based technologies to meet the needs of diverse end users and the demands of manufacturers has recently attracted a lot of attention. Additionally, great efforts have been made to accomplish sensitive, low-cost detections. To further ease the financial burden on end users, researchers have demonstrated multiplexing paper-based POCT devices. Sadly, despite intensive research and development efforts on paper-based biosensors, the results are primarily qualitative or semi-quantitative and still need to be improved. By using a variety of cutting-edge engineering and production techniques, these issues may be handled. Investigating the type of paper and introducing cutting-edge technology for reliable mass manufacture are crucial and promising for the commercial viability of these POCT devices. It is hoped that more thorough research and analysis of paper-based biosensors will open the door for their use in individualized diagnosis, which might eventually reduce the burden of disease and improve people's quality of life.

Acknowledgments

The authors thank the Director, CSIR—Council of Scientific and Industrial Research–Advanced Materials and Process Research AMPRI Bhopal, India, for his interest and encouragement in this work. The fellowship provided to Arpana Parihar under the scheme DST-WoS-B scheme is duly acknowledged. Raju Khan would like to acknowledge Science and Engineering Research Board SERB for providing funds in the form of the IPA/2020/000130 project.

References

[1] Parihar A, Ranjan P, Sanghi S K, Srivastava A K and Khan R 2020 Point-of-care biosensor-based diagnosis of COVID-19 holds promise to combat current and future pandemics *ACS Appl. Bio Mater.* **3** 7326–43

[2] Ranjan P, Parihar A, Jain S, Kumar N, Dhand C, Murali S and Khan R 2020 Biosensor-based diagnostic approaches for various cellular biomarkers of breast cancer: a comprehensive review *Anal. Biochem.* **610** 113996

[3] Singhal A, Parihar A, Kumar N and Khan R 2022 High throughput molecularly imprinted polymers based electrochemical nanosensors for point-of-care diagnostics of COVID-19 *Mater. Lett.* **306** 130898

[4] Bhardwaj T, Ramana L N and Sharma T K 2022 Current advancements and future road map to develop assured microfluidic biosensors for infectious and non-infectious diseases *Biosensors* **12** 357

[5] Chadha U *et al* 2022 Recent progress and growth in biosensors technology: a critical review *J. Ind. Eng. Chem* **109** 21–51

[6] Kuri P R, Das P and Goswami P 2020 Fundamentals of Biosensors *Advanced Materials and Techniques for Biosensors and Bioanalytical Applications* (Boca Raton, FL: CRC Press) pp 1–28

[7] Clark L C Jr 1956 Monitor and control of blood and tissue oxygen tensions *ASAIO J.* **2** 41–8

[8] Heineman W R and Jensen W B 2006 Leland C. Clark Jr. (1918–2005). *Biosens. Bioelectron.* **8** 1403–4

[9] Clark L C Jr and Yons C L 1962 Electrode systems for continuous monitoring in cardiovascular surgery *Ann. N.Y. Acad. Sci.* **102** 29–45
[10] Updike S J and Hicks G P 1967 The enzyme electrode *Nature* **214** 986–8
[11] Nguyen H H, Lee S H, Lee U J, Fermin C D and Kim M 2019 Immobilized enzymes in biosensor applications *Materials* **12** 121
[12] Shukla S K, Govender P P and Tiwari A 2016 Polymeric micellar structures for biosensor technology *Advances in Biomembranes and Lipid Self-Assembly* 1st edn (Cambridge, MA: Academic) pp 143–61
[13] Malhotra BD and Ali MA 2018 Nanomaterials in Biosensors: Fundamentals and Applications. *Nanomaterials for Biosensors.* 1–74 PMCID: PMC7152100.
[14] Chen C and Wang J 2020 Optical biosensors: an exhaustive and comprehensive review *Analyst* **145** 1605–28
[15] Cali K, Tuccori E and Persaud K C 2020 Gravimetric biosensors *Methods Enzymology* vol 642 (New York: Academic) pp 435–68
[16] Vasuki S, Varsha V, Mithra R, Dharshni R A, Abinaya S, Dharshini R D and Sivarajasekar N 2019 Thermal biosensors and their applications *Am. Int. J. Res. Sci. Tech. Eng. Math.* 262–4
[17] Perez D J, Patino E B and Orozco J 2022 Electrochemical nanobiosensors as point-of-care testing solution to cytokines measurement limitations *Electroanalysis* **34** 184–211
[18] Harish V, Tewari D, Gaur M, Yadav A B, Swaroop S, Bechelany M and Barhoum A 2022 Review on nanoparticles and nanostructured materials: bioimaging, biosensing, drug delivery, tissue engineering, antimicrobial, and agro-food applications *Nanomaterials* **12** 457
[19] Vidic J and Manzano M 2021 Electrochemical biosensors for rapid pathogen detection *Curr. Opin. Electrochem.* **29** 100750
[20] Baracu A M and Gugoasa L A D 2021 Recent advances in microfabrication, design and applications of amperometric sensors and biosensors *J. Electrochem. Soc.* **168** 037503
[21] Popov A, Aukstakojyte R, Gaidukevic J, Lisyte V, Kausaite-Minkstimiene A, Barkauskas J and Ramanaviciene A 2021 Reduced graphene oxide and polyaniline nanofibers nanocomposite for the development of an amperometric glucose biosensor *Sensors* **21** 948
[22] Dzyadevych S and Renault N J 2014 Conductometric biosensors *Biological Identification* 1st edn.; R P Schaudies (Cambridge, MA: Elsevier) pp 153–93
[23] Soldatkin O O, Kucherenko I S, Siediuko D V, Kucherenko D Y, Dzyadevych S V and Soldatkin A P 2021 Development of enzyme conductometric biosensor for dopamine determination in aqueous samples *Electroanalysis* **33** 2187–95
[24] Walker N L, Roshkolaeva A B, Chapoval A I and Dick J E 2021 Recent advances in potentiometric biosensing *Curr. Opin. Electrochem.* **28** 100735
[25] Liv L, Çoban G, Nakiboğlu N and Kocagöz T 2021 A rapid, ultrasensitive voltammetric biosensor for determining SARS-CoV-2 spike protein in real samples *Biosens. Bioelectron.* **192** 113497
[26] Li J, Si Y, Park Y E, Choi J S, Jung S M, Lee J E and Lee H J 2021 A serotonin voltammetric biosensor composed of carbon nanocomposites and DNA aptamer *Microchim. Acta* **188** 1–8
[27] Khaliliazar S, Toldrà A, Chondrogiannis G and Hamedi M M 2021 Electroanalytical paper-based nucleic acid amplification biosensors with integrated thread electrodes *Anal. Chem.* **93** 14187–95
[28] Seo S E, Tabei F, Park S J, Askarian B, Kim K H, Moallem G, Chong J W and Kwon O S 2019 Smartphone with optical, physical, and electrochemical nanobiosensors *J. Ind. Eng. Chem.* **77** 1–11

[29] Maddali H, Miles C E, Kohn J and O'Carroll D M 2021 Optical biosensors for virus detection: prospects for SARS-CoV-2/COVID-19 *Chem. Bio. Chem.* **22** 1176–89
[30] Song M, Yang M and Hao J 2021 Pathogenic virus detection by optical nanobiosensors *Cell Rep. Phys. Sci.* **2** 100288
[31] Nagy-Simon T, Hada A M, Suarasan S and Potara M 2021 Recent advances on the development of plasmon-assisted biosensors for detection of C-reactive protein *J. Mol. Struct.* **1246** 131178
[32] Sharma A, Majdinasab M, Khan R, Li Z, Hayat A and Marty J L 2021 Nanomaterials in fluorescence-based biosensors: defining key roles *Nano-Struct. Nano-Objects* **27** 100774
[33] Liu G, Feng D Q, Qian Y, Wang W and Zhu J J 2019 Construction of FRET biosensor for off-on detection of lead ions based on carbon dots and gold nanorods *Talanta* **201** 90–5
[34] Calabretta M M, Zangheri M, Calabria D, Lopreside A, Montali L, Marchegiani E, Trozzi I, Guardigli M, Mirasoli M and Michelini E 2021 Paper-Based Immunosensors with Bio-Chemiluminescence Detection *Sensors (Basel)* **21** 4309
[35] Zangheri M, Di Nardo F, Calabria D, Marchegiani E, Anfossi L, Guardigli M, Mirasoli M, Baggiani C and Roda A 2021 Smartphone biosensor for point-of-need chemiluminescence detection of ochratoxin A in wine and coffee *Anal. Chim. Acta* **1163** 338515
[36] Kushwaha A S, Kumar A, Kumar R and Srivastava S K 2018 A study of surface plasmon resonance (SPR) based biosensor with improved sensitivity *Photonics Nanostructures-Fundam. Appl.* **31** 99–106
[37] Blackburn T J, Tyler S M and Pemberton J E 2022 Optical spectroscopy of surfaces, interfaces, and thin films *Anal. Chem.* **94** 515–58
[38] Hossain B, Paul A K, Islam M A, Rahman M M, Sarkar A K and Abdulrazak L F 2022 A highly sensitive surface plasmon resonance biosensor using SnSe allotrope and heterostructure of BlueP/MoS_2 for cancerous cell detection *Optik* **252** 168506
[39] Gong F *et al* 2021 Pulling-force spinning top for serum separation combined with paper-based microfluidic devices in COVID-19 ELISA diagnosis *ACS Sens.* **6** 2709–19
[40] Martinez A W, Phillips S T, Butte M J and Whitesides G M 2007 Patterned paper as a platform for inexpensive, low-volume, portable bioassays *Angew. Chem.* **119** 1340–2
[41] Mahadeva S K, Walus K and Stoeber B 2015 Paper as a platform for sensing applications and other devices: a review *ACS Appl. Mater. Interfaces* **7** 8345–62
[42] Cate D M, Adkins J A, Mettakoonpitak J and Henry C S 2015 Recent developments in paper-based microfluidic devices *Anal. Chem.* **87** 19e41
[43] Fu L M and Wang Y N 2018 Detection methods and applications of microfluidic paper-based analytical devices *TrAC, Trends Anal. Chem.* **107** 196e211
[44] Wu M R, Lai Q Y, Ju Q, Li L, Yu H D and Huang W 2018 Paper-based fluorogenic devices for *in vitro* diagnostics *Biosens. Bioelectron.* **102** 256e266
[45] Noviana E, McCord C P, Clark K M, Jang I and Henry C S 2020 Electrochemical paper-based devices: sensing approaches and progress toward practical applications *Lab Chip* **20** 185–5
[46] Morbioli G G, Mazzu-Nascimento T, Stockton A M and Carrilho E 2017 Technical aspects and challenges of colorimetric detection with microfluidic paperbased analytical devices (mPADs)—a review *Anal. Chim. Acta* **970** 1e22
[47] Ge L, Yu J H, Ge S G and Yan M 2014 Lab-on-paper-based devices using chemiluminescence and electrogenerated chemiluminescence detection *Anal. Bioanal. Chem.* **406** 5613e5630

[48] Chinnadayyala S R, Park J, Le H T N, Santhosh M, Kadam A N and Cho S 2019 Recent advances in microfluidic paper-based electrochemiluminescence analytical devices for point-of-care testing applications *Biosens. Bioelectron* **126** 68e81

[49] Hasanzadeh M and Shadjou N 2016 Electrochemical and photoelectrochemical nano-immunesensing using origami paper based method *Mater. Sci. Eng.* C **61** 979e1001

[50] Liu X, Gao X, Yang L, Zhao Y and Li F 2021 Metal–organic framework-functionalized paper-based electrochemical biosensor for ultrasensitive exosome assay *Anal. Chem.* **93** 11792–9

[51] Liu J, Xing Y, Xue B and Zhou X 2022 Nanozyme enhanced paper-based biochip with a smartphone readout system for rapid detection of cyanotoxins in water *Biosens. Bioelectron.* **205** 4099

[52] Huang L, Xiao W, Xu T, Chen H, Jin Z, Zhang Z, Song Q and Tang Y 2021 Miniaturized paper-based smartphone biosensor for differential diagnosis of wild-type pseudorabies virus infection versus vaccination immunization *Sensors Actuators* B **327** 128893

[53] Boonkaew S, Yakoh A, Chuaypen N, Tangkijvanich P, Rengpipat S, Siangproh W and Chailapakul O 2021 An automated fast-flow/delayed paper-based platform for the simultaneous electrochemical detection of hepatitis B virus and hepatitis C virus core antigen *Biosens. Bioelectron.* **193** 113543

[54] Davidson J L *et al* 2021 A paper-based colorimetric molecular test for SARS-CoV-2 in saliva *Biosensors Bioelectron.* X **9** 100076

[55] Singhal C, Dubey A, Mathur A, Pundir C S and Narang J 2018 Paper based DNA biosensor for detection of chikungunya virus using gold shells coated magnetic nanocubes *Process Biochem.* **74** 35–42

[56] Zhang M, Liu J, Shen Z, Liu Y, Song Y, Liang Y, Li Z, Nie L, Fang Y and Zhao Y 2021 A newly developed paper embedded microchip based on LAMP for rapid multiple detections of foodborne pathogens *BMC Microbiol.* **21** 197

[57] Loo S W and Pui T S 2020 Cytokine and cancer biomarkers detection: the dawn of electrochemical paper-based biosensor *Sensors* **20** 1854

[58] White D, Keramane M, Capretta A and Brennan J D 2020 A paper-based biosensor for visual detection of glucose-6-phosphate dehydrogenase from whole blood *Analyst* **145** 1817–24

[59] Farshchi F, Saadati A, Fathi N, Hasanzadeh M and Samiei M 2021 Flexible paper-based label-free electrochemical biosensor for the monitoring of miRNA-21 using core–shell Ag@Au/GQD nano-ink: a new platform for the accurate and rapid analysis by low cost lab-on-paper technology *Anal. Methods* **13** 1286–94

[60] Noori R, Perwez M, Mazumder J A and Sardar M 2020 Development of low-cost paper-based biosensor of polyphenol oxidase for detection of phenolic contaminants in water and clinical samples *Environ. Sci. Pollut. Res.* **27** 30081–92

[61] Fakhri N, Abarghoei S, Dadmehr M, Hosseini M, Sabahi H and Ganjali M R 2020 Paper based colorimetric detection of miRNA-21 using Ag/Pt nanoclusters *Spectrochim. Acta, Part* A **227** 117529

[62] Lin Y H and Yeh Y C 2021 Rapid synthesis of microwave-assisted zinc oxide nanorods on a paper-based analytical device for fluorometric detection of L-dopa *Colloids Surf.*, B **207** 111995

[63] Rezk A R, Qi A, Friend J R, Li W H and Yeo L Y 2012 Uniform mixing in paper-based microfluidic systems using surface acoustic waves *Lab Chip* **12** 773–9

[64] Kumar A, Parihar A, Panda U and Parihar D S 2022 Microfluidics-based point-of-care testing (POCT) devices in dealing with waves of COVID-19 pandemic: the emerging solution *ACS Appl. Bio Mater.* **5** 2046–68

[65] Liu X, Mwangi M, Li X, O'Brien M and Whitesides G M 2011 Paper-based piezoresistive MEMS sensors *Lab Chip* **11** 2189–96

[66] Parihar A, Parihar D S, Ranjan P and Khan R 2022 Role of microfluidics-based point-of-care testing (POCT) for clinical applications *Advanced Microfluidics-Based Point-of-Care Diagnostics* (Boca Raton, FL: CRC Press) pp 39–60

[67] Pomili T, Donati P and Pompa P P 2021 Paper-based multiplexed colorimetric device for the simultaneous detection of salivary biomarkers *Biosensors* **11** 443

[68] Mahato K, Purohit B, Kumar A and Chandra P 2020 Based biosensors for clinical and biomedical applications: emerging engineering concepts and challenges *Comprehensive Analytical Chemistry* vol 89 (Amsterdam: Elsevier) pp 163–88

[69] Nnachi R C, Sui N, Ke B, Luo Z, Bhalla N, He D and Yang Z 2022 Recent progress on biosensors for rapid detection of bacterial pathogens in water, food and environment *Environ. Int.* **166** 107357

[70] Bhardwaj T, Ramana L N and Sharma T K 2022 Current advancements and future road map to develop assured microfluidic biosensors for infectious and non-infectious diseases *Biosensors* **12** 357

[71] Parihar A, Pandita V, Kumar A, Parihar D S, Puranik N, Bajpai T and Khan R 2021 3D printing: advancement in biogenerative engineering to combat shortage of organs and bioapplicable materials *Regen. Eng. Transl. Med.* **8** 173–99

[72] Parihar A, Singhal A, Kumar N, Khan R, Khan M and Srivastava A K 2022 Next-generation intelligent MXene-based electrochemical aptasensors for point-of-care cancer diagnostics *Nano-Micro Lett.* **14** 1–34

[73] Jena S, Gupta A, Pippara R K, Pal P and Adit 2019 Wireless sensing systems: a review *Energy Environ. Sustain* 143–92

[74] Singhal A, Sadique M A, Kumar N, Yadav S, Ranjan P, Parihar A and Kaushik A K 2022 Multifunctional carbon nanomaterials decorated molecularly imprinted hybrid polymers for efficient electrochemical antibiotics sensing *J. Environ. Chem. Eng.* **10** 107703

[75] Ranjan P, Sadique M A, Parihar A, Dhand C, Mishra A and Khan R 2022 Commercialization of microfluidic point-of-care diagnostic devices *Advanced Microfluidics-Based Point-of-Care Diagnostics* (Boca Raton, FL: CRC Press) pp 383–98

[76] Öndeş B, Akpınar F, Uygun M, Muti M and Uygun D A 2021 High stability potentiometric urea biosensor based on enzyme attached nanoparticles *Microchem. J.* **160** 105667

[77] Abrego-Martinez J C, Jafari M, Chergui S, Pavel C, Che D and Siaj M 2022 Aptamer-based electrochemical biosensor for rapid detection of SARS-CoV-2: nanoscale electrode-aptamer-SARS-CoV-2 imaging by photo-induced force microscopy *Biosens. Bioelectron.* **195** 113595

[78] Kumar D N, Pinker N and Shtenberg G 2020 Porous silicon Fabry–Pérot interferometer for *N*-acetyl-β-D-glucosaminidase biomarker monitoring *ACS Sens.* **5** 1969–76

[79] Tessaro L, Aquino A, de Carvalho A P A and Conte-Junior C A 2021 A systematic review on gold nanoparticles based-optical biosensors for Influenza virus detection *Sensors Actuators Rep.* **3** 100060